PHYSICAL EDUCATION FOR CHILDREN

BUILDING THE FOUNDATION

PHYSICAL EDUCATION FOR CHILDREN

BUILDING THE FOUNDATION

Carl Gabbard

Elizabeth LeBlanc

Susan Lowy

College of Education,
Texas A & M University

PRENTICE-HALL, INC., ENGLEWOOD CLIFFS, NEW JERSEY 07632

Library of Congress Cataloging-in-Publication Data

Gabbard, Carl, 1948–
    Physical education for children.

    Includes bibliographies and index.
    1. Physical education for children.   2. Physical
education for children—Study and teaching.
3. Movement education.   I. LeBlanc, Elizabeth,
1937–   .   II. Lowy, Susan, 1950–   .   III. Title.
GV443.G15   1987   613.7'042   86-25458
ISBN 0-13-667023-7

Editorial/production supervision
    and interior design: Virginia L. McCarthy
Cover design: Photo Plus Art
Cover photo: GSC Sports Inc.
Manufacturing buyer: Harry P. Baisley
Page layout: Meg Van Arsdale

© 1987 by Prentice-Hall, Inc.
A Division of Simon & Schuster
Englewood Cliffs, New Jersey 07632

Printed in the United States of America

10 9 8 7 6 5 4 3 2 1

ISBN 0-13-667023-7   01

Prentice-Hall International (UK) Limited, London
Prentice-Hall of Australia Pty. Limited, Sydney
Prentice-Hall Canada Inc., Toronto
Prentice-Hall Hispanoamericana, S.A., Mexico
Prentice-Hall of India Private Limited, New Delhi
Prentice-Hall of Japan, Inc., Tokyo
Prentice-Hall of Southeast Asia Pte. Ltd., Singapore
Editora Prentice-Hall do Brasil, Ltda., Rio de Janeiro

CONTENTS

v

Section II
CURRICULUM, PLANNING, TEACHING

Section III
PROGRAM CONTENT

APPENDIXES

PREFACE

Physical Education for Children: Building the Foundation is designed for under-graduate students, teachers, and parents seeking an understanding and course of action related to the psychomotor development of children. The primary focus of the text is upon the development of movement skills and health-related fitness among children described within three proficiency and performance levels iden-tified as Levels I, II, and III. This is a departure from the traditional age/grade association with curricular content and task complexity. Our premise is that all children are different, and they come to the classroom with varying amounts of experience; thus individuals in the same age group and grade may perform at dif-ferent proficiency levels. Information is also provided that relates to curriculum and use of the "foundation" in the form of more advanced activities known as the Level IV–VI program.

Section I is devoted to an understanding of the "Basis for the Foundation." Chapter 1 introduces the reader to the philosophy and purposes of physical ed-ucation for children, emphasizing current trends and practices. Chapter 2 focuses upon an extensive description of general child development and the contributions of physical activity to growth and "total" development. Chapter 3, "The Scientific Basis for Motor-Skill Acquisition," presents scientific information related to how children perform and acquire motor skills. The primary focus of this chapter is on the practical implications of a relatively recent (1975) and strongly supported motor-performance and learning theory, namely, *schema theory*. Chapter 4 deals with an explanation of physical fitness components and assessment. In addition to pre-senting movement themes, the authors believe that the discussion of health-related fitness is among the strongest assets of the text.

Section II focuses on "Curriculum, Planning, and Teaching." Chapter 5 de-scribes the curricular model suggested, encompassing the use of fitness activities, developmental movement themes, and the integration of game, rhythm, and gymnastic activities into the curriculum. Implementation of the model is presented in the form of yearly, theme, and daily lesson plan formats, along with examples. Chapter 6 deals with organization and instruction. A unique instructional strategy model is provided to present a comprehensive description of the instructional process. Chapter 7 focuses upon the factors related to class management and discipline; practical suggestions and techniques are provided. Chapter 8, "Evaluation," presents a comprehensive discussion of both evaluation and techniques that teachers can use to help them not only understand children better but also their own instructional effectiveness.

Section III is devoted to "Program Content." Chapters 9 through 12 provide a thorough discussion of the fundamental movement themes, each with a subsection for movement description, observation, variability, and enhancement activities. Each theme is accompanied by an enhancement chart identifying a selection of rhythms/dance, game, and gymnastic activities that are developmentally categorized into levels of difficulty. Chapter 13 is an activity-oriented chapter focusing upon the description and implementation of health-related fitness activities into the curriculum.

Section IV (Chapters 14 through 16) describes methods for teaching games, rhythms/dance, and gymnastics. Each chapter also includes charts designating developmentally appropriate activities used to enhance theme development.

Finally, the Appendices present the complete AAHPERD (American Alliance for Health, Physical Education, Recreation and Dance) health-related fitness norms, information on how to construct a sit-and-teach apparatus, and procedures for skill-related fitness screening.

ACKNOWLEDGMENTS

As with any text, many individuals contributed to its conception and completion. First, we wish to express our appreciation to the many colleagues and educators who provided the foundation upon which our ideas were conceived. We are especially indebted to Richard Schmidt for providing the basis for "movement variability" and identifying the need to translate scientific theory into information applicable (and practical) at the teaching level. We are also grateful to the reviewers who provided numerous helpful comments that added strength and credibility to the text.

Our sincere thanks are extended to those who made the text come alive; the many wonderful children (and adults) who appeared in the illustrations; the photographer Diana Sultenfus, and Jim Raatz, who provided the line drawings. Special thanks go to Emily Baker and the people at Prentice-Hall for believing in us, and to the many typists and secretaries who helped prepare the manuscript.

Most importantly, we cannot close these acknowledgments without thanking our families for their patience and willingness to share life's precious time with our endeavor.

Carl, Betty, Susan

1

PHYSICAL EDUCATION FOR CHILDREN

Numerous significant strides and innovations have occurred over the past two and a half decades in physical education programs for children. Indications are strong that the most exciting and profound changes, however, are still unfolding. This is due, perhaps in part, to the national exposure that the profession is presently experiencing, based upon better communication to the public of the values of such programs and, most important, the establishment of a stronger knowledge base supported by years of specific scientific inquiry. These "happenings," which have unfolded over the last five years or so, have endowed the profession of teaching physical education to children with the recognition that it is an integral and irreplaceable part of the total school curriculum and child-development process.

DIRECTIONS IN PHYSICAL ACTIVITY PROGRAMS FOR CHILDREN

As with any educational discipline in which scientific inquiry is continuously occurring and enhancing the body of theoretical and practical knowledge, aspects of physical activity programs for children have been and are currently experiencing some very exciting and positive changes. Two areas that are currently experiencing a transition–due to what may be described as the result of cooperation and unification between the scientific community (researchers) and practitioners–are physical fitness and curricular approach. Both sides advocate a somewhat dramatic shift in philosophy from more traditional practices.

In 1980, the American Alliance for Health, Physical Education, Recreation and Dance (AAHPERD) introduced a new concept for nationwide physical fitness: the *AAHPERD Health-Related Physical Fitness Test Program*. The test, designed to screen children and youth ages 5 through 17 on items related to one's health status (discussed in detail in Chapter 4), advocates a focus upon the development and maintenance of those components basic to health. Aside from the valuable information related to child growth and development, the philosophy behind the program deemphasizes the importance of "skill-related" fitness (for example, speed, coordination, balance, agility) that characterized the majority of physical fitness batteries for children before 1980.

Another wave currently growing in popularity and related to curricular approach is "developmental physical education" and the use of "skill themes." Morris (1980) describes developmental physical education as the sequential ordering of movement tasks presented to children, so that each task takes into account the developmental status of every child. Corresponding to this philosophy is the use of skill themes as described in two excellent texts, one by Graham, Holt-Hale, McEwen, and Parker (1980) and another by Gallahue (1982).

The theme approach is not a new idea in elementary physical education. Prior to 1980, its use was described in movement-education texts by Stanley (1977), Gilliom (1970), Krueger and Krueger (1977), and Kirchner, Cunningham, and Warrell (1978). These programs have been described by Gallahue (1982) as movement analysis models that primarily utilize the movement concepts (that is, effort, space, and relationships) originally proposed by Rudolf Laban. Gallahue also notes that the use of movement concepts has value, but like the content areas of physical education (activities such as dance, games, sport, gymnastics), they should serve as vehicles by which skills are developed and refined. Graham and others (1980) define a theme as a series of movements based on a skill from which variations are developed. A major aspect of the philosophy supporting both the Graham and colleagues and Gallahue curricular models, and the one to be described in this text, is that planning, especially for preschool and primary-level children, should not focus primarily around dance, game, and gymnastic activities; rather it should be upon specific themes corresponding to our knowledge of the developmental behaviors and needs of children. Gallahue (1982) states:

Current programs focus upon the development and maintenance of health-related fitness.

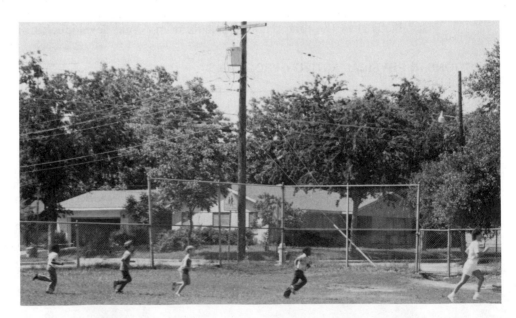

. . . the developmental model is defined as that approach to physical education which aims to educate children in the use of their bodies so that they can move efficiently and effectively in a wide variety of fundamental movements and be able to apply these basic abilities to a wide variety of movement skills that may or may not be sport related. At the heart of the developmental model is the focus on developmentally appropriate movement experiences that promote increased skill development at all levels. Games, sports, dances, and the like serve as a vehicle for improving skill.

The primary use of dance, game, and gymnastic activities rather than specific themes has value and still is a popular and widely used approach. This philosophy, considered the traditional "activity" approach, is reflected in many popular texts and curriculum guides in which allotments (or percentages) of time are suggested for activities to be taught during the year. Also connected to this approach is the use of units that focus upon pieces of equipment such as hoops, beanbags, ropes, and balls. Graham and colleagues (1980) note that children are frequently taught dance, game strategies, or complex gymnastic stunts before they are able to perform the associative skills needed for efficient performance. Many teachers who use activities primarily tend to focus their attention upon the activity as a total fun and learning experience, rather than on proficiency of skill performance. This example is of course not meant to attach a characteristic label on all teachers using the activity approach to teaching children, nor does it suggest the total elimination of such practices. Dance, game, and gymnastic activities, even at the preschool-primary level, play an integral role in the development, refinement, and utilization of fundamental skills and movement awarenesses. The authors of this text suggest only that careful attention be paid to the appropriate application of "activities"; we are not questioning their existence.

The Teacher

Along with the many changes in philosophy and curriculum concerning children and physical education over recent years have come changes associated with the teacher and teacher preparation. From the early years of supervised recess (and other less desirable conditions) has evolved a sophisticated elementary physical education specialist. The specialist is generally an individual who has been educated in the growth, development, and psychology of children as well as in physical education and the psychomotor behaviors of children. Currently, a strong trend in hiring the specialist exists in many parts of the country, mainly because of the exposure and national acceptance that the profession has attained. The acceptance of physical education as an integral part of the "basic" school curriculum in most parts of the nation has brought about the logical response that an unspecialized individual simply is not adequately prepared to direct physical education programs for children. State and local governing agencies are noticeably tightening the preparation requirements for individuals who wish to teach children motor skills and direct physical fitness activities. If a specialist cannot be hired, most state education agencies and universities provide consultative services and resources to school districts. Many universities, realizing that elementary classroom teachers may be responsible for all curriculum areas including physical education, are preparing future teachers with at least a minimum knowledge in physical education for children. Another frequently observable trend is the use of hired teacher "aides" and parent volunteers to supplement the specialist or regular classroom teacher. Unfortunately, some school districts have abused the use of teacher aides by allowing them to be primarily responsible for an entire program; however, their use under the guidance of a specialist can be a definite asset.

Public Law 94–142

Public Law 94–142 (Federal Education for All Handicapped Children Act of 1975) provided public education with a term and concept known as *mainstreaming*. Mainstreaming is the inclusion of children with handicaps into the regular instructional classes and activities with all other children. Among the requirements of the law are:

1. Free and appropriate public education that emphasizes special education and related services for all handicapped children with the "least restrictive environment";
2. The development of an annual individualized education program (I.E.P.) for each handicapped child;
3. A statement explaining the extent to which the child is able to participate in the regular classroom.

The implications of mainstreaming to physical education are strong and far-reaching. Basically it means that handicapped children may be scheduled in regular physical education classes, if that is the least restrictive environment. Provision for instruction in physical education is clearly defined in the elements of special education. It is noted that each handicapped child be afforded the opportunity to participate in the regular physical education program unless the child is enrolled full-time in a separate facility, or needs a specially designed program as prescribed in the I.E.P. For the physical education teacher, this means possibly individualizing specific portions of instruction to cope with the limitations of each handicapped child. Many states and universities now require that future elementary school teachers (regardless of specialization) possess a basic knowledge of the characteristics of exceptional children and that those majoring in physical education take at least one course in adaptive physical education (that is, adapting

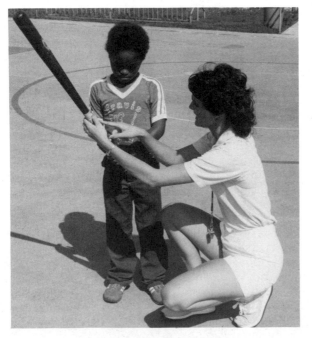

The professional educator provides individual challenges to meet the needs of all children.

physical activities to accommodate the limitations of specific and general handicapped conditions).

Since 1975, tremendous strides have been made in providing educational opportunities, including physical education, to handicapped youngsters. Along with the much needed physical education experiences afforded the exceptional child, mainstreaming has provided both handicapped and nonhandicapped children a positive experience of exposure to each other. (For further information concerning adaptive physical education and the handicapped child, the reader is directed to the reading list at the end of this chapter.)

THE VALUES AND PURPOSES OF PHYSICAL EDUCATION

Educators generally agree that the primary purpose of education is to help each child develop to his or her fullest potential. With this commitment to individualized and equal education has emerged a revitalized push to educate the "total" child. Educators and parents are being enlightened to an increasing base of information that has strengthened the role of physical education in the elementary curriculum and provided a new dimension to "total" child development. The physical activity programs of today are based upon a vast body of knowledge supported by a number of professional disciplines including medicine, psychology, child development, and education.

The components of total child development are generally accepted as being the three domains of behavior: psychomotor, cognitive, and affective. It is through the development and stimulation of these behaviors that the values and purposes of physical activity programs are given credence. Figure 1–1 illustrates some of

Figure 1–1 The contributions of physical activity to child development.

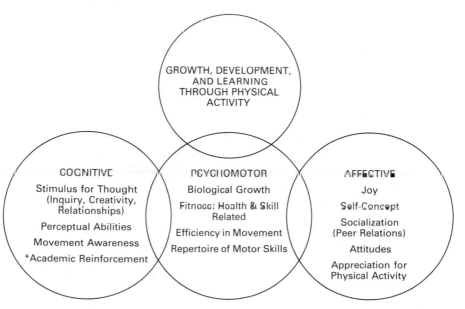

*Term referring to reinforcement of academic concepts using specific movement activities

the contributions of physical activity to child development as represented by three interrelated circles (that is, behavioral domains). This interrelationship also represents a philosophy that supports the belief that a functioning, happy, "total" individual is one who has attained an acceptable level of behavior in each domain, and in many situations, elements from all three must be utilized for the individual to function effectively. Unlike most educational programs, *movement*, being the child's natural learning medium, is in a unique position to contribute to the development of all three domains and do so effectively!

The following section presents a brief introduction into the contributions (that is, values and basis of purpose) of physical education to the psychomotor, cognitive, and affective development of children. Chapter 2, "Child Development and Physical Activity," presents a more detailed treatment of information within the behavioral domains.

Psychomotor Development

Psychomotor behavior includes those responses related to fitness and motor activity, as well as the components of physical growth and development responsible for such functions. It is generally accepted that physical education contributes more to growth and psychomotor development than any other discipline. The merits of physical acitivity for children in terms of normal growth, development, and health-related physical fitness are supported by a large body of research (Bailey, 1976; Malina, 1969; Elliot, 1966; Rarick, 1973). The majority of information suggests that physical activity at an early age is not only necessary for normal growth and development but also enhances the chances of a physically fit adult life.

By using the medium of movement, the physical educator not only has the opportunity to enhance the physical quality of individual lives but to provide for the learning and practice of motor skills essential for a child to attain desirable goals of motor proficiency and recreation.

PHYSICAL ACTIVITY CONTRIBUTES TO THE DEVELOPMENT OF THE FOLLOWING PSYCHOMOTOR BEHAVIORS AND COMPONENTS:

Physical growth and development
Health-related physical fitness
Motor-skill proficiency
Recreational endeavors

Cognitive Development

Primarily composed of the thought processes, such as problem solving, comprehension, evaluation, and creativity, the *cognitive* domain has received the most recognition of all the educational domains. Jean Piaget, one of the most renowned child psychologists, gives a great deal of recognition to the importance of movement and play in the stimulation of cognitive behavior, especially during the child's early years. Exploration, discovery, and problem solving, all attainable in the physical education setting, have been found most appropriate for the stimulation of cognitive development. A strong interaction exists between movement and cognitive stimulation; children "learn to move," and to the physical educator's credit, "learn through movement." The motor-skill learning mechanism is, in part, a cognitive process. Success is dependent largely upon an understanding (awareness) of the environment, how the actions are to be performed, and reflection of the outcome. Movement and play are stimulating and motivating mediums that offer an exciting dimension to the learning environment. Learning through movement entails thinking and an understanding of *why* as well as *how*.

Gallahue (1982) notes that there are two primary aspects of cognitive development that may be dealt with in movement programs: *perceptual-motor concepts* and the development and reinforcement of *academic concepts*. Evidence suggests that the acquisition of both types of concepts may be enhanced through selected movement experiences (Zaichkowsky, Zaichkowsky, & Martinek, 1980). Perhaps one of the most supportive and recognized studies related to this area is the Vanves experiments (MacKenzie, 1974; Bailey, 1976). Conducted in Vanves, France, after French doctors and educators became concerned with "overloaded" academic programs, the now famous "1/3 time" program was established (one-third to academics, one-third to physical education, and one-third to art, music, and supervised study). A series of experiments over a 10-year period using control groups indicated that children in the experimental program had better academic performance and were less susceptible to stress, in addition to exhibiting superior levels of fitness, health, discipline, and enthusiasm.

Although a direct relationship between motor activity experience and academic achievement has not been found, strong indirect implications have been presented. Most educators believe that motor acitivities play an important role in cognitive and perceptual development. With both of these attributes being essential in academic success, the possible link between motor activities and academic achievement may be indirectly drawn. It is perhaps a stronger case for the connection if one assumes that the "total" child possesses a positive attitude not only about himself or herself but also toward learning, which improves the child's chances for classroom achievement. Movement experiences can stimulate motivation and aid in the development of a positive self-concept, both of which are contributing factors in a learning environment.

PHYSICAL ACTIVITY CONTRIBUTES TO THE DEVELOPMENT OF THE FOLLOWING COGNITIVE BEHAVIORS:

Perceptual awareness
Problem solving/strategy
Creativity
Vocabulary
Understanding and communication of concepts and ideas

Affective Development

A desirable goal of all educational programs in general should be the development of individuals who can interact effectively with others as well as with themselves. The *affective* domain, responsible for social and emotional behaviors, has received perhaps less attention from educators than the other domains even though the very basis of society and our own personal success depends upon its development. There are many who believe that the moral values of our society (especially among the youth) are decaying and that more moral education should be stressed at the early educational levels. Physical education, through individual and group activities, can foster desirable attitudes about the self, which in turn allow one to understand better the feelings of others. A good physical education setting is a natural learning laboratory in which children interact with individuals, groups, and authority figures. Through properly directed movement experiences, children can confront and develop such positive traits as honesty, courtesy, respect for others, cooperation, fair play, respect for authority and rules, as well as develop healthy assertiveness. A number of research studies support the premise that an adequate level of motor-skill ability is important to the child and the ongoing relationship with peers. Most children place great emphasis and value on motor-skill performance. Cratty (1970) indicates the importance of children distinguishing themselves in this area by stating, "For the educator to ignore the marked influence that game success has on the social acceptance of children and adolescents is to ignore an important dimension of the value system with which youngsters are surrounded." In order to achieve the maximum potential of development and citizenship, emphasis must be placed on values, social interactions, and self-concept during the formative years.

PHYSICAL ACTIVITY CONTRIBUTES TO THE DEVELOPMENT OF THE FOLLOWING GENERAL AFFECTIVE BEHAVIORS:

Pleasure
Self-concept
Socialization
Positive attitudes
Self-discipline

REFERENCES

CRATTY, B. (1970). *Perceptional and motor development in infants and children*. London: Macmillan, p. 228.

BAILEY, D. A. (1976). The growing child and the need for physical activity. In J. G. Alvenson & G. M. Andrew (Eds.), *Child in sport and physical activity*. Baltimore, MD: University Park Press, pp. 81–93.

ELLIOT, G. M. (1966). The effects of exercise on structural growth. *Journal of Canadian association, HPER, 36*, 21.

GALLAHUE, D. L. (1982). *Developmental movement experiences for children*. New York: Wiley.

GILLIOM, B. C. (1970). *Basic movement education for children: Rationale and teaching units*. Reading, MA: Addison-Wesley.

GRAHAM, G., HOLT-HALE, S. A., McEWEN, T., & PARKER, M. (1980). *Children moving: A reflective approach to teaching physical education*. Palo Alto, CA: Mayfield.

KIRCHNER, G., CUNNINGHAM, J., & WARRELL, E. (1978). *Introduction to movement education* (2nd ed.). Dubuque, IA: Wm. C. Brown.

KRUEGER, H., & KRUEGER, J. (1977). *Movement education in physical education: A guide to teaching and planning*. Dubuque, IA: Wm. C. Brown.

MACKENZIE, T. (1974). 1/3 time physical education. *Saskatchewan Movement and Leisure, 1,6*.

MALINA, R. M. (1969). Exercise as an influence upon growth. *Clinical Pediatrics, 8,16*.

MORRIS, G. S. D. (1980). *Elementary physical education: Towards Inclusion*. Salt Lake City: Brighton.

RARICK, G. L. (Ed.). (1973). *Physical activity: Human growth and development*. New York: Academic Press.

STANLEY, S. (1977). *Physical education: A movement orientation* (2nd ed.). Toronto: McGraw-Hill Ryerson Limited.

ZAICHKOWSKY, D. L., ZAICHKOWSKY, L. B., & MARTINEK, T. J. (1980). *Growth and development: The child and physical activity*. St. Louis: C. V. Mosby.

SUGGESTED READINGS

HOFFMAN, H. A., YOUNG, J., & KLESIUS, S. E. (1981). *Meaningful movement for children*. Boston: Allyn & Bacon.

KRUEGER, H., & KRUEGER, J. (1982). *Movement education in physical education: A guide to teaching and planning*. Dubuque, IA: Wm. C. Brown.

ADAPTIVE PHYSICAL EDUCATION AND THE HANDICAPPED

ADAMS, R. C., DANIEL, A. N., & ROLLMAN, L. (1982). *Games, sports, and exercises for the physically handicapped* (3rd ed.). Philadelphia: Lea & Febiger.

CROWE, W. C., AUXTER, D., & PYLER, J. (1981). *Principles and methods of adapted physical education and recreation* (4th ed.). St. Louis: C. V. Mosby.

MILLER, A. G., & SULLIVAN, J. V. (1982). *Teaching physical activities to impaired youth*. New York: Wiley.

SEAMAN, J. A., & DePAUW, K. P. (1982). *The new adapted physical education*. Palo Alto, CA: Mayfield.

SHERRILL, C. (1981). *Adapted physical education and recreation* (2nd ed.). Dubuque, IA: Wm. C. Brown.

2

CHILD DEVELOPMENT AND PHYSICAL ACTIVITY

Human development may be viewed as a process in which psychomotor, cognitive, and affective factors all interact and contribute to total individual development. Physical activity can have a profound effect on the development of these behavioral domains (thus enhancing total development), for movement is the child's natural learning medium. Physical educators should have a thorough understanding of total child development so the structuring of both physical activities and the learning environment can provide an adequate stimulus for the developmental process.

TOTAL DEVELOPMENT

As already mentioned, child development has been conceptualized into three behavioral domains: psychomotor, cognitive, and affective. The psychomotor domain consists of physical and motor abilities based upon biological (growth) and motor (functioning) processes. Cognitive (intellectual) functions include thought processes, language, and memory, all of which contribute to perceptual-motor and academic abilities. The affective domain encompasses those aspects related to feelings, self-concept, and social interaction. These three domains interact in the development of the child and should not be viewed as independent mechanisms.

Children grow, develop, and learn through physical activity. Movement plays a very important role in the "total" developmental process. Movement serves as a vehicle by which children explore, challenge, and conquer the environment around them. To view physical education as relevant only to the psychomotor domain is to place severe limitations on a potentially valuable medium for development. In this age of accountability and individualized education, physical education teachers must be able to justify the values of physical activity sessions as

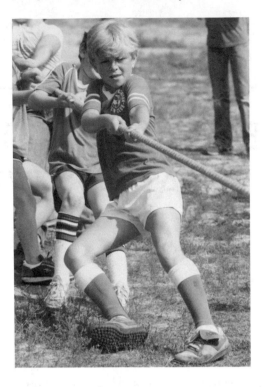

more than learning to throw a ball or folk-dance. The sections of this chapter entitled Psychomotor Development, Cognitive Behavior, and Affective Behavior and Physical Activity focus upon the contributions (and implications) of physical activity to those specific behavioral domains.

General Child Development Terminology

Development refers to changes in the individual's level of functioning. Whether in the psychomotor, cognitive, or affective domain, the level of functioning is a product of heredity, growth, maturation, and one's experiences (that is, environmental effects).

Heredity, represented by 46 chromosomes (23 pairs; consisting of thousands of genes), refers to qualities that are fixed at birth and account for many individual traits and characteristics. Heredity is partially or strongly responsible for height, time of tooth eruption, eye and hair color, body build, personality, and intelligence, to name a few. These traits and characteristics may, however, be modified by environmental factors. Zaichkowsky, Zaichkowsky, and Martinek (1980) refer to the example of body build. Although build is determined primarily by heredity, it is possible to alter one's body build by using weight training, steroids, and specific diets. The same interaction of environment with heredity may be observed in the intelligence of individuals.

Growth, often used interchangeably with "development" and "maturation," usually refers to an increase in body size such as height or arm circumference. The term may also refer to a change in quantity, such as a growth in one's vocabulary. Although maturation may be a factor in growth (but not necessarily), environmental factors and learning may also contribute.

Maturation is associated with qualitative changes that enable an individual to progress from one level of functioning to a higher level. Primarily innate (that is, genetically determined) and resistant to external influences, maturation interacts strongly with learning and environmental factors to influence development of the child. The fixed order of progression in which humans develop is strongly associated with maturation. Locomotion, for example, develops in a very consistent sequence (sit, stand, walk, run) and at approximate ages. The pace and rate of appearance may vary (usually dependent upon environmental influences), but the sequence generally does not.

Experience, perhaps the most influential factor because it can be easily manipulated (compared with the other factors), refers to those factors within the environment that may prompt changes in various developmental characteristics through the learning process. Learning may be described as a relatively permanent change in behavior attributable to experience or practice, as opposed to natural biological processes. Although the environment affects development in numerous ways, its principal effect is its influence on learning. Learning, however, is not the only environmental influence that may affect developmental change. Other strong influences are diet, child-rearing practices, and the physical environment (for example, poverty).

Adaptation is the process of altering one's own behaviors to interact effectively with the environment. Gallahue (1976) uses the term to describe the complex interplay between the child and the environment. The developmental aspects of maturation and the child's experience are interwoven to create behavior.

Developmental Stages

Human development is often classified and studied by stages describing age-related changes in behaviors and growth. Table 2-1 presents the various stages with approximate age range of each corresponding educational level.

Especially during the young years, certain developmental tasks and milestones such as walking, talking, and puberty are attained by all normal children within a general age range. Many educators view the accomplishment of certain developmental tasks as predictive in nature, that is, predictive of later success or failure. Such a viewpoint would also dictate that the child must achieve a specific task by a certain "time." One should be careful, however, when judging age-related behavior, especially during the early years, and in comparison to other behaviors. Individual developmental structures and experiences (or lack thereof) may, and generally do, account for most behavioral differences within specific age groups.

Table 2-1   Developmental Stages

STAGE	APPROXIMATE AGE RANGE	EDUCATIONAL LEVEL
Prenatal	Conception to birth	—
Neonate	Birth to 1 month	—
Infancy	1 month to 2 years	—
Early childhood	2 to 6 years	Preschool to first grade
Middle childhood	6 to 9 years	First to fourth grade
Late childhood	9 to 12 years	Fourth to seventh grade
Adolescence	12 to 18 years	Seventh to secondary completion

Piaget's Theory of Child Development

Perhaps the most elaborate and fully articulate view on child development theory available is that of Jean Piaget. Piaget theorizes that children pass through a series of behavioral stages from infancy to adolescence. Passage through the stages is the result of adaptation to the environment and organized structures of thought. Piaget (1963) has identified four stages of intellectual development: (1) the sensorimotor period [0 to 2 years], (2) the preoperational period [2 to 7 years], (3) concrete operations stage [7 to 11 years], and (4) the period of formal operations [11 and beyond].

As in the situation with most theories using the "age-stage" relationship, the various time periods designated for this model are only approximate. Individual differences may account for the child moving out of a specific stage sooner or remaining longer than is predicted. What follows is a summary of Piaget's theory as adapted from Yussen and Santrock (1978), Winnick (1979), and interpretations of primary sources by the authors. Because of Piaget's repeated reference to behaviors that involve movement (and motor development) during the sensorimotor period, additional emphasis has been directed there.

Important to the understanding of Piaget's theory of development are the terms *schema, assimilation, accommodation,* and *adaptation.* A schema (not to be confused with Schmidt's Schema theory discussed later, although there are some similarities) refers to the basic unit for an organized pattern of sensorimotor functioning. Examples of schemata include sucking, tossing a ball, and grasping. A schema often functions in conjunction or in sequence with other schema, as when the child combines grasping, throwing, and releasing. When a schema is retained in memory, it may be utilized as programmed or altered to meet the demands of a changing environment. According to Piaget, when children deal with the environment in terms of their current schema (from memory), they exhibit the process of *assimilation.* In this situation, the child utilizes existing schema to perform a task. *Accommodation* refers to the process of modifying basic schema structure to the demands of the environment. For example, the child may use a different type of grip than previously used to handle the shape of a new toy. For Piaget (1963), cognitive development is an *adaptation*—the balance between assimilation and accommodation.

Sensorimotor Period (0 to 2 years)

Most of the following make direct reference to movement and motor development.

1. *Simple reflexes* (0 to 1 month)
   During this period the neonate coordinates sensation and action-reflexive (involuntary) behaviors, many of which began in the prenatal period. He or she also develops the ability to produce behaviors that resemble reflexes but are voluntary in nature. Thus begins the emergence of some voluntary movement structuring.

2. *Habits and Primary Circular Reactions* (1 to 4 months)
   Reflexive behavior is gradually replaced by voluntary movements. Where the child sucked on a bottle after being orally stimulated, the child now sucks even if no bottle (stimulus) is present; thus a "habit" is structured. A primary circular reaction is based upon the child's wish to reproduce an interesting or pleasurable event, such as sucking the fingers. During this period the child's body still remains the center of attention.

3. *Secondary Circular Reactions* (4 to 8 months)
   During this period the child becomes more object-oriented, thus focusing on the surrounding environment. The infant imitates simple actions, but they are limited to those the infant is already able to produce. Primary circular reactions are repeated and prolonged by secondary reactions.

4. *Coordination of Secondary Reactions* (8 to 12 months)
   The infant is now able to combine previously learned schemata in a coordinated fashion. The perceptual motor act is now present. The child may observe a toy and grasp it simultaneously. This period marks the separation of means and goals in accomplishing simple feats; hence the presence of *intentionality*. For example, the child may move one doll to reach and play with another one, or manipulate a stick (the means) to bring a toy within reach (the goal).

5. *Tertiary Circular Reactions, Novelty, and Curiosity* (12 to 18 months)
   Piaget refers to this period as beginning the developmental starting point for curiosity and interest in novelty. Infants are intrigued by new events and the things that they can make happen. Tertiary reactions are schemes in which the infant explores new possibilities with objects. This reaction is the first to be concerned with novel events; thus it is an excellent mechanism for trial-and-error learning.

6. *Internalization of Schemes* (18 months to 2 years)
   At this time there is a shift in mental functioning from the sensorimotor plane to the ability to use primitive symbols. A symbol is described here as a sensory image or word that represents an event. This function allows the child to think about concrete events without directly acting or perceiving. One of Piaget's examples refers to a child that opened a door slowly to avoid disturbing a piece of paper lying on the floor. Presumably the child had an image of the paper and what would happen to it if the door were to open rapidly. It should also be mentioned that during this period one of the infant's most significant sensorimotor accomplishments occurs, namely, *object permanence*. Object permanence is the understanding (awareness) that the self is distinct from other objects in space and those objects exist even when no longer in direct perceptual contact. For example, after the rubber duck falls from the playpen and is out of sight, the child searches for it.

Preoperational Period (2 to 7 years)

This period, which extends from preschool to early middle childhood, is subdivided into two stages: the preconceptual stage (2 to 4 years) and intuitive stage (4 to 7 years). Although still an egocentric, the child, during the preconceptual stage, begins to discover both the environment and self through movement and play. The child must deal with each thing individually for he or she does not possess the ability to group objects. The intuitive stage presents the child as using symbolic language without really understanding the meaning of it. Piaget perceives these limitations as the child's inability to conserve (that is, understand that the basic properties of objects often remain unchanged even after the superficial appearance is altered) and the child's failure to order objects in a series and classify them.

Concrete Operations Stage (7 to 11)

During this period the child's thought processes crystallize into more of a system. Children begin to think in a logical manner, and although they cannot yet abstract, they think in terms of the concrete or actual experience. One of the major changes from the preoperational period is the shift from egocentrism to *relativism*. Relativism is the ability to think from various perspectives and to think simultaneously about two or more aspects of a problem. *Reversibility* is also acquired; this is the capacity of relating an event or a thought to a total system of interrelated parts in order to conceive the event from start to finish, or vice versa. A major limitation of concrete thinking is that the child has to be able to perceive an object before thinking in this way. Many times children fail to distinguish between their representation of events and the actual event.

Period of Formal Operations (11 years and beyond)

According to Piaget, in this last stage, as the child enters into adolescence, he or she has achieved the most advanced level of cognition. The child now thinks and reasons beyond the world of actual, concrete experiences. Cognition is logical, and systematic problem solving is used. The child is able to create many hypotheses to account for some event and then test them in a deductive fashion (that is, against empirical data; scientifically).

Implications

Piaget's writings make several references to "action-oriented" activities that involve movement and play; thus his developmental theory has ramifications for every dimension of the play paradigm. Through play (structured and unstructured movement activities), the child is given the opportunity to test novel physical, cognitive, emotional, and social patterns that cannot be accommodated in the real world, thus a buffered form of learning. Once the patterns have been tested through play, they become part of one's memory bank; hence, from a cognitive perspective, play permits the development of intelligence (Levy, 1978). Play also gives the child the opportunity to practice and expand on existing knowledge.

The reader is directed to Winnick (1979) for a more detailed review of Piaget's theory as it relates to play and child development.

Characteristic Behaviors of Children

Because the primary thrust of this text is the psychomotor characteristics and needs of children, the following tables, which contain cognitive and affective behavioral characteristics, have been included to provide a more complete understanding of the "total" child. As with other generalizations of behavior related to age and/or educational level, information noted here is approximate, and individual children may deviate considerably, especially in affective behaviors (many of which are based upon one's emotions). (See Tables 2–2 through 2–5.)

Table 2-2 Characteristic Behaviors of Children 3 to 4 Years Old (PRESCHOOL)

Cognitive Characteristics	Affective Characteristics
Increasing ability to express thoughts and ideas verbally	Egocentric in nature, often quarrelsome, and has difficulty sharing and getting along with others
Unable to sit still for more than a short period of time	Fear of heights, failure, and new situations
Constantly exploring the environment by trial and error	Likes to imitate
Fantastic imagination and fantasy play	Shy and self-conscious
Use of numbers without comprehending concept of quantity	Attitudes formed through family and group play
Can follow directions if not more than two ideas are given	Moral foundation is established
Period of transition from self-satisfying behavior to socialized behavior	Physical aggression decreases; verbal aggression increases
Questions, requests, and commands characterize communication	Likes to play individually or in small groups
	Needs constant encouragement
	Learns appropriate sex role

Table 2-3 Characteristic Behaviors of Children 5 to 6 Years Old (KINDERGART[E]N GRADE)

Cognitive Characteristics	Affective Charact[eristics]
Learning to count, read, and write	Seeks individual attention
Short attention span	Dependence and independence
Uses such concepts as size, volume, numbers, and weight logically	Possible apprehension toward school
Average first grader reading well by midterm	Tends to be very serious
Interest in what the body can do; often asks "why" about movements	Temper tantrums may occur
Expression of personal ideas and views	Sensitive and individualistic
Teamwork is beginning to be understood	Child wants to help
Highly creative	Expresses affection toward others
Eager to learn and please adults	Competition begins to be enjoyed
Interests include songs, fairy tales, television, movies, rhythmic games, and gymnastic-type activities	Sense of humor
Desires to repeat activities that are known and can perform well	Impatient when waiting for his or her turn
	Enjoys rough-and-tumble activity
	Small-group activities are handled well; poor large-group member
	Responds well to authority, "fair" punishment, and discipline

Table 2-4 Characteristic Behaviors of Children 7 to 8 Years Old (SECOND AND THIRD GRADE)

Cognitive Characteristics	Affective Characteristics
Precise speech production, auditory memory, and discrimination abilities are equal to adults	Shows a need for peer and adult approval as well as being individualistic
Enjoys challenges	Better cooperation in group play
Improvement in use of language and elocution	Likes physical contact
Longer attention span	Wants to excel in skills
Develops ability to plan with and for others	Becoming socially conscious
Capable and willing to accept increased personal responsibilities	Enjoys doing well and being admired for it
	Is a poor loser
	Will admit doing wrong
	Girls and boys begin playing their own games
	Fear of being embarrassed
	Displays jealousy over parent

Table 2-5 Characteristic Behaviors of Children 9 to 12 Years (FOURTH THROUGH SIXTH GRADE)

Cognitive Characteristics	Affective Characteristics
Capable of abstract thinking and problem solving	Able to control emotions
Attention span lengthens greatly	More self-reliant
Intellectual curiosity increases	Fears being different
Communication continues to be refined, including a vocabulary increase and sentence-structure complexity	Sensitive to criticism
	Increasing independence and identity to peer group
	Boys and girls enjoy team sports; boys concerned with physique and skill; want to display strength
	Personal appearance and activities involving graceful and creative movements are of interest to girls
	Some rejection of adult standards
	Demonstrates less affection
	Constantly worries
	Need for ego to be bolstered
	Peer acceptance is more important than adult acceptance
	Anger is more easily aroused
	Are admired for their sports abilities
	Emotions teeter between love and hate

SYCHOMOTOR DEVELOPMENT

This section is devoted to the child development area generally known as *motor development*. Motor development refers to those abilities deemed essential in motor-skill functioning. It is also an investigative area that primarily observes motor-skill characteristics (performance and relationship to growth) across periods of time.

The following pages focus upon three subdivisions of psychomotor development: physical growth and development, development of motor skills, and perceptual-motor development. A fourth base of essential information, "physical fitness," will be discussed separately in a later chapter. Preceding the discussion of the three subdivisions is a brief explanation of general growth and development trends and terminology. It should be noted that each of the three areas discussed has an extensive scientific information base and that a thorough discussion of each is beyond the scope of this book. It is the authors' intention to provide the reader with sufficient knowledge with which to understand the mechanisms, capabilities, and abilities of children's motor-skill functioning.

General Trends and Terminology

Cephalocaudal and Proximodistal. These terms refer to the orderly and predictable sequences of physical development. *Cephalocaudal* is physical development that proceeds longitudinally from the head to the feet. This is a gradual progression of increased muscular control moving from the muscles of the head and neck to the trunk, and then to the legs and feet. This phenomenon is characteristic in the developing fetus; the head forms and then the arms and legs. Muscular control is exhibited in the same sequential order. *Proximodistal* development proceeds from the center of the body to its periphery, that is, growth and muscular control occur in the trunk and shoulders before the wrist, hand, and fingers. Both of these trends (that is, of motor control) may be observed in the young child. Preschool children are usually more coordinated in the upper torso of the body before the lower extremities are mastered (cephalocaudal), just as children during early attempts at writing tend to utilize gross shoulder movements before fine-motor cursive forms are achieved.

Mass to Specific (Gross to Fine) Motor Control. Corresponding to cephalocaudal and proximodistal development, *mass to specific motor control* refers to the child's muscular control first over the large muscles before the child is able to differentiate between parts and move them independently. The handwriting example previously described fits this trend as well; during the early attempts, the child uses more parts of the body than are needed.

Bilateral to Unilateral Trend. During the early periods of motor control, movements tend to be *bilateral*; that is, the young child uses either or both hands to manipulate objects. Gradually, preference for and control of a given hand or foot emerge (*unilateral*).

Differentiation and Integration. These two related processes are associated with the increase in motor functioning that stems from neural development. *Differentiation* is associated with the gradual progression from mass (gross) motor control to the more refined specific (fine) movements made by developing individuals. *Integration*, on the other hand, refers to the intricate interviewing of neural mech-

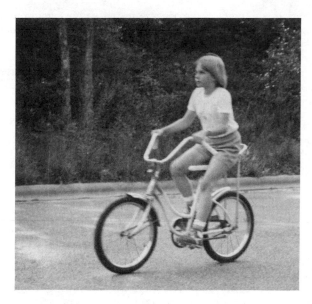

Riding a bicycle is an ontogenetic skill.

anisms of various opposing muscle groups into a coordinated interaction with one another.

Phylogenetic and Ontogenetic. *Phylogenetic* skills are movement behaviors that tend to appear somewhat automatically and in a predictable sequence. Such behaviors as reaching, grasping, walking, and running are presumably resistant to external environmental influences. *Ontogenetic* behaviors are those that are influenced by learning and the environment: swimming, bicycling, roller skating, and so forth.

Maturation and Experience. A relevant question in the study of motor development concerns the influence of *maturation* and *experience* (that is, instruction, practice, equipment) in the acquisition of motor skills. Several studies have been conducted to determine whether instruction and practice can significantly affect children's motor skill acquisition or whether maturational factors appear to predominate. The majority of the investigations conducted have used young twins; one twin is given advanced opportunities for practice, whereas the other one receives no instruction or additional practice.

McGraw (1935) concluded in his famous study of twins, Johnny and Jimmy, that, for any task, there appeared to be critical periods when it was most susceptible to change through practice. The author also indicated (as have others: Gesell, 1928; Shirley, 1931; Hilgard, 1932) that phylogenetic skills (that is, those acquired automatically: creeping, walking, running) are more maturationally structured and less subject to modification through practice than are ontogenetic activities (activities culturally influenced: swimming, bicycling, skating). However, Espenschade and Eckert (1980) stated that one phylogenetic skill, throwing, does seem to be more influenced by practice. Gallahue (1982) pointed out that, in follow-up studies of their original twin investigations, both Gesell and McGraw found that the trained twin exhibited more confidence in the skills in which he or she had previous special assistance; this suggests a possible benefit from training.

Winnick (1979) concluded from the research literature the following generalizations regarding the effects of early training on skill acquisition:

1. The role of maturation is important, particularly in the early years, in motor development, and skill acquisition. Training rarely transcends maturation, and especially not before neural mechanisms have reached a certain state of readiness. Maturation enables efficient learning to take place.
2. It is important to provide children opportunities to practice those behaviors for which the child is ready.
3. Instruction enhances the development of motor abilities, provided the child's maturational level is high enough to benefit from such experiences.

Individual Differences and Readiness.   Although the sequence of motor-skill development is predictable, the rate of appearance may be quite variable. Each child is unique in that he or she has a timetable for development. It is not uncommon to observe deviations from the "average" by as much as six months in the onset of numerous motor skills. This phenomenon is closely related to the child's "readiness" to learn new skills. Readiness may be defined as "a condition of the individual that makes a particular task an appropriate one for him to master" (Oxendine, 1968). Several factors, such as maturation, prior experience, and motivation, promote readiness. Much of our educational methodology is based upon the principles of readiness, that is, preparing individuals for more complex tasks. This same principle should be observed in physical education by developing a foundation of psychological and perceptual-motor readiness, at the same time allowing the child to take full advantage of his or her present maturational level.

Physical Growth and Development

Physical growth and development refers to quantitative and functional changes in the nervous, skeletal, and muscular systems. What follows is a brief review of the physical characteristics of each system.

Nervous System Development

The nervous system includes the brain, spinal cord, and the peripheral nerves that innervate (stimulate) the muscles. There are approximately 10 billion neurons (cells) present in the brain at birth; however, numerous structural and functional changes occur as one ages. With differentiation and integration, cells become larger, myelinated, and interconnections are built up among themselves. *Myelination,* or the development of myelin, that is, a white, fatty tissue that forms a sheath around the cell, is primarily responsible for the effectiveness of transmission of nerve impulses. Myelin coats the nerve, serving as an insulation against misdirected nerve impulses, thus allowing for increased speed of muscle action and more precise movement. For the most part, myelination is completed by the tenth or eleventh year (Cratty, 1979).

The brain, in terms of total weight, is the organ nearest that of an adult value at birth: 25 percent. This is increased to 90 percent of its final adult weight by 5 years of age.

The *midbrain* (located in the lower part of the brain) is the portion of the brain most fully developed at birth. Its early developmental importance is in its control of many reflexes exhibited in infants (which disappear with increased development of the cerebral cortex).

The *cerebral cortex* controls voluntary motor responses and is necessary for the acquisition of language, abstract thinking, and virtually all cognitive processes. Development is almost entirely complete by the time the child is four. The motor portion of the cortex that is responsible for control of the upper body (trunk, arms,

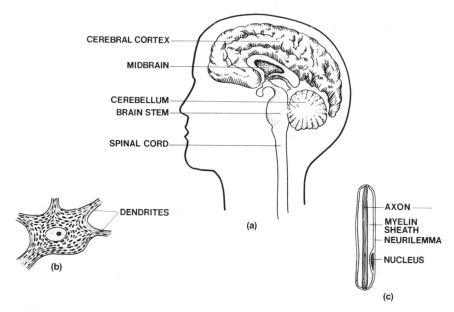

Figure 2-1   (a) A representation of major sections of the brain; (b) a
nerve fiber; (c) a cell body.

hands) is highly developed by 6 months of age; however, the portion that controls
the legs develops later (associated with cephalocaudal development).

Also important to the development of motor control and performance are
the number of *dendrites* (a branched part of the neuron that conducts impulses
toward the cell body), which increase with age. An increase in dendrites and con-
necting fibers from the associative areas of the cortex (responsible for integrating
sensory information and organizing muscular responses) allow for such functions
as executing complex motor tasks. Immature development of the cortex severely
limits the perceptual and motor abilities of the child.

The last portion of the brain to develop is the *cerebellum*. One of the major
functions of the cerebellum lies in its temporal (timing) control or regulation of
movement, more specifically voluntary skilled movements. Another functional role
is maintaining equilibrium of the body. This is accomplished through interaction
with the vestibular apparatus in which information is then transmitted to various
muscles responsible for maintaining stability.

Skeletal Development (and body weight)

The skeletal structure of the body originates as soft cartilage tissue before it
hardens. Beginning during the prenatal period and extending into late adoles
cence, this process is known as *ossification*. As with other growth and developmental characteristics, the onset and rate of ossification may differ considerably
among individuals. The long bones, such as the radius and femur, have a primary
center of growth in the middle of the bone called *diaphysis* and one or more secondary centers at each end identified as *epiphyses* (Fig. 2–2). Growth occurs both
from the center toward the ends and from the ends toward the center. Because
the bones of a developing child are not completely ossified, they are relatively soft
and flexible. Hence they can absorb more strain without fracturing.

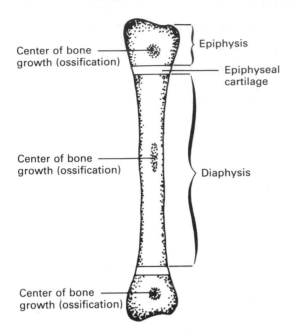

Center of bone growth (ossification)

Epiphysis

Epiphyseal cartilage

Center of bone growth (ossification)

Diaphysis

Center of bone growth (ossification)

Figure 2-2   The growth of long bones.

Figures 2–3 to 2–6 present growth patterns of height and weight for individuals 2 to 18 years of age. Arnheim and Pestolesi (1978) indicate that even though children may vary considerably in height and weight, they usually follow a consistent pattern from birth to maturity. The growth patterns for height and weight are generally characterized by alternating phases of faster and slower growth. A very rapid tissue growth occurs during the first two years and gradually decreases by age 5. A leveling off then takes place until the adolescent growth spurt. Females

Figure 2-3   Boys' stature by age percentiles. (Source: National Center for Health Statistics, U.S. Department of Health, Education, and Welfare, June 1976.)

Figure 2-4   Girls' stature by age percentiles.

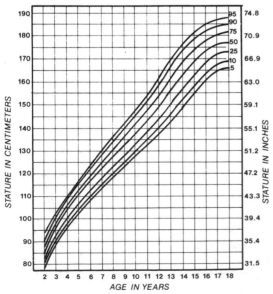

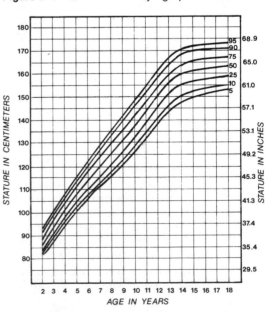

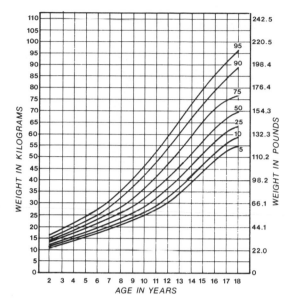

Figure 2-5 Boys' weight by age percentiles.

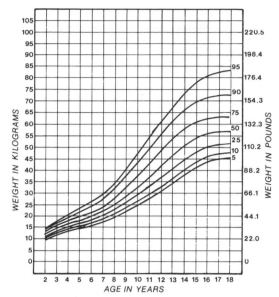

Figure 2-6 Girls' weight by age percentiles.

begin their adolescent growth spurt at approximately 9 years of age and reach a peak during the twelfth or thirteenth year. Females are slightly taller than males between the ages of 12 to 14; however, males then become increasingly taller. Males begin approximately two years later (11 years) and reach their peak during the fourteenth or fifteenth year. Weight gain follows approximately the same growth pattern as height, with females reaching a peak at about 12 years and boys at 14 years of age (Corbin, 1980). Growth in height is generally completed by age 16 for females and at age 18 for males. Although fluctuating levels may occur in body weight throughout adulthood, growth generally ceases in the early twenties.

Muscular Development

There are three types of muscle: smooth, cardiac, and skeletal. *Smooth muscle* tissue forms the muscular portion of the internal organs and functions automatically (involuntarily). The muscular portion of the heart consists of *cardiac* muscle, which operates under the involuntary control of the brain. *Skeletal* muscle is unlike either cardiac or smooth muscle in that contractions are voluntarily controlled (that is, brought about by a stimulus from the brain via motor nerves innervating the muscle fiber). Skeletal muscle consists of muscle fibers (that increase in size but not number) that are bound together by a connective tissue that fuses at each end of the muscle to form a fascia (tendon) that is normally attached to a bone. During normal development, muscles grow along with bones, increasing in length and breadth with age. Development generally occurs in a cephalocaudal direction; that is, muscles near the head develop prior to those located in the lower extremities.

An increase in muscle size, whether from normal growth or stimulated by human influence (for example, exercise, drugs), is called *hypertrophy*. Muscle weight increases approximately 40 times from birth to maturity, which means that the average 12-year-old child has nearly doubled the amount of muscle tissue present at age 6.

Generally, as the child increases in age and grows larger, strength increases. The majority of studies examining strength and children have assessed static strength (that is, pounds of pressure exerted against a reasonably immobile surface) using a grip dynamometer (which assesses grip strength). Results indicate similar scores for boys and girls, with approximately a 65 percent increase between the ages of 3 and 6 years (Metheny, 1941). Meredith (1935) revealed that between the ages of 6 and 18 years, boys increased 359 percent, while a similar study noted an increase of 260 percent for girls in the same age range. Cratty (1979) indicated that boys doubled their grip strength between 6 and 12 years, while the girls increased by more than 2.5 times. Although girls reveal slightly lower strength performance scores at almost all age levels, there is a markedly significant difference between the sexes after the onset of puberty, with the boys being superior (Corbin, 1980). Researchers explain this difference (which appears in almost all strength tests) by the secretion of testosterone (a hormone), which is accompanied in males by significant (compared to females) increases in muscle weight and size of muscle fibers.

A more detailed coverage of muscular performance and other components of fitness are presented in Chapter 4.

Development of Motor Skills

With the development of certain physical characteristics, as described in the previous section, and with maturity, the child develops the capability of performing motor skills. Although the bulk of our behaviors are learned, one should remember that maturational factors (for example, the readiness of neural mechanisms) set a limit as to what skills and how many can be acquired. As previously noted (and the focus of this review) the acquisition of a motor skill is primarily dependent upon an orderly progression of development.

Phases of Motor Behavior

Table 2–6 presents a summary of the phases of motor behavior along with examples of behavioral characteristics and approximate corresponding developmental stages.

Table 2-6   Phases of Motor Behavior

DEVELOPMENTAL STAGE (APPROXIMATE)	PHASE	CHARACTERISTIC BEHAVIOR EXAMPLES
Prenatal-Infancy (−5 mo. to 1 year)	Reflexive	Sucking, grasping, flexion, extension, postural adjustments
Infancy (0 to 2 years)	Rudimentary	Rolling, sitting, crawling, creeping, standing, walking, grasping
Early Childhood (2 to 7 years)	Fundamental movement (and perceptual efficiency)	Locomotor, nonlocomotor, manipulative movements, movement awarenesses
Middle-late Childhood (8 to 12 years)	Specific	Refinement of fundamental skills and movement awarenesses; use of foundation in specific dance, game (sport), gymnastic, and aquatic activities
Adolescence Adulthood (12 to adult years)	Specialized	Recreational- or competitive-level activities

Reflexive Behavior. The *reflexive* phase of motor behavior begins with the unborn child and continues into the first year of life. Reflexes are involuntary (that is, uncontrolled) actions triggered by various kinds of external stimuli. They are usually associated with survival or primitive motor responses such as sucking and grasping. Because the full complement of reflexes is well documented in terms of appearance, longevity, and disappearance, they are often used as indicators of an infant's neurological maturity and soundness. Reflexive behavior mirrors the relative immaturity of the nervous system. As the system matures (that is, increased development of the cerebral cortex and associated areas), reflexes are gradually phased out and voluntary control is phased in. Many survival reflexes such as sneezing and coughing stay with us through life.

Rudimentary Phase. During the rudimentary phase, which begins shortly after birth and terminates at approximately 2 years of age, voluntary behavior and muscle control gradually develop in a cephalocaudal-proximodistal direction (that is, head, neck, and trunk to feet, and trunk area to periphery). Some characteristic behaviors during this phase are crawling, creeping, walking, and voluntary grasping.

Fundamental-Movement Phase. As the title of this text implies, "Building the Foundation" should be of primary concern to educators. The fundamental-movement-skill areas of locomotion, nonlocomotion (stability), manipulation, and perceptual efficiency (movement awareness) are the foundation upon which more complex skills are acquired and executed proficiently. For normal children, almost all of the skills and awarenesses associated with their fundamental areas should be acquired with some degree of proficiency by the end of the early childhood period (approximately 7 years of age).

The study of children's fundamental motor patterns, especially in the locomotor- and manipulative-skill areas, has been and continues to be a topic of primary interest among researchers and practitioners. Leaders in this area—such as Wickstrom (1983) and McClenaghan and Gallahue (1978)—have provided information relative to the developmental progression in the acquisition of fundamental-movement abilities. This information has enabled the practitioner to understand better the movements of children. The observation of children's proficiency in movement usually involves a description (and assessment) of a series of movements organized in a particular time-space sequence, known as a *movement pattern*.

A *fundamental* skill (using a fundamental movement pattern) is a common motor activity with a general goal such as running, jumping, throwing, or catching. Each of these skills is identified in the various categories (that is, locomotor, nonlocomotor, and manipulative) of fundamental skills. Descriptions of the various developmental stages of specific skills are typically identified as ranging from *immature* (or *initial*) to *mature*, or *minimal* form to *sport-skill* form. All of these identify the performance traits of children aged 2 to 7. Fundamental skills are the foundations for more advanced and specialized motor activities, known as *sport skills*. Sport skills are mature fundamental motor patterns that have been adapted to the special requirements of a particular advanced movement activity such as pitching a baseball (throwing), jumping hurdles (leaping), or swinging a golf club (striking). All advanced skill movements retain most of the characteristics found in basic patterns, hence the importance of a solid and varied fundamental-movement foundation.

Figure 2–7 presents an illustration of the foundation of fundamental skills

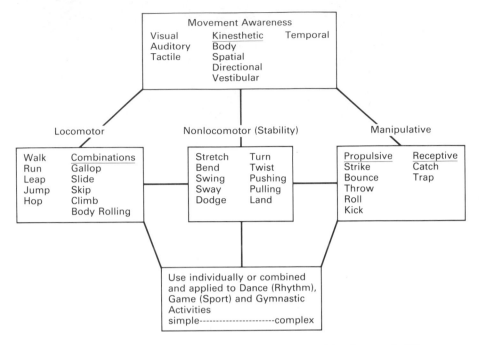

Figure 2-7 The foundation of movement awarenesses and fundamental skills.

and movement awareness and their relationship to more complex movement activities. The skills and awarenesses in each area are not intended to be exhaustive; however, they do represent those commonly identified in the literature.

Generally, by 7 years of age, normally developing children have acquired to some degree of proficiency all of the basic postural and locomotor movement skills. Table 2–7 lists the sequence of human locomotion.

Locomotor skills, essential for human transportation, are identified as skills that move the individual through space from one place to another. Most locomotor skills develop as a result of a certain level of maturation; however, practice and experience are essential to reach mature proficiency. The gallop, slide, and skip are more difficult because they are combinations of other fundamental patterns.

Nonlocomotor skills, known also as *stability* skills, are movements executed with minimal or no movement of one's base of support (for example, twisting, bending, swaying). The ability to execute these skills parallels mastery of locomotor skills.

Manipulative skills involve the control of objects primarily with the hands and feet. There are two classifications of manipulative skills: *receptive* and *propulsive*. Receptive skills involve the receiving of objects (for example, catching, trapping), whereas propulsive skills characteristically include imparting force to objects (throwing, striking, kicking).

Movement awarenesses include those abilities necessary for conceptualization and effective response to sensory information needed to execute a desired motor task (for example, body, spatial, and rhythmic awareness). Chapters 9 through 12 present a thorough discussion of skills and awarenesses that are characteristic of both preschool-age children and older youngsters.

Table 2-7   Sequence of Human Locomotion

MOVEMENT	PERFORMANCE TRAITS	APPROXIMATE AGE
Rolling	voluntary—stomach to back	3–4 months
	back to stomach	5–6 months
Sitting	voluntary—no support	6–8 months
Crawling		
(body drag)		7 months
Creeping		
(abdomen clear)		8–10 months
Climbing		
stairs (mature pattern)		8–10 months
(descending)		4 years
Standing	pull-up to	8–9 months
	no support	9–12 months
Walking	forward	9–15 months
	backwards	16–19 months
	up steps	18–21 months
Running	attempts	18 months
	true "flight"	2–3 years
	smooth	4–5 years
Leaping		
(extension of running)	one foot take-off/opposite foot landing	3–4 years
Jumping	one foot take-off	1½–2 years
	two foot take-off	2–2½ years
	skillful	5 years
Hopping		3 years
(take off and land on same foot)	skillful	6 years
Galloping		4 years
(walk-leap)	skillful	6½ years
Sliding		4 years
(gallop executed sideways)	skillful	6½ years
Skipping		4 years
(step-hop)	skillful	6½ years

Specific Phase.   The skills and awarenesses that the child acquires during the fundamental-movement phase gradually become more refined in the forms of adaptability and accuracy. By the fourth grade (8 to 9 years), social development has stimulated the child's interest in refining those skills used in popular game, dance, and gymnastic activities. During the latter part of this phase, (approximately 9 to 12 years; fourth to sixth grade), many of the fundamental competencies are utilized (and continuously refined) in more complex specific dance, game (primarily sport), and gymnastic activities. Fundamental kicking variations, for example, may be refined and adapted to the game of soccer or football (the progression usually begins with lead-up and modified game activities). A number of locomotor and stability skills can be combined to execute more advanced forms of gymnastics and dance.

Specialized Skills.   During adolescence and continuing through adulthood, most specific abilities can be refined and adapted to the point of specialization. These are largely dependent upon practice and interest. Such skills as the triple jump or pole vault are considered specialized. Both skills consist of a combination of fundamental abilities that require advanced levels of perceptual and physical efficiency for optimal performance.

Perceptual-Motor Development

The perceptual-motor process may be described as the monitoring and interpretation of sensory data and the subsequent response to information in terms of some behavior.

Humans have available certain sensory receptors (modalities) that serve to provide information about the environment, their own bodies, and their relationship to each other. These receptors are activated either by external stimuli (light, sound, and so forth) or by the body itself (kinesthetic). Sensations that are derived from such activation are mediated and transmitted through the sensory mechanisms to the central nervous system. Perception, which occurs primarily in the brain, enables the individual to interpret sensory information (stimuli) by associating it with past experiences (memory) and making judgments. These internal judgments are based in large part upon the individual's past experience, which in turn provides the foundation for a motor response (See Fig. 2–8). Perception cannot be viewed as separate or independent from the cognitive or psychomotor domain. Perception should be considered a function that can be learned and modified by varying the environment. Most learning and development are inherently linked to sensori-perceptual processes, which in effect provide the foundation upon which all related behaviors are built.

The often used term *perceptual-motor development* refers primarily to changes or improvements in the child's capacity to perceive and respond to stimuli as a function of age. As the child develops there is an accompanying increase in sensori-perceptual capacities that allow for greater control of motor behavior. Behaviorally, this means that the child will gradually acquire more complex skills and through practice will perform them proficiently.

Williams and DeOreo (1980) note that as children grow older, three major developmental changes in the sensori-perceptual processes take place: (1) a shift in the hierarchy of the dominant sensory systems, (2) an increase in intersensory communication, and (3) an accompanying improvement in intrasensory discrimination.

The first developmental change is characterized by a shift from the primary use of tactile (touch) and kinesthetic (sense of body position) input to the use of visual information for the regulation of motor behavior. This change in the sensori-perceptual process constitutes development from a crude information-processing capacity (tactile), to the most advanced of all sensory systems in terms of speed

Figure 2-8 The perceptual-motor process.

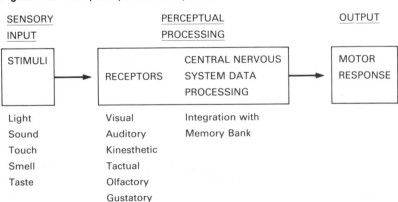

and precision: the visual modality. Williams and DeOreo illustrate this shift in behavior with the following jump-rope example. A 4-year-old who is attempting to jump a rope being swung by two adults is generally unable to use the visual information from the swinging rope to coordinate bodily movements. The child must first establish an individual pattern of movement and then the rope may be added as those turning the rope aid in the coordination of the task. This behavior suggests that the child is relying on bodily cues (tactile-kinesthetic awareness) to perform the motor task and cannot as yet use available visual information. By the time most children are 7 or 8 years of age, they have little or no problem in coordinating their bodily movements with the swinging of a rope; thus, as a result of visual input utilization, more rapid and precise judgments can occur resulting in a greater degree of success.

The second developmental change in the sensori-perceptual processes is that of improved *intersensory* communication. This means that as the child grows older he or she is using more of a multisensory functioning, that is, using several sensory modalities for information in regulating motor behavior. For example, the child interrelates auditory with visual information, visual with tactile, and, finally, what is *felt* with both what is observed and heard. In comparison to the 7- or 8-year-old who was superior to the 4-year-old in the use of visual information while jumping rope, the child at this level has developed a capacity for interrelating visual information (swinging rope) to the sounds of the rope as it hits the surface. This level of perceptual-motor development is characterized by a definite trend toward the use of multisensory sources for information and away from isolated functioning of the sensory systems.

The third change in the sensori-perceptual mechanisms is an increase in the discriminatory capabilities of the individual sensory modalities. This change seems to appear simultaneously with improved intersensory communication. At this time the individual sensory modalities become increasingly refined and develop a more detailed capacity for differentiation and discrimination. As a result of this improvement in *intrasensory* functioning, the child is able to make finer discriminations about stimuli, resulting in more efficient motor performance. The child attempting to jump rope at this level possesses greater discriminatory powers than those (children) described previously; thus he or she is able to make better judgments relating to the speed, direction, and movement of the swinging rope.

The developmental changes that have been described form a major portion of the perceptual-motor control upon which effective motor responses are based.

Components of the Perceptual-Motor System: Movement Awarenesses

Kinesthetic Perception

Sometimes referred to as the "sixth sense," *kinesthetic perception* is a comprehensive term encompassing the memory and awareness of movement. Unlike the visual, auditory, and tactile sensory modalities that receive information from outside the body, the kinesthetic system is supplied with data from the muscles, tendons, joints, and the vestibular (balance) system. Defined as "awareness of movement and body position," this modality is basic to all movement. Every time an individual moves, sensory information is sent to the cerebral cortex, keeping it informed about the spatial characteristics (positions) of various body parts. This information is used by the brain to decide on programmed movements and to regulate motor behavior.

Kinesthetic perception, like the other sensory modalities, does not operate independently, but integrates with information from other sources to provide the brain with a more complete description of the external and internal environment. It should be stressed that the *visual modality* is a critical source of information to kinesthetic perception. The combination of the two sources dominates the learning and acquisition of motor skills.

Although kinesthetic perception has been described as basic to all movement, the following movement awarenesses have been identified as subdivisions of the modality: body awareness, spatial awareness, directional awareness, and vestibular awareness. It should be stressed that, because each awareness is dependent to a great degree upon each other, they are inseparable in the perceptual-motor process. Some researchers have combined all of the terms into one or two categories, such as body awareness or spatial awareness; however, it is our view that by presenting and understanding the "parts" a better understanding of the "whole" can be gathered, both as a theoretical and, most importantly (and a purpose of this text), as a teaching model.

Body Awareness. Sometimes referred to as "body concept" or "body knowledge," *body awareness*, involves the following:

1. Awareness of body parts and their relationship to each other (location and name)
2. Awareness of the capabilities and limitations of body parts
3. Knowledge of how to execute movements efficiently.

As children increase in age, they become increasingly more cognizant of their body parts in terms of location, name, relationship to one another, capabilities, and limitations. With this knowledge they gradually improve their ability to perform desired movements efficiently. It has been suggested by some child-development experts that only as children begin to define the dimensions of their body (parts and positions) are they able to differentiate among corresponding sectors of the space in which they desire to move. Williams and DeOreo (1980) point out that since the body is a three-dimensional object contained within space, it is conceivable that young children might rely heavily on bodily identifications and dimensions as reference points for initial judgments about dimensions of their desired movement space.

One of the first body awareness characteristics that the child develops is the ability to label body parts. Although essentially an academic function, it is included with kinesthetic perception because of its major thrust and importance to this modality. Research indicates that by the time children are 5 years of age, they are able to identify approximately 55 percent of their body parts accurately; 100 percent accuracy is usually achieved by 12 years (Williams, 1973).

Spatial Awareness. Awareness of the position (orientation) of objects in three-dimensional space is termed *spatial awareness*. An extension of body awareness, this perception relies on and can be considered a primary element of the visual modality as well. However, spatial awareness as defined here refers to the child's perception of spatial relationships, which are based upon visual information and involve egocentric and objective localization of objects in space. *Egocentric localization* can be described as the ability to locate objects in space in relation to oneself. This behavior is characteristic of preschool children who determine the location of an object relative to where their own body is positioned. *Objective localization*, which follows egocentric perception, refers to locating the position of two or more objects in relation to each other. Such behavior is exhibited by older children who can locate an object relative to its nearness to other objects but not in relationship to the location of their own bodies. With the knowledge of space and one's body, the child then has the information upon which to project the body effectively.

Directional Awareness. An extension of body and spatial awareness, *directional awareness* consists of two awareness components: laterality and directionality.

The basis for directional awareness derives from laterality. *Laterality* refers to the conscious internal awareness of the two sides of the body. It may also be described in kinesthetic terms as a "sense of feel" for the various dimensions of the body with regard to their location and direction. Through movement experiences, children become increasingly aware that their bodies have two distinct sides—right and left—and although similar in size and shape, these sides occupy decidedly different positions in space. Children with a good sense of laterality do not need to rely on cues such as a ribbon or watch around their wrist or a ring on their finger to provide information about left and right. Zaichkowsky and others (1980) note that children generally develop laterality at around 3 to 4 years, and they then begin to attach the verbal labels of left and right to the sides of the body. However, the ability to label correctly the two sides is usually not fully developed until approximately 7 years of age. It is during the time when the two sides of the body are being differentiated that preferences in the use of one of the eyes, hands, or feet over the other appears (that is, lateral dominance). *Handedness* (that is, preference for left or right hand), which appears as early as age 4 (at this age approximately 84 percent of children are right-handed), may not become permanently established until the age of 9 or 10 (Williams & DeOreo, 1980). Before that time, one is likely to observe some unstable periods of preferential hand use. During the years between 5 and 8, this inconsistency seems more apparent. A preference for one foot over the other appears to be established by the age of 5 years and remains quite stable. Williams and DeOreo (1980) note that children do not exhibit the same degree of lateralization in the use of the eyes as they do for a hand or foot, at any age. Approximately 20 to 25 percent of children at any age up to 10 fail to reveal a clear-cut eye preference. By 9 to 11 years, a stronger preference is shown; however, some children may never establish a definite eye preference. Research concerning eye-hand preferences indicates some interesting information for the movement specialist. It appears that 5- and 6-year-olds exhibit

Directional awareness allows the child to understand the dimensions of space.

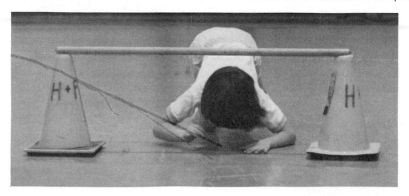

a definite mixed preference (that is, the preferred eye is on the side opposite the preferred hand); 7- and 8-year-olds are divided (mixed and pure [same side]); and the majority of children 9 to 11 years reveal eye and hand preferences on the same side of the body (Williams & De Oreo, 1980).

Directionality, the second component in directional awareness, refers to the ability to identify dimensions of external space. It is through laterality and directionality that children are able to understand the concepts of space (direction) and to project their bodies left-right, up-down, in-out, front-back, and over-under. These dimensions in external space exist only as they relate to the individual's body position at any given time in space.

Vestibular Awareness.   As previously mentioned, kinesthetic perception derives information from within the body itself through the muscles, tendons, joints, and vestibular system. The vestibular apparatus (located in the inner ear) provides the individual with information about the body's relationship to gravity; thus it serves as the basis for *balance* and a "sense of body position." Williams and De Oreo (1980) have summarized the overall functions of the vestibular system as follows:

1. Maintenance of upright posture and equilibrium using the antigravity muscles of the trunk and body for control and postural reflexes;
2. Aid the muscles of the eyes in maintaining visual fixation during bodily movements;
3. Mediation of the body-sighting reflexes (balance) using muscles of the head, neck, and shoulders;
4. To merge with receptors from the muscles, joints, and tendons to appraise the central nervous system of the body's spatial orientation;
5. To contribute to the overall perception of bodily movement (kinesthetic sense).

Balance, designated as a skill-related fitness component (as opposed to health-related), refers to the ability to maintain one's equilibrium in relation to the force of gravity. Balance depends primarily upon vestibular awareness; however, basic reflexes and unconscious as well as conscious abilities interrelate to make postural adjustments. Postural balance that occurs as a result of reflexes responding to gravity allows us to maintain upright posture and perform simple tasks such as holding the head erect, sitting, standing, and walking. Balancing tasks are generally considered as either *static* or *dynamic*. Static balance refers to the ability to maintain equilibrium while the body is stationary, such as the ability to stand on one foot, tiptoe, or balance on a stabilometer or balance board. *Dynamic* balance is the ability of the body to maintain and control posture during movement. Dynamic balance tasks generally employ walking on balance beams of different heights and

Table 2-8   Selected Balance Abilities

TYPE OF BALANCE	TASK	APPROXIMATE AGE
STATIC	Balances on one foot 3–4 seconds	3 years
	Balances on one foot 10 seconds	4 years
	Supports body in basic inverted position	6 years
DYNAMIC	Walks on 1-inch straight line	3 years
	Walks on 4-inch-wide beam using alternating steps	3 years
	Walks in 1-inch circular (line) pattern	4 years
	Walks on 2- or 3-inch beam (alternating steps)	4½ years
	Hops (traveling) proficiently	6 years

widths. Because of its complexity, balance is difficult to isolate and measure; however, some practical methods of assessment such as the ability to walk across a balance beam or stand on one's toes are fair indicators of gross equilibrium. Table 2–8 presents some basic developmental abilities with various balancing tasks.

Although the child's ability to balance begins to stand out after 2 years of age, it is not until approximately the fifth year that the child possesses the neurological maturity necessary to acquire such skills as roller skating and riding a bicycle (Espenschade & Eckert, 1980).

Visual Awareness

Many regard vision and kinesthesis (that is, kinesthetic perception) as the two most important senses relating to motor skills. When vision is present, and it is in most motor-skill actions, visual awareness tends to dominate the other senses and may even be used to calibrate information being received from other senses (Marteniuk, 1976). Gallahue (1976) notes that an estimated 80 percent of all information we perceive comes from the visual modality.

Although all types of visual information are utilized in the execution of motor skills, we will only review a selection of those considered primarily relevant and applicable as aspects of instruction.

Spatial Awareness. Discussed under kinesthetic awareness, those aspects of spacial awareness concerning relationships or spatial orientation (for instance, making judgments about the positional changes of objects in space) are closely related to the level of visual complexity that the child possesses. Kerr (1982) reports that the final stages of this complexity are reached by the majority of children by approximately 9 years of age.

Depth and Distance Perception. The perception for spatial relationships involves the ability to distinquish the relationships among distance, depth, and direction. Although the terms are quite similar, DeOreo and Williams (1980) do note a difference. *Depth perception* refers to the space between two objects in space, whereas *distance perception* refers to the space between the individual and object. A more general definition identifies depth (and distance) perception as the ability to judge relative distances in three-dimensional space. Basically two aspects of vision—binocular and monocular—provide clues for the perception of depth and distance. *Binocular vision,* the forerunner of depth perception, refers to the ability to focus both eyes accurately on an object to produce a three-dimensional view. *Monocular vision* involves the perception of single-image cues such as those viewed on television or the changing size of objects as we or they move. By the age of 6 or 7 years, children can judge depth as accurately with reduced information, that is, monocular cues, as with binocular cues. With growth, the two types of information become more integrated, thus more efficient. Sage (1977) suggests evidence based on empirical data that depth perception can be improved through training.

Figure-Ground Discrimination. *Figure-ground discrimination* (perception) refers to the ability to distinquish an object from its surrounding background. This perception, as with most meaningful motor-skill performances, necessitates that the child be able to concentrate and to give selective attention to a visual stimulus. Such is the situation when the child attempts to focus upon and catch a white ball that has been hit into the white and blue sky. The child must concentrate and select a limited number of stimuli (ball) from a vast background.

Many factors (including lack of concentration and neurological immaturity) may allow the ball to be lost against the background. Gallahue (1968) suggests that both lack of contrast (for example, a white ball and white or lighted background) and a distracting complexity of figure-ground patterns (for example, attention being focused elsewhere) can affect motor-skill performance, especially up to the age of 10 years.

Form Discrimination.   *Form discrimination* involves the ability to recognize differences in shapes and symbols. Very much related to this aspect of visual recognition is *perceptual constancy*; that is, the ability to perceive and recognize an object despite variations in its presentation. These variations may include shape identification from various angles and color recognition (even if partially diminished). Children experiencing problems with this ability are usually unable to match or clearly differentiate similar and dissimilar designs, letters, and objects.

Form discrimination is essential for academic success. Children must learn that two- and three-dimensional forms belong to certain categories (circles, squares, triangles, and so forth) regardless of size, color, texture, or angle of observation. Gallahue (1976) notes that 3- and 4-year-olds tend to rely on form (or shape) rather than color for object identification, whereas by age 6 or 7, children utilize color and form information in a more integrated manner.

Visual-Motor Coordination.   The ability to coordinate visual abilities with movements of the body is termed *visual-motor coordination*. This aspect of movement combines both visual and kinesthetic perceptions with the ability to make controlled and coordinated bodily movements usually involving eye-hand or eye-foot integration. Development of these actions generally follows the proximodistal (midline to periphery), cephalocaudal (head to toes), and gross to fine motor order. Fine motor tasks, such as lacing shoes or writing, involve the synchronization of small muscles of the hand or foot, which in turn are coordinated with vision. Table 2–9 presents a selection of fine visual-motor behaviors characteristically exhibited by children 3 to 8 years of age.

The successful performance of almost all gross-motor skills requires the integration of visual information with kinesthetic awareness and mechanisms of the motor system. When attempting gross-motor skills such as kicking, throwing, or striking, children must be able to judge accurately the speed and distance of the approaching object, the force to be applied, and the direction of projection. In kicking, for example, visual information is relayed to the brain that gives information about the location of the approaching object. This information integrates with the motor system in the form of a motor program, which enables the child to kick the oncoming ball; this is, of course, a very simplified explanation of a very complex process.

An essential component in the performance of several gross visual-motor tasks is the perception and interception of moving stimuli (catching, striking). Children between the ages of 5 and 10 vastly improve their ability to track moving stimuli (balls, objects) traveling at a variety of speeds and from various angles. Morris (1980) indicates that by 5 or 6 years of age, children can efficiently track a ball traveling on a horizontal plane. By age 7 or 8, children perceive a ball traveling downward or upward more easily, and by age 9 they can track an object moving in an arc.

Williams (1967) conducted one of the most recognized developmental studies of perception of a moving object. Children 6 to 11 years of age had to judge the speed and direction of a projected ball and move as quickly as possible to a location where they thought the ball would land (it landed on a canvas ceiling above the

Table 2-9   Selected Fine Visual-Motor Characteristics of Children 3 to 8 Years Old

AGE (IN YEARS)

3	4	5	6	7	8
Uses hand constructively to direct visual responses	Visual manipulation; does not need support of hands	Understands horizontal and vertical concepts	Copying tasks come easily	Prefers pencil over crayons	Can copy a diamond shape
Skillful manipulations	Discoveries made in depth perception	Copies squares and triangles	Fair ability to print	Ability to make uniform size letters, numbers, etc.	Attempts cursive writing
Draws lines with more control	Laces shoes	Increase in fine finger control		Drawing of person more accurate	Uniformity in alignment of letters
Can copy circles and crosses	Buttons large buttons	Colors within the lines			
Stacks 1-inch cubes	Orients movements from center of periphery	Fairly accurate cutting abilities			
Writing utensils handled like adults	Draws a recognizable picture with some detail	Draws a recognizable person			
Strings beads					
Cuts with scissors					

child's head). Results indicated that children 6 to 8 years of age were not capable of integrating their motor behavior with visual information; they reacted quickly, but inaccurately. The 9-year-old children seemed to perceive the complexity of the task; they reacted slower, but were significantly more accurate in their judgments. It was the 11-year-old group, however, that demonstrated a mature interphase between the perceptual and motor aspects of the task by responding quickly and accurately. It may be assumed from this and other studies of this nature that complex spatial perceptions involving perceptual anticipation of rapidly moving objects with locomotor movements and manipulative responses are not mature in children until late childhood (Cratty, 1979). Such evidence would make it impractical to expect but a few children 6 to 8 years to catch a well-hit fly ball on a Little League field.

Temporal Awareness

Temporal awareness involves the timing mechanism within the body. As previously mentioned, all movements involve spatial temporal characteristics (movement in space within a time structure). The child with a well-developed time dimension generally performs a series of movements in a coordinated manner. Gallahue (1976) describes the following components of temporal awareness:

1. Synchrony—the ability to get the body parts to work together smoothly.
2. Rhythm—the process of executing many synchronous acts in a harmonious pattern.
3. Sequence—the proper order of actions required to perform a skill.
4. Eye-hand and eye-foot coordination—the end result of the above components working in an integrated manner.

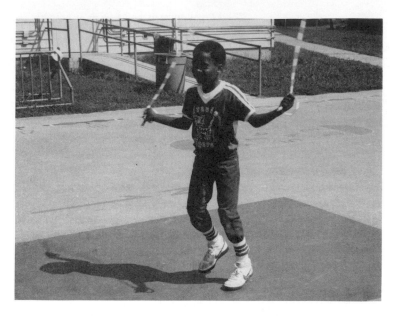

Jumping rope requires a well-developed time structure.

Rhythm, referred to as rhythmic awareness and an instructional theme (along with eye-hand and eye-foot under "temporal awarenesses") in this text, is a basic component of all coordinated movement, and it plays an important role in the everyday lives of children. Rhythm may also be described as the measured release of energy consisting of repeated units of time.

Auditory Awareness

Auditory perception is dependent upon learning and involves the ability to discriminate, associate, and interpret auditory stimuli (Winnick, 1979). Despite the fact that auditory awareness is one of the most common means by which humans receive information, it has been given little attention in physical education and motor development as compared to other sensory modalities. The importance of an awareness of sound is obvious, however, and awareness of sound may be improved through movement programs. The following are components that appear to be relevant to the instructional program.

Auditory Discrimination. This refers to the ability to distinquish between different frequencies and amplitudes of sounds.

Auditory Figure-Ground Perception. Similar to visual figure-ground, this perception involves selecting relevant stimuli from a background of general sounds. This awareness necessitates that the child attend to relevant stimuli in situations where irrelevant sounds are present. A commonly used example describes the problem that a football player may have in trying to distinguish the quarterback's signals over the noise emanating from the crowd and opposing players.

Sound Localization. This refers to the ability to localize the source or direction of sound in the environment. Without direct visual information, children having problems with this ability would find it difficult to determine the direction of a honking horn or a teacher calling in a playground.

Temporal Auditory Perception.   This aspect of auditory awareness involves the ability to perceive and discriminate variations of sounds presented in time. This perception includes distinction of rate, emphasis, tempo, and order, which are those awarenesses generally needed to perform rhythmic activities using auditory stimuli.

Tactile Awareness

Tactile awareness (that is, sense of touch) refers to the ability to interpret sensations from the cutaneous (skin) surfaces of the body. Through touch and manipulation of objects, children learn to understand their environment. During early development, children learn to distinquish hot from cold, sharp from dull, wet from dry, and so on. Tactile perception enables the child to cope with and understand his or her world on relatively tangible terms. Previously described as being prevalent during the early stages of perceptual motor development (that is, primary use of tactile-kinesthetic information) and a less sophisticated mode of information input as compared to other modalities, tactile awareness can be quite effective when combined with other modalities.

Along with assisting the child in the development of fine motor skills such as drawing, cutting, and coloring, tactile perception enhances manipulative abilities by providing information relative to contact with objects. Children first learning to walk on a balance beam usually visually guide their movements by looking at their feet and then progress to guidance by "sense of feel." Some movement specialists suggest that we allow children to perform more activities barefoot (and on various surfaces) in support of tactile stimulation as a learning medium.

Gallahue (1976) describes two aspects of tactile awareness relative to the teaching of young children: tactile discrimination and tactile memory. *Discrimination,* the earliest form of tactile development, involves the ability to distinguish through touch, differentiate between objects, and match objects by tactile information. With tactile discrimination children develop a corresponding vocabulary such as hard, soft, rough, and smooth. *Tactile memory* refers to the ability to discriminate and apply verbal labels to tactile information.

Intersensory Integration

The presentation of perceptual modalities as separate components as described in this and other texts should not convey the overall perceptual-motor process as less than very complex. The functioning of any one modality (or component within) is interrelated and accommodated by the other sensory systems. In the instance of kinesthetic perception, for example, four awarenesses were identified, all of which are interrelated and dependent upon each other for efficient movement. At the same time, visual, auditory, and tactile cues may integrate to enhance information input and facilitate processing. Figure 2–9 illustrates the intersensory integration that results in movement.

COGNITIVE BEHAVIOR AND PHYSICAL ACTIVITY

As previously noted, one of the most recognized theorists in cognitive development in children is Jean Piaget. In his many works, repeated references related to movement (and play) experiences are given. This same belief that motor activity in the form of play contributes to intellectual development has also been mentioned by such noted modern educators as Dewey and Montessori, as well as the

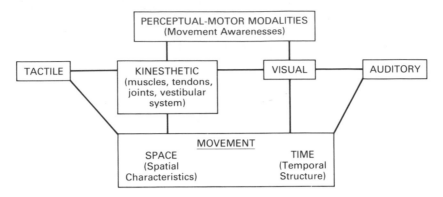

Figure 2-9 Intersensory integration and movement.

ancient Greek philosophers Plato and Socrates. It is with this type of support that educators have recognized the contributions of early movement experiences to the cognitive and perceptual development of children. One could assume that if motor activities play an important role in cognitive and perceptual development, and if both of these attributes are essential in academic success, then an indirect relationship should exist between motor activities and academic achievement. It should be stressed, however, that the relationship is indirect, for few recognized empirical studies have demonstrated that physical activity directly enhances cognitive abilities. Two of the indirect mediums between movement experiences and academic success are *motivation* and *self-concept*. Through movement experiences both of these behavioral influences may be improved. Many researchers have assumed these behavioral influences enhance the total learning attitude of the child and improve the chances for classroom success.

Zaichkowsky, Zaichkowsky, and Martinek (1980) note that if educators wish to enhance cognitive skills through movement experiences, the experiences must be "specifically" structured so that they tax the perceptual modality, encourage social interaction, and stimulate cognition.

What follows are some examples of how movement experiences may stimulate and enhance the cognitive skills in children:

1. The use of games and other movement activities should encourage problem solving rather than replication from demonstration. In these instances, the child is allowed the opportunity to think creatively, logically, and to seek discoveries. Games and other movement-oriented activities may be designed to enhance specific cognitive skills such as attention, memory, and sequencing (see Cratty 1971, 1972, 1973 in "Suggested Readings").
2. Basic to the cognitive development of children is *perception*. Through the various sensory modalities children interact with the environment and challenge information. Movement activities stimulate the perceptual mechanisms of the body as the child develops an awareness for body, space, time, and force. The acquisition of these awarenesses and factors of movement fosters conceptualization, that is, cognitive understanding.
3. Although very little hard research is available at this time, many researchers and teachers believe that *self-concept* is intricately related to academic success and therefore cognitive development. Because participation in movement programs may en-

hance the child's self-concept, it is suggested that teachers recognize both the physical and the emotional characteristics of their pupils.

4. Another increasingly popular medium between movement activities and academic achievement is *academic reinforcement*. This type of learning medium, generally utilized by elementary classroom teachers, involves the use of specifically structured movement activities to enhance specific academic concepts (usually the basics in language arts, math, science, and social studies). Research comparing the uses of specific movement-oriented programs and traditional classroom methods has indicated both superiority for "movement" groups in information gained (Humphrey, 1967; Penman, Christopher, & Wood, 1976; Bledsoe, Purser, & Frantz, 1974) and in the retention of material over a period of time (Gabbard & Shea, 1979).

Some of the possible reasons for the success of movement activities in cognitive development (and academic achievement) are listed below:

1. *Motivation.* Very simply, children are interested in movement; they become attentive and eager to participate; therefore the learning process is enjoyable.

2. *Fun.* Not to be overlooked when combined with motivation, together they are prime factors in the learning and retention of information. Children possess a high regard for movement experiences that are fun; therefore any negative thoughts concerning "academics" may be diminished.

3. *Active participation.* Active games and other movement experiences motivate children who have typically short attention spans and get them involved in the discovery-learning process.

4. *Multisensory approach.* This approach refers to the concept that during movement activities the child will utilize more modes of sensory input, namely kinesthetic and tactile awareness, than the child may experience sitting in the classroom. Students generally learn using the visual and auditory modalities. During academic-reinforcement activities, it is quite easy to incorporate visual and auditory stimuli as well as increase kinesthetic and tactile information input (some kinesthetic and tactile awarenesses are involved in most classroom instruction).

5. *Reinforcement.* Humphrey (1974) contends that academic reinforcement actually reinforces attention to the learning tasks, thus keeping the child involved in the activity.

6. *Retention.* This is perhaps the product of all the factors mentioned; motor-learning specialists have claimed for years that retention of motor-skill learning is higher than "academic" verbal-based learning because of the motivation and processes of neuromuscular feedback (Sage, 1971).

AFFECTIVE BEHAVIOR AND PHYSICAL ACTIVITY

Another important contribution of physical activity to child development is in the *affective domain*. Affective development as discussed here refers to children's increasing ability to interact with others as well as to understand themselves. Because children's feelings about themselves are markedly affected by the actions and reactions of others, the two cannot be perceived as separate. Few would deny that physical activity contributes to a child's social growth, attitudes, and self-concept, for most of the young child's social contacts are in a play setting. Physical education classes are often referred to as laboratories in which children experience a multitude of social and psychological encounters.

Three major aspects of affective development that are particularly relevant to the physical education setting are: socialization, self-concept, and the development of attitudes.

Socialization

A general definition of *socialization* is that it is a process whereby children learn to interact with others (also known as *peer relations*) and understand what kind of behavior is expected or appropriate in different contexts. A major portion of the socialization process for children involves *play* (a term encompassing all pleasurable physical activity). Play is a primary vehicle by which children learn about themselves and how to interact with their peers. One of the benefits of physical activity is that, in the play environment, children are afforded the opportunity to progress through a ladder of socialization. In general, the following stages of socialization and peer relations may be observed in children.

1. *Egocentric stage* (0 to 2 years). Also described as the stage of solitary play, this is when the child is the center of the universe, engrossed in his or her own activities with limited contact with others.
2. *Parallel play* (3 to 4 years). During this stage children generally play alongside, but not with, others for extended periods of time. Limited play between two children usually involves the use of the same toys or play apparatus; for example: follow-the-leader–type activities.
3. *Small-group play* (5 to 6 years). Although still enjoying solitary and parallel-play situations, children at this level have the ability and desire to play in small groups of two to four with simple activities of low organization for increasing periods of time. The ability to work with others usually increases at the same time that children learn how to share space, equipment, and ideas, and become less and less egocentric.
4. *Large-group play* (7 to 8 years). At this age, most children are eager and capable of participating in large groups (with increasing role complexity) such as found in many dance and team-sport activities. Children at this level are less egocentric and increasingly interested in becoming proficient in motor-skill activities (especially popular team sports) that require more complex behavior and group cooperation.

As with other behavioral characteristics with corresponding age ranges, one should be cognizant of the possible differences between individual children, especially in the psychological realm. Many children (and adults) may never feel "adequate" or "comfortable" when placed in the role of a functioning part of a small- or large-group situation, as commonly found in many game, dance, and sport activities. It is important that teachers attempt to understand both the sociopsychological (psychological behavior in a social setting, which includes emotion and expression) difference among children and their physical and motor-performance variations.

Self-Concept

Self-concept, unquestionably one of the most important components of a child's psychological makeup, refers to one's perceptions and evaluations of the self. Perceptions, or judgements, relative to the self may include personal evaluations about behaviors (for example, academic, motor skills, emotional, physical appearance), or an assumption related to how others perceive those characteristics. Children's successes and their developing tolerance of failures provide a strong influence on self-concept. Many of these events occur in play situations, for movement is one of the primary ways in which children explore and discover themselves and their capabilities. Through movement, children are provided the opportunity to express emotions and identify with a group.

As evidenced by the "hero-type" worship that many young children show for popular athletes, proficiency in motor skills has a great influence on self-concept. Numerous studies have indicated a definite link between high positive peer-group acceptance and motor-skill proficiency, as well as a lower acceptance of the less proficient, overweight child (especially among males). There are, however, other influencing factors involved in peer-group acceptance: attitudes toward others (for example, the bully), intelligence to attempt the challenge, and the teacher's acceptance of the individual. The teacher who allows any child to be chosen last, for example, or openly criticizes poor performance may be adding to a child's already negative self-image. Children with a negative self-concept have a tendency to reveal one of two behaviors; they either become more introverted (turn into themselves) or live up to their negative self-image by establishing themselves as failures. These negative feelings about self are often acted out in aggressive behavior.

Gallahue (1976) has described the following factors as components that enhance success in physical activities and allow for the development of a positive self-concept.

Developmentally Appropriate Activities

Activities should be used that meet the needs, interests, and capabilities of children at various development stages. Six- and 7-year-olds are not adolescents or adults, and they should not be expected to perform as examples. Forcing children to attempt activities that are beyond their perceptual-motor, physical, and emotional capabilities is not conducive to success; rather, in most cases, failure occurs. Developmentally appropriate activities should be used as a means of enhancing a realistic concept of abilities.

Sequencing of Tasks

Vital to the success of most motor skills, especially more complex ones, is the *sequencing* (that is, difficulty progression) of motor tasks. It seems perfectly logical, for example, to first instruct children on how to perform a tripod or frogstand followed by a headstand, handstand, and cartwheel. Motor learning theory would support the practice of teaching the basics first as well as having children experience success at initial skill learning before attempting more difficult tasks. Children who experience high frequency of failure during early learning stages may give up or not try as hard during future attempts. Competition should not be introduced too early in the learning process and certainly not until the necessary skills can be performed with an acceptable degree of proficiency. Competition necessitates that there be a winner, which is related to success, and in the true sense of competition there must be a loser. Generally speaking, competition for children in kindergarten and first grade should be restricted to self-testing; that is, how many successive bounces before loss of control rather than a relay race involving dribbling a ball. For most young children, failure is a confusing aspect when they attempt to relate the result to self-concept.

Adventure Activities

A third way in which physical education programs may have an impact on self-concept is by participation in adventure activities—activities that enhance self-confidence. Such experiences as climbing, swinging on a rope, balancing, crawling, or hanging by the knees challenge the child's courage and imagination while fulfilling the need for mastery that comes from success.

Reasonable Expectations

Teachers can also have an influence on the development of self-concept by helping children establish reasonable expectations of their abilities. Children need to attain goals to feel successful and to establish a positive attitude about their own abilities.

Programmed activities or tasks should not, however, be too low as to not stimulate a challenge and provide discovery. Once reasonable success is secured, new goals should be established in order to maintain a level of challenge. Frost (1972) supports this notion by stating that "when tasks are too easy and success too cheap, little development takes place. When tasks are too difficult and achievement impossible, frustration and reinforcement of a negative self-concept are likely to follow."

Encouragement

Another area in which movement programs may influence a child's developing self is through direct communication to the child. As previously mentioned in the definition of self-concept, an important aspect involves how children perceive others perceive them. Thus communication of how we feel about the child's accomplishments is very important. Positive remarks and praise, although very effective, should be used appropriately so the child does not perceive your actions

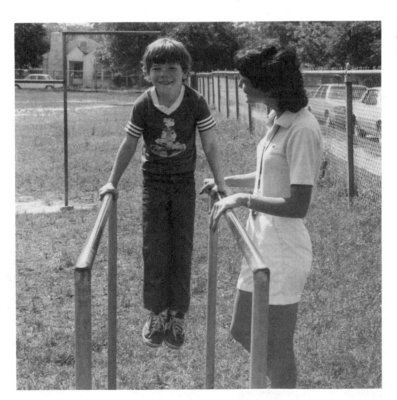

Praise is important in the development of a positive self-concept.

as a "game" of constant and sometimes meaningless statements. Children develop self-confidence through accomplishments and from words, attitudes, and judgments of those around them. Many times the way in which the teacher says things makes a difference as well. Instead of negative feedback such as "That was all wrong" or "I do not think you can do this task," teachers should attempt to be more neutral by stating, "You are almost there," and "You are really working hard; perhaps this task is too difficult until we accomplish more basics." If more negative remarks are necessary (in unusual situations such as display of bad behavior), the child should be communicated to individually and not in the presence of others.

Other techniques and methods that may influence self-concept and be incorporated in the physical education program include the use of individualized movement instruction and teaching strategies that enhance self-reliance, self-discovery and individual success.

Attitudes

Physical educators have for years acknowledged the development of positive attitudes as a desirable outcome of movement experiences. Attitudes toward physical activity, as in other instances, generally involve feelings of a like or dislike for something. Children form positive attitudes about physical activity if they perceive such experiences as pleasurable or beneficial to the self. The "fun" component is an essential ingredient in the development of positive attitudes, especially with young children. One of the major goals of physical educators should be to establish positive attitudes toward physical fitness. These attitudes will motivate children to be conscious of the benefits of physical activity that are important to them now as well as throughout life. Although not supported by conclusive scientific evidence, positive attitudes toward physical activity carry into adulthood and enhance the quality of one's life, and most physical educators would agree with that statement. It is also assumed that many children who are described as "overweight" or "clumsy" and possess a low self-concept tend to be less "pro" exercise as adults. Teachers of children have a tremendous, if not critical, task before them in establishing positive attitudes that may enhance substantially the quality of mental and physical well-being of individuals. Such practices as using physical activity as punishment (running laps or doing sit-ups), or presenting daily fitness activities in a traditional, boring manner (for example, daily mass calisthenics) are not conducive to establishing positive attitudes. We often hear remarks of former athletes who state that they will never run again because of the memories it brings back related to training. Fortunately, children possess a zest for physical activity; however, they also relate desired movement experiences with events found pleasurable. It is therefore the responsibility of physical educators to build positive attitudes toward physical activity with pleasurable experiences.

REFERENCES

ARNHEIM, D. D., & PESTOLESI, R. H. (1978). *Elementary physical education: A developmental approach*, 2nd ed. St. Louis: C. V. Mosby.

ARNHEIM, D., & SINCLAIR, W. A. (1979). *The clumsy child: A program of motor therapy*. St. Louis: C.V. Mosby.

BLEDSOE, C. J., PURSER, D. J., & FRANTZ, R. N. (1974). Effects of manipulative activities on arithmetic achievement and retention. *Psychological Reports, 35,* 247–252.

CORBIN, C. (1980). *A textbook of motor development*. Dubuque, IA: Wm. C. Brown.

CRATTY, B. J. (1979). *Perceptual and motor development in infants and children* (2nd ed.) Englewood Cliffs, NJ: Prentice-Hall.

ESPENSCHADE, A., & ECKERT, H. (1980). *Motor*

development, 2nd ed. Columbus, OH: Chas. E. Merrill.

FROST, R. B. (1972). Physical education and self-concept. *Journal of Physical Education, 36,* 25.

GABBARD, C. & SHEA, C. (1979). Influence of movement activities on shape recognition and retention. *Perceptual and Motor Skills, 48,* 116–118.

GALLAHUE, D. L. (1968). The relationship between perceptual and motor abilities. *Research Quarterly, 39,* 948–952.

GALLAHUE, D. L. (1976). *Motor development and movement experiences for young children (3–7).* New York: Wiley.

GALLAHUE, D. L. (1982). *Developmental movement experiences for young children.* New York: Wiley.

GESELL, A. (1928). *Infancy and human growth.* New York: Macmillan.

HILGARD, J. R. (1932). Learning and maturation in preschool children. *Journal of Genetic Psychology, 41,* 36–56.

HUMPHREY, J. (1974). *Child learning.* Dubuque, IA: Wm. C. Brown.

HUMPHREY, J. (1967). The use of the active game learning medium in the reinforcement of reading skills with fourth-grade children. *Journal of Special Education, 1,* 369.

KERR, R. (1982). *Psychomotor learning.* Philadelphia: Saunders College Publishing.

LEVY, J. (1978). *Play behavior.* New York: Wiley.

MARTENIUK, R. G. (1976). *Information processing in motor skills.* New York: Holt, Rinehart & Winston.

McCLENAGHAN, B. A., & GALLAHUE, D. L. (1978). *Fundamental movement: A developmental and remedial approach.* Philadelphia: Saunders, 1978.

McGRAW, M. B. (1935). *Growth: A study of Johnny and Jimmy.* New York: Appleton-Century.

MEREDITH, H. V. (1935). The rhythm of physical growth: A study of 18 anthropometric measures on Iowa City males ranging in age between birth and 18 years. *University of Iowa Stud. Child Welfare, II,* 3.

METHENY, E. (1941). The present status of strength testing for children of elementary school and preschool age. *Research Quarterly, 12,* 115–130.

MORRIS, G. S. D. (1980). *Elementary physical education: Towards inclusion.* Salt Lake City: Brighton.

NATIONAL CENTER FOR HEALTH STATISTICS. (1976). U.S. Department of Health, Education and Welfare, *25,* June 26, 3.

OXENDINE, J. B. (1968). *Psychology of motor learning.* Englewood Cliffs, NJ: Prentice-Hall.

PENMAN, K. A., CHRISTOPHER, J. R., & WOOD, G. (1976). Using gross motor activity to improve language arts concepts by third-grade students. *Research Quarterly, 48,* 134–137.

PIAGET, J. (1963). *The origins of intelligence in children* (M. Cook, Trans.). New York: W. W. Norton & Co., Inc.

SAGE, G. H. (1971). *Introduction to motor behavior: A neuropsychological approach.* Reading, MA: Addison-Wesley.

SHIRLEY, M. M. (1931). *The first two years: A study of twenty-five babies: Vol. 1. Postural and locomotor development.* Minneapolis: University of Minnesota Press.

WICKSTROM, R. L. (1983). *Fundamental motor patterns.* Philadelphia: Lea & Febiger.

WILLIAMS, H. G. (1967). *The perception of moving objects by children.* Unpublished study, University of California, Los Angeles, Perceptual-Motor Learning Laboratory.

WILLIAMS, H. G. (1973). Perceptual-motor development in children. In C. Corbin (Ed.), *A textbook of motor development.* Dubuque, IA: Wm. C. Brown.

WILLIAMS, H. G., DEOREO, K. (1980). Perceptual-motor development: A theoretical overview. In C. Corbin (Ed.), *A textbook of motor development,* 2nd ed. Dubuque, IA.: W. C. Brown.

WINNICK, J. P. (1979). *Early movement experiences and development-habilitation and remediation.* Philadelphia: Saunders.

YUSSEN, S. R., & SANTROCK, J. W. (1978). *Child development: An introduction.* Dubuque, IA: Wm. C. Brown.

ZAICHKOWSKY, D. L., ZAICHKOWSKY, L. B., & MARTINEK, T. J. (1980). *Growth and development: The child and physical activity.* St. Louis: C. V. Mosby.

SUGGESTED READINGS

GALLAHUE, D. L. (1982). *Understanding motor development in children.* New York: Wiley.

KELSO, S. & CLARK, J. (Eds.). (1982). *The development of movement control and co-ordination.* New York: Wiley & Sons.

KEOGH, J., & SUGDEN, D. (1985). *Movement skill development.* New York: Macmillan.

KERR, R. (1982). *Psychomotor learning.* Philadelphia: Saunders College Publishing.

MALINA, R. M. (1975). *Growth and development—The first twenty years.* Minneapolis: Burgess.

RARICK, G. (Ed.). (1973) *Physical activity: Human growth and development.* New York: Academic Press.

RIDENOUR, M. (1978). *Motor development: Issues and applications.* Princeton, NJ: Princeton.

SHEPHARD, R. J. (1982). *Physical Activity and Growth.* Chicago: Year Book Medical Publishers.

THOMAS, J. (Ed.). (1984). *Motor development during childhood and adolescence.* Minneapolis: Burgess Publishing.

WILLIAMS, H. G. (1983). *Perceptual and motor development.* Englewood Cliffs, NJ: Prentice-Hall.

3

THE SCIENTIFIC BASIS FOR MOTOR-SKILL ACQUISITION

SCHEMA THEORY

One of the recent major developments in elementary physical education has been the use of *schema theory* as a basis for teaching and understanding the acquisition of motor skills by children. Few theories of motor-skill learning have had as great an impact or as much support from the scientific community. As with other scientific notions, it has been the role of the practitioner to gather what is believed to be the "best" scientific information available and develop teaching/learning models to facilitate application in a practical setting. This process of "theory into practice," joining the scientific with the practical, is the subject of this section (see Gabbard, 1984).

Understanding the Theory

Schema theory (Schmidt, 1975, 1977) proposes an explanation of how individuals learn and perform a seemingly endless variety of movements. Basically, the theory proposes that humans store in memory past movement experiences. This storage of "movement elements" and their relationship to each other are called *movement schema*. The theory suggests that the motor programs we store in memory are not specific records of the movements to be performed; rather, they are a set of general rules (schemas) to guide performance. An individual calls up his or her schema to program (in a sense, "piece together") movements. Schema theory suggests an explanation (which other theories do not) for two characteristics of human performance. First, individuals rarely repeat a set of movements precisely in the same manner. If a separate program were required for each movement variation performed, our storage capabilities would be quickly surpassed. Second, individuals are capable of programming movements to fit seemingly novel situations. An example of schema theory in practice is the performance of an individual playing shortstop in baseball or guard in basketball. The shortstop can field a ball from numerous positions—many novel (not practiced)—and return the ball to first base, just as the basketball player can shoot successfully from almost any (unrehearsed) position on the court. Schema theory treats motor programs in much the same manner as concepts are treated in verbal learning. The motor program begins with the cognitive domain and perception of incoming information. The child who has practiced throwing far, hard, soft, or short has a good cognitive sense of what may be in the middle. The same sense of prediction is assumed to be applicable to other movement situations. Abstractions are derived from a large number of similar instances that may represent the relationship among various guidelines needed to identify a particular instance of the concept or produce a particular segment of the movement. The motor schema (concept) for a general skill area (e.g., throwing, jumping) is bounded by dimensions related to space, time, and force. Each dimension represents a continuum that may (depending upon experience) be very limited or quite diverse. The more particular instances generated by the individual, the more abstract the schema becomes. The motor schema enables the individual to select the appropriate level from each dimension to program a task that may be either known or novel. The basketball player calls upon a program consisting of a relationship among distance the ball has to travel, required muscular force, arm speed, and angle of release, all of which may change from one attempt to the other.

One of the most fundamental applications and aspects of schema theory is that the learning of a skill can be facilitated by "variability in practice." The theory predicts that practicing a variety of movement outcomes within the same general skill area will provide a widely based set of experiences upon which a schema can be built. Schema theory predicts that individuals with high variability within an area should show superior performance over those with limited experiences. For example, the child who is limited to throwing experiences, using an overhand pattern only, would not be as adept to the performance of a novel throwing task outside that pattern as the child who has had experiences throwing from various positions. Generally, schema research supports what researchers have assumed for a long time: If the task is "closed" (that is, the number of movements is somewhat fixed, as in bowling or swinging a golf club), it is more conducive to practice that one movement pattern than to practice variations. If the task is classified as "open"

"Variability in practice" is the key to a diversified motor-skill foundation.

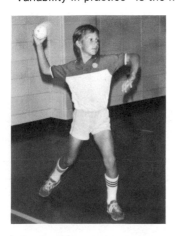
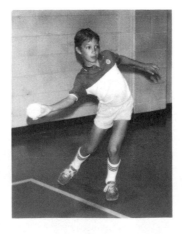
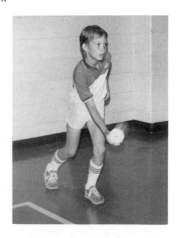

(that is, the movement responses are somewhat unpredictable, such as playing shortstop in baseball or guard in basketball), it is much better to practice a variety of responses because one never knows what specific movements will be required. It may also be assumed that the more "open" a task is, the more effective will be variable practice.

A strong body of research findings (with variable practice conditions) using children support the predictions of this theory, namely that variability in practice is a strong variable in determining transfer to a novel motor response of the same class (Shapiro & Schmidt, 1981).

Implications and Applications

Of course the strongest practical implications of this theory would be in the area of elementary school physical education, because it is at this age when basic motor skills are being established. (Kerr, 1982)

. . . . practice variability is a positive factor in motor learning, especially so for children's motor learning. (Schmidt, 1982)

Schema theory (and variability in practice) strongly suggests developing a solid foundation consisting of a variety of motor-skill experiences early in life. Variability in practice is predictively more effective for children than for adults simply because young individuals have considerably more to learn. Generally, schema theory supports the practice of problem solving during early years rather than the instruction of specific sport skills. With the establishment of a broad motor foundation (schema), children should be in a better position to acquire and apply specific skills, especially in an "open" environment (where conditions vary frequently). Schema theory suggests a progression from a general base to more specific concepts.

Variability In Practice

Schmidt (1977) suggests that if attempting to apply concepts of the schema theory, variability within the same class of movements (for example, throwing) should be structured to maximize the motor program dimensions of space (spatial), time, and force. Figure 3–1 presents an illustrative example of the theoretical process of se-

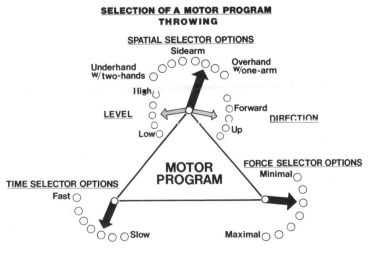

Figure 3–1 A schematic representation of the selection of a motor program for throwing.

lection of a motor program for throwing. What follows is an explanation of those concepts when used in the practice situation.

Spatial

The *spatial* dimension is best enhanced through movement-pattern variability. Within the schema class of throwing, for example, this dimension may contain variations ("elements") of the overhand, sidearm, and underhand patterns. Each of these can be performed with one of two hands, or both, at different levels from the ground (squatting, while jumping, and so forth), and with impetus toward various directions.

Time

The *time* dimension contains information upon which to judge at what speed the spatial (movement) pattern should be activated. Experiences should be provided that develop the continuum that ranges from slow motion to fast.

Force

Another dimension along which the motor program might be varied is the amount of *force* that is exerted. Related to time, mass (size), and weight, this dimension can be greatly enhanced with the use of manipulative objects and implements. Experiences that vary the force requirements, such as throwing (using the overhand pattern) to a target from varied distances, and using various size (mass) and weighted balls (weight), should enhance throwing schema and allow increased transfer to a novel task. Table 3–1 presents an outline of practice variation that may be implemented after basic mechanical principles are introduced.

Table 3–1 Throwing

	SPATIAL	
	Movement Pattern Variations	
Two hands:	One hand (right/left):	
Underhand (from front	underhand	
and either side)	sidearm	
Overhand (overhead, chest	overhand	Vary base of support
pass, from either side)	variations	(narrow to wide)
	Directions/Pathways/Levels	
	Throw up, down, forward, to side, at an angle	
	Throw while:	
	squatting or sitting (low level)	
	jumping or leaping (high level)	
	Throw while moving in various directions:	
	forward sideways	
	backward diagonally	

TIME	*FORCE*
Slow to fast	Throw objects of various sizes and weight
Throwing balls at a stationary target	(e.g., whiffleball, fleeceball, softball,
Throwing balls at a moving target	football, frisbee, playground ball)
Throwing while moving a target	Throw hard for distance
(stationary/moving)	Throw soft to medium
To a rhythmic beat	Combine distance and accuracy

OTHER FACTORS AFFECTING MOTOR–SKILL ACQUISITION

Along with the practical implications of motor-learning theory such as those previously discussed, other factors may enhance or negatively affect the learning of motor skills by children. With a knowledge of these factors, the teacher is in a better position to optimize individual as well as group-learning conditions.

Selective Attention

Critical to the learning of any task is the ability to attend selectively (concentrate) to a specific stimulus while ignoring other simultaneously presented information. The ability to concentrate on one specific feature while performing a task can be difficult for many children. Such may be the situation when a child is attempting to kick or strike a ball, especially if the teacher instructs the child to concentrate not only on specific parts of the movement but also to attend visually to the flight of the object. The experienced performer has less difficulty in attending to multiple sources of information; however, when instructing children it is best to present relative information separately, or within the capabilities of the individual child. Ideally, the teacher must provide an environment that helps the child attend to the most relevant information he or she can process and respond to. For optimal learning, the physical environment should be free of distractions such as irrelevant noises, visual displays, and extra equipment. Instructions should be clearly and concisely transmitted so that they emphasize the most relevant points of the task. Many teachers fail to realize that potential failure by the child may be caused either by an overload of information or the fact that the child is not focusing on the parts of the task, but rather on the result of a demonstration.

Motivation and Interest

Motivation and *interest* are ever-present factors in the performance and learning of a skill. Motivation is often described as an intrinsic need or desire to perform or learn that prompts one to satisfy that need or desire. Because motivation is intrinsically based, the teacher does not actually motivate the learner, but instead provides conditions that may result in an increased or decreased state of motivation. In reference to motor performance, one of the most frequently utilized motivational constructs is *arousal*. Thus a better description of motivation would be that it is an internal factor that *arouses* and directs a person's behavior (Stallings, 1982). Although motivation and arousal are positive factors in the learning of a skill, research indicates that too much or too little arousal may not be conducive to motor performance and learning. The child has to be aroused to a level of desiring to learn; however, a high degree of arousal, causing anxiety or stress, may not allow the individual to attend to the task optimally. Teachers need to be effective in eliciting arousal, and this may be accomplished through various conditions: providing interesting activities, knowledge of results, realistic goal setting, and degree of success.

As already stated, interest is an ever-present contributing factor to the learning situation. An innovative teacher not only has knowledge of the traditional activities that interest children but is also aware of their current concerns and stimulates new areas of interest. With movement experiences, the stimulation of interest is usually a natural phenomenon and it is the "unstructured" (that is, flexible) teacher who makes the most of these opportunities. Important to the stimulation of interest is making the activity and learning meaningful to the child, which may best be accomplished by individualizing the learning situation.

Feedback/Knowledge of Results

Feedback refers to all the information that a child receives relative to his or her performance. Feedback may be internal or external, and it might occur during or after the performance of a task. *Internal feedback,* the stimuli coming from within the body, primarily originates with the kinesthetic senses (from receptors in muscles, tendons, joints, and the inner ear). *External feedback* may involve any one or combination of external sources: the five senses or a person such as the teacher. Fitts and Posner (1967) theorize that feedback has three functions (1) to motivate, (2) to change immediate performance, and (3) to reinforce learning. The importance of feedback to the learning process cannot be overemphasized. Teachers should think of feedback as more than knowledge of results, for appropriate information *during* and *after* the task is important for reinforcing correct behavior and possibly modifying incorrect responses.

Although most feedback in physical education is external and produced by the teacher using verbal cues or manual guidance, activities should be presented that encourage internal feedback as well. This may be provided through the introduction of simple skills, which allow for immediate and recognizable results, such as jumping, running, kicking, and throwing. More complex activities, such as learning to dance or performing certain gymnastic stunts, may not be easily analyzed by the child; therefore feedback should be provided during, as well as after, the performance. The teacher should remember that children respond best when they are continuously aware of the performance and results of their efforts. The alert teacher will provide the child with appropriate external feedback and present conditions (activities) that stimulate internal awareness.

Whole and Part Learning

Whole and part learning refers to the presentation and learning of skills in their entirety or in parts, which are then combined to form the complete skill. Important considerations for the teacher will be the complexity of the skill and the abilities of the child. A commonly utilized method (if the task is not too complex) is to begin by teaching the whole and then, if the child is having difficulty, identifying the problem and working on the part(s). Generally it is agreed that complex skills, such as specific dance, track and field, or swimming skills, be taught to students in their logical parts before being presented in their entirety. Because most skills taught to young children are fundamental movements (and not a combination of skills), the whole method is usually appropriate.

Retention and Overlearning

Retention refers to our capacity to remember. It usually entails the ability to repeat an act correctly over a period of time. In terms of motor performance, retention refers specifically to the extent of motor-skill proficiency remaining after a period without practice. Influencing factors on the retention of a skill are *review periods* and *overlearning.* When children are permitted to practice (review) motor skills in spaced intervals, they retain the information longer. Overlearning refers to the continuation of practice on a motor skill after attaining a criterion level of performance, usually determined by the teacher. Overlearning enhances refinement of skill performance and retention by allowing the learning that has taken place to "set" or "consolidate" (that is, a strengthening of the connection between the sensory and motor apparatus). The teacher should, if possible, allow for adequate practice of skills presented; this needs to be a strong consideration during planning. If the physical education periods are relatively short, (about 15 to 30 minutes) skills from previous periods should be reviewed and, if possible, combined with new skills presented. Children should also be encouraged to practice on their own time, such as during recess or after-school hours.

REFERENCES

FITTS, P. & POSNER, M. (1967). *Human perfor-mance.* Belmont, Calif.: Brooks/Cole Publisher.

GABBARD, C. (1984). Teaching motor skills to chil-dren: Theory into practice. *The Physical Educator, 41,* 69–71.

KERR, R. (1982). *Psychomotor learning.* Philadelphia: Saunders College Publishing.

SCHMIDT, R. A. (1975). A schema theory of discrete motor skill learning. *Psychological Review, 82,* 225–260.

SCHMIDT, R. A. (1982). *Motor control and learning:* Champaign, Illinois: Human Kinetics.

SCHMIDT, R. A. (1977). Schema theory: implications for movement education. *Motor Skills: Theory into Practice, 2,* 36–48.

SHAPIRO, D. C. & SCHMIDT, R. A. (1981). The schema theory: recent evidence and developmental implications. In J. A. S. Kelso & J. E. Clark (Eds.), *The development of movement control and coordination.* New York: Wiley.

STALLINGS, L. M. (1982). *Motor learning: from theory to practice.* St. Louis: C. V. Mosby.

SUGGESTED READINGS

CONNALLY, K. J. (Ed.) (1970). *Mechanism of motor skill development.* New York: Academic Press.

CORBIN, C. (1980). *A textbook of motor development.* Dubuque: W. C. Brown.

CRATTY, B. J. (1979). *Perceptual and motor develop-ment in infants and children.* Englewood Cliffs, NJ: Prentice-Hall.

GALLAHUE, D. L. (1982). *Understanding motor devel-opment in children.* New York: Wiley.

KELSO, S. & CLARK, J. (Eds.) (1982). *The develop-ment of movement control and coordination.* New York: Wiley & Sons.

KEOGH, J. & SUGDEN, D. (1985). *Movement skill de-velopment.* New York: Macmillan.

THOMAS, J. (Ed.) (1984). *Motor development during childhood and adolescence.* Minneapolis: Burgess Pub-lishing.

THOMAS, M. R. (1979). *Comparing theories of child development.* Belmont, CA.: Wadsworth Publishing.

WILLIAMS, H. G. (1983). *Perceptual and motor devel-opment.* Englewood Cliffs, NJ: Prentice-Hall.

YUSSEN, S. & SANTROCK, J. (1978). *Child develop-ment.* Dubuque, Iowa: Wm. C. Brown.

ZAICHKOWSKY, D. L., et al. (1980). *Growth and de velopment - The child and physical activity.* St. Louis: C. V. Mosby.

4

PHYSICAL FITNESS

Just as with the acquisition of specific motor skills, physical fitness does not occur by chance. In even the most active physical education programs, fitness components such as cardiovascular endurance, upper body strength/endurance, and flexibility may not be acquired at acceptable levels. Specific and general physical fitness activities should be a part of every daily plan during the "Fitness Phase" of the lesson. Chapters 5 and 13 present a detailed discussion related to this phase of the daily lesson.

FITNESS AND COMPONENTS

The term *fitness* has taken on numerous meanings over the years. General definitions have included such concepts as the ability to function normally without undue fatigue, and being able to enjoy leisure-time activities without debilitating physical stress. In recent times, the term has been divided into two distinct categories: skill-related and health-related fitness.

Skill-Related Fitness

Skill-related fitness (sometimes referred to as *performance fitness*) includes those qualities that provide the individual with the ability to participate in sport activities. This type of fitness assessment is usually found in most physical fitness tests (for example, 50-yard dash, shuttle run, broad jump). The results reflect a person's quality of performance of a specific motor task.

Components of Skill-Related Fitness
Speed. This is the ability to move from one place to another in the shortest possible time. It is primarily innate yet it can be improved through practice for technique and movement efficiency.

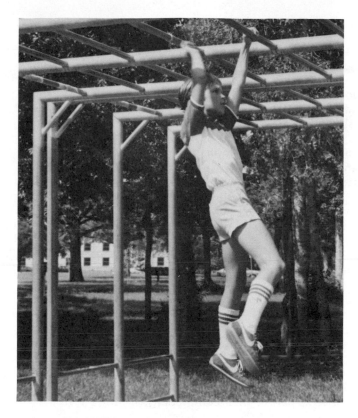

Agility.   This is the ability to change direction or body position rapidly and proceed with another movement. Agility is interrelated with speed, strength, balance, and coordination. Agility, like speed, is partially innate yet it can also be improved through practice. The acquisition of agility is very important to success in game activities requiring dodging, changing of direction, and quick starts and stops.

Coordination.   This is the ability to integrate motor and sensory systems into an efficient pattern of movement. Essential to good eye-hand, eye-foot, and rhythmic movements, coordination is vital to success in most movement activities, including those performed as part of daily functioning.

Power.   This is the combination of strength with explosiveness (speed); maximum muscular force released at maximum speed. Power is a fundamental factor in jumping, throwing, kicking, and striking. Power is improved through increases in strength and practice.

Balance.   This is defined as the ability to maintain one's body position and equilibrium in both static and dynamic movement situations.

Health-Related Fitness

Over the last 15 years Americans have expressed a strong interest in health and physical activity. It has been estimated that participation in fitness activities has doubled during this period and appears to be on the upswing (President's Council on Physical Fitness and Sports, 1980). Much of this trend has been stimulated by some new and convincing evidence that regular exercise in combination with proper diet and abstention from smoking and using potentially dangerous drugs will increase greatly one's quality of health.

Health-related fitness refers to "those aspects of physiological and psychological functioning which are believed to offer the individual some protection against degenerative type diseases such as coronary heart disease, obesity, and various musculoskeletal disorders" (Falls, 1980).

Fitness Components and Effects on Growth and Development

Cardiovascular Endurance.   Identified as the most important component in health-related fitness, cardiovascular endurance is the ability of the heart, lungs, and vascular system to function efficiently for an extended period of time. Directly related to this function is *physical working capacity*. A heart and circulatory system that is functioning at a higher level, thus delivering more blood, is also making more oxygen available to working muscles. This process increases the child's ability to work at a greater intensity and over a longer period of time without debilitating fatigue.

Research studies have reported the indication of early symptoms of coronary heart disease such as arteriosclerosis present in children as young as 2 years of age (Albinson & Andrews, 1976; Rose, 1973; Wilmore & McNamara, 1974). Such diseases, found to be related to diet and level of physical activity (exercise), have been shown to decrease with changes in lifestyle that should start as a preventative health program during early childhood. The American Heart Association (1980) recently stated that "people of all ages should be encouraged to develop a physically active lifestyle as part of their comprehensive program of heart disease prevention."

Body Composition.   *Body composition* is defined as the relative percentages of fat and lean body mass. Generally, children who are 10 to 20 percent over recommended "weight for height" charts are considered overweight. The *obese* category represents those who are 20 percent over recommended values. A more scientific method of determining body fat, recommended by the American Alliance for Health, Physical Education, Recreation and Dance, is measuring skinfolds using calipers (see "Assessment" section in this chapter).

The American Medical Association has estimated that at least 40 percent of school-aged children are overweight. Convincing evidence exists to show that "most" fat children will have to fight their problem for the rest of their lives (Corbin, 1973; Eden, 1975; Heald, 1966). Kaufman (1975) reports "there is strong evidence that if an individual is obese as a child, he has a 90 percent chance of being obese as an adult." Much of the problem has come from parents who have been resistant to helping their young child, believing that the youngster will "grow out of it"; fortunately, these attitudes about "body fat" seem to be changing.

Not only does obesity mean decreased endurance and work capacity, but it also means that children exhibiting these characteristics usually consume a diet high in saturated fats and cholesterol, thus increasing the probability of coronary heart disease and atherosclerosis (Stein, 1981).

The physical education instructor can make a significant contribution to decreasing the obese child's problem only if the parents cooperate. Increased physical activity levels increase caloric expenditure (decrease weight); however, a controlled diet is of equal, if not more, importance. After the child's fitness assessment, physical educators should consult with the parents and suggest a remedial program to be carried out at home.

Muscular Strength.   *Muscular strength* is the ability of the bo̶ imum force against an external resistance. Strength in its purest fo̶ to exert one maximum effort (for example, lifting a heavy weight, ̶ ing, kicking). *Static strength* refers to exerting maximum force on object, such as employed with isometric exercises.

The relevance of strength to skill-related performance is rather ̶ ̶̶̶̶ ̶ ̶ ̶ ̶ ̶ w-ever, its importance in general health is less apparent. Stronger muscles give better protection to the joints, which they cross, and, as a result, the child is less susceptible to strains and sprains. Better muscle tone has been shown to aid in the prevention of some common postural problems, including low back syndrome, that approximately 80 percent of the population experiences at some point in their lives (Falls, 1980).

Muscular Endurance.   *Muscular endurance* is the ability of a muscle or groups of muscles to sustain repetitive contractions over a long period of time. Muscle endurance is generally related to muscular strength but differs in the emphasis. Strength is exhibited by a greater overload with fewer contractions and is specific to the muscles exercised. Muscular endurance activities have less overload and involve a greater number of contractions. Examples of muscular endurance activities are pull-ups, sit-ups, push-ups, and the flexed- or straight-arm hang. Muscular endurance is also related to posture and muscular fatigue, for it is generally agreed that muscles that are easily fatigued and/or strained cannot support proper spinal alignment. Muscular-endurance-type activities enable children to build greater resistance to muscular fatigue, which in turn allows them to work and play for longer periods of time.

Flexibility.   *Flexibility* is the degree to which a joint may move through its maximum possible normal range of motion. Flexibility can be improved with movement experiences. From a health viewpoint, lack of adequate flexibility often contributes to postural problems. These problems are usually a result of shortening of muscles and/or connective tissue around a joint owing to inactivity. Together with strength, adequate flexibility is a major contributor to the prevention of back problems, primarily caused by a shortening of connective tissue in the lower back and thighs, and weakened abdominal muscles.

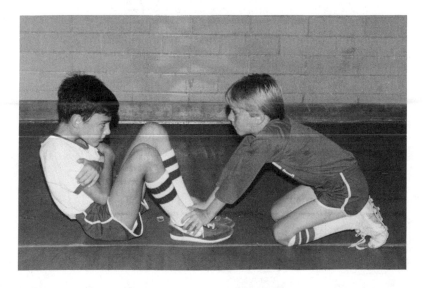

Although most children present adequate levels of flexibility because of their active nature, a decrease in the range of motion may prevent the child from performing many motor skills efficiently. It has also been observed that many active children can have poor hamstring flexibility because of high activity and insufficient stretching.

Basic Benefits of Health-Related Physical Activity

1. Increases physical working capacity.
2. When combined with proper diet, vigorous activity is a positive contributor toward the control of body fat and coronary heart disease.
3. Vigorous activity contributes to the development of skeletal growth through increased mineralization. Inactivity for prolonged periods causes demineralization, thus brittleness in bones.
4. Muscular strength, endurance, and flexibility promote good posture and are conducive to efficient movement patterns.
5. Physical activity results in more energy and thus contributes to greater individual productivity for physical as well as mental tasks.
6. The development of health-related components contributes to better performance in many skill-related activities.
7. Being fit helps in the development of a desirable self-concept.

POSTURE

Most experts agree that early detection and correction of deviate postural conditions are important to the quality of one's life. Posture, like all human characteristics, not only involves individual differences but also variation within the individual. Generally, good posture is judged when one is standing behind a plumb line and the body segments appear in good alignment over the base of support (Figs. 4-1 and 4-2). Physical fitness and posture are closely interrelated, for each contributes somewhat to the other. Proper alignment promotes efficiency of movement, whereas fitness provides muscle tone that supports segmental alignment.

Figure 4-1 Figure side view.

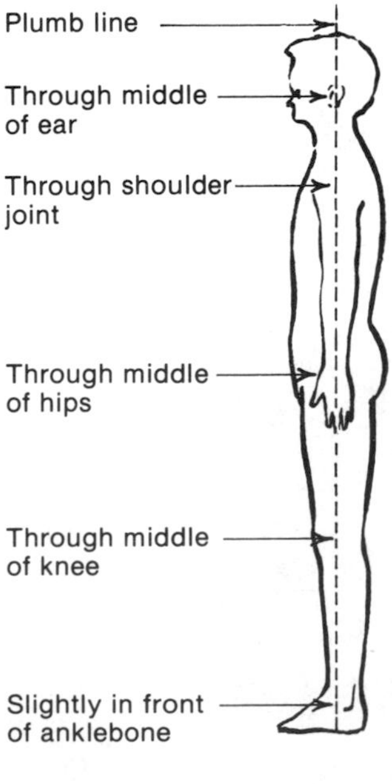

Plumb line

Through middle of ear

Through shoulder joint

Through middle of hips

Through middle of knee

Slightly in front of anklebone

Figure 4-2 Figure rear view.

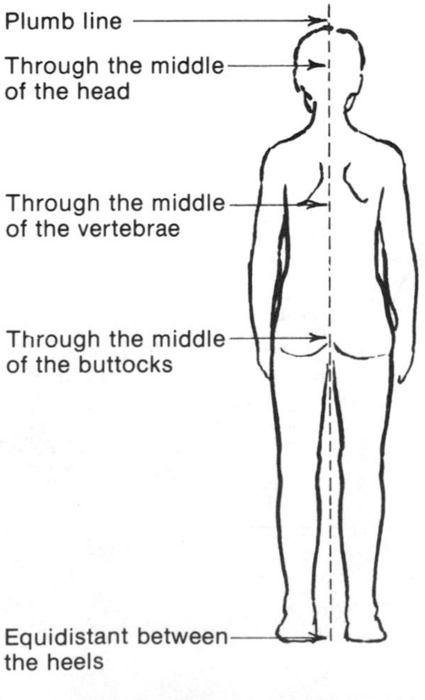

Plumb line

Through the middle of the head

Through the middle of the vertebrae

Through the middle of the buttocks

Equidistant between the heels

Problems and Common Conditions

Poor posture prolonged over a long period of time encourages the muscles to adapt to the incorrect position, therefore making it increasingly difficult to correct the condition(s). Early screening, starting at the preschool or kindergarten level, is recommended. Some of the causes of postural deviations are chronic television viewing, sitting in awkward positions (in desks, chairs, on the floor), improper diet, inadequate lighting, excess weight, and poor muscle tone (especially in the abdominal region). Most common postural conditions can be observed and corrected with proper exercise; however, the physical educator (or nurse) should take into account his or her professional limitations. Cases that appear less than normal (especially signs of scoliosis) should be brought to the attention of the child's parents along with a recommendation that professional medical advice be sought.

Conditions

Lordosis (swayback).   *Lordosis* is characterized by an exaggerated forward curvature of the lower back and prominence of the sacrum and buttocks (Fig. 4–3). Many young children, especially females (3 to 5 years of age), exhibit slight characteristics of this condition that are due to immaturity, but these are usually resolved between the ages of 7 and 9. Weak abdominal muscles may be the cause; however, the problem could be a fixed structural deformity such as slipped vertebrae or spondylolisthesis.

Kyphosis (round back).   *Kyphosis* is associated with an exaggerated curvature of the upper back. This condition places a strain on the upper back musculature, thus shifting the weight of the body to the front of the feet (Fig. 4–4).

Scoliosis (lateral curvature of the spine).   *Scoliosis* is a lateral curvature of the spine that can take either of two forms: a C- or S-shaped curve (Fig. 4–5). Scoliosis is a very debilitating condition if undetected and untreated, and signs of scoliosis should be reported to parents and medical personnel immediately.

Figure 4-3 Lordosis (swayback).

Figure 4-4 Kyhosis (round back)

Figure 4-5 Scoliosis (C and S curves).

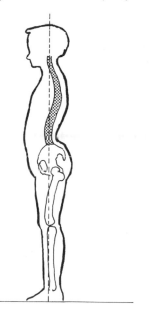
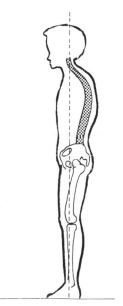
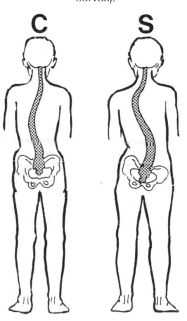

Postural Assessment

The school nurse usually coordinates the assessment program with the help of the physical education and/or classroom teacher. A number of methods are available such as screens and tape, but one of the most popular and convenient ways is with a plumb line or string with a weight on one end hung in a doorway. It is suggested that children wear leotards, or shorts and halters, and that an adult female be present for screening girls.

The following type of posture assessment chart is recommended because of its specific screening characteristics (Fig. 4-6).

Figure 4-6   Posture assessment chart.

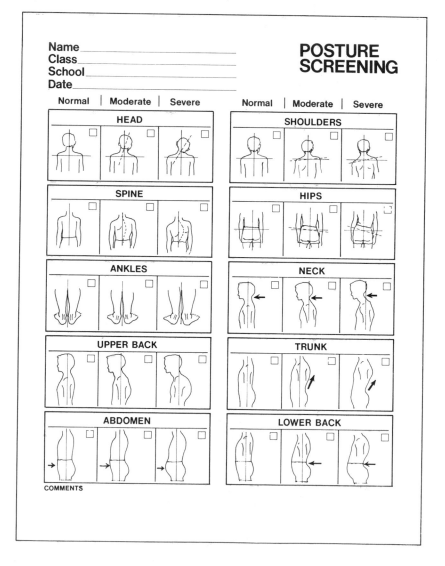

Recommended exercises and activities conducive to the development of good posture can be found in Chapter 13, "Physical Fitness Activities."

Fitness Assessment

In response to current trends, children's needs, and scientific evidence, the American Alliance for Health, Physical Education, Recreation and Dance (AAHPERD) introduced the *AAHPERD Health-Related Physical Fitness Test* in 1980. Its focus, upon health-related components, emphasizes the need for a basic health-fitness program for children: test items and norms are designed for individuals 5 to 17 years of age.

H. B. Falls, who headed the AAHPERD Task Force on Youth Fitness, refers to the test as a "return to the basics." He adds that the components have been shown by research and/or clinical practice to be significantly related to health and that "adequate function in these components can have a positive effect on one's quality of life throughout childhood and adult years" (Falls, 1980).

Components and test items are as follows:

1. Cardiorespiratory function
   Mile run or 9-minute run;
   1.5-mile run, or 12-minute run, is optional for individuals 13 years or older
2. Body Composition (leanness/fatness)
   Sum of triceps and subcapular skinfolds (norms start at 6 years);
   triceps skinfold is used if only one site is selected
3. Abdominal and low back-hamstring musculoskeletal function (two tests):
   a. Modified, timed sit-ups (60 seconds)
   b. Sit and reach

(Procedures and norms may be found in the Appendix)

Although not many test batteries of the skill-related type are available for primary-grade children (and should not be used as the primary fitness assessment), the teacher may wish to screen individuals to identify underachievers. With the high interest today in sports and skill-related fitness components (speed, agility, power) associated with them, teachers will find such activities highly motivating. If underachievers are identified, a remedial program for such individuals should be conducted. Table 4–1 suggests average performance levels for children 5 to 9 years of age on selected skill-related tasks. Testing procedures may be found in the Appendix.

Table 4-1 Average Levels of Performance for Children 5–9 Years of Age

	BOYS AND GIRLS				
Age	Flexed-arm Hang (sec)*	Shuttle Run (sec)	Standing Long Jump	Softball Throw	40-yd. Dash (sec)
5	8	13.9	3'1"	24'	8.4
6	9	13.7	3'4"	26'	8.3
7	10	13.0	3'7"	36'	8.2
8	11	12.6	3'11"	45'	7.8
9	12	12.1	4'5"	56'	7.4

*The flexed-arm hang is an assessment of muscular strength/endurance; therefore it may also be identified as health related.

Table 4-2 Fitness Tests

NAME OF TEST	LEVEL	ITEMS	SOURCE
AAHPERD—Health-Related Physical Fitness Test (1980)	Ages 5–17	(Described in text) 1-mile or 9-min run 1.5 mile or 12-min run/(13 yrs or older) Skinfolds 1-min bent-knee sit-up Sit and reach	AAHPERD, 1900 Association Dr., Reston, Va. 22091
Texas Physical and Motor Fitness Development Program: Evaluation (1983)	Ages 5–9	1-mile or 9-min walk/run 1-min bent-knee sit-up/static push-up Sit and reach Shuttle run Standing long jump Also included are: Dynamic balance/static balance Kicking/throwing/catching Body awareness Posture	The Governor's Commission on Physical Fitness, 400 North Lamar, Suite 101, Austin, Texas 78756

AAHPERD Youth Fitness Test (1976 Edition)	Grades 5–12	Pull-ups (boys)
		Flexed-arm hang (girls)
		Sit-ups
		Shuttle run
		Standing long jump
		50-yd dash
		600-yd run or options
		   1-mile or 9-min run (10–12 yrs)
		   1.5-mile or 12-min run (13 yrs or older)
			AAHPERD, 1900 Association Dr., Reston, Va. 22091

Texas Physical Fitness-Motor Ability Test (1973)	Grades 4–12	Chin-ups (boys) Flexed-arm hang (girls) Dips Sit-ups 9-min or 1-mile run 12-min or 1.5-mile run (grades 7–12) 50-yd dash or 8-sec run 15-sec shuttle or zigzag run Vertical or standing long jump	The Governor's Commission on Physical Fitness, 400 North Lamar, Suite 101, Austin, Texas 78756

Table 4–2 is a list of recommended test batteries suitable for children. Manuals and other information (norms, awards) may be secured at the addresses provided.

General Testing Guidelines

1. Be sure that each child participating in the testing has had a recent physical and that no restrictions on vigorous activity are indicated. This may be accomplished by checking with the school nurse, checking the records yourself, or asking the parents in written form.

2. Precondition the children at the beginning of the year (prior to the first test session). A suggestion is to describe one test item daily and allow practice over a couple of days during the fitness activity. It is recommended that the teacher hold off on the first testing until *at least* the tenth class meeting. The second testing should be no earlier than the last week of April and no later than the first week of May to allow for make-up tests, formulation of awards, and recording.

3. Provide enough motivation so children exhibit their maximum possible effort. Motivation can be stimulated with an effective discussion about the importance of fitness as well as with extrinsic rewards.

4. Record results on the child's cumulative record.

5. Send home test results along with a description of the items and the purpose of each.

Use the information about each child to accommodate his or her needs. If a deficiency is indicated, outline a program for the child that can be used at home as well as at school. Use extra help if available (aides, parent volunteers, others).

Data Forms

Recording and dissemination of results may take many forms, usually dependent upon funds, number of children, school or system organizational structure, and personal preference. No matter what form the record may take, it should: (1) be transmitted to parents and, preferably, by the child, in an interpretable form, and (2) be cumulative (recorded from test to test, year to year).

The cumulative record, ideally on heavy weight cards, should indicate performance on each test item administered during the year; usually two full batteries are given yearly, at least four months apart. The more popular dates are mid-September and late April.

Computers, very much a part of our everyday life, have been put to great use in many elementary fitness programs. Computers are especially popular in larger school systems, but they are by no means just advantageous to them. Major assets of computers are efficiency with large populations and versatility in the form of analysis and printed results. Some of the benefits of using a computer, along with a reduction in hours of manual calculations, are: generating systemwide norms, making comparisons between scores (individuals and/or classes), and generating printed results (tables and/or graphs) that are more understandable to teachers, parents, and children.

The following are examples of (1) a cumulative fitness record (Table 4-3), (2) individual profiles for parents and child (Tables 4-4 and 4-5), and (3) a computerized fitness printout (Figure 4-7). For skill-related items, norms and percentages from recommended tests may be used, or if for screening purposes (see Table 4-1), the raw score and Satisfactory or Unsatisfactory should be placed in the appropriate boxes.

A brief explanation (description and purpose) of test items and interpretation should be included on a second sheet if sent home to the child's parents.

A Trend Toward Total School Involvement

Along with the recent awareness and concern about cardiorespiratory fitness and prevention of coronary heart disease, a number of prevention programs designed specifically for children in grades K-6 have emerged. Such programs, referred to as the "total school fitness involvement" concept, characteristically consist of a combined program of physical assessment, exercise, health education, and diet.

One very successful program, "Sunflower Project,"[1] involving children, teachers, and parents, altered the school curriculum in several ways to accomplish stated objectives. A family fitness program was initiated which involved individuals

[1] For information on this program, contact Mrs. Donna Osness, Project Director, Shawnee Mission, Instructional Program Center, 6649 Lamar, Shawnee Mission, Kans. 66202.

Table 4-3 Cumulative Fitness Record

NAME _____

Grade	K		1		2		3		4		5		6	
Date	Fall	Spr	Fall	Spr	Fall	Spr	Fall	Spr	Fall	Spr	Fall	Spr	Fall	Spr
Age														
Height (in/cm)														
Weight (lb/kg)														
Posture														
Rating														

Component	SC	%	SC	%	SC	%	SC	%	SC	%	SC	%	SC	%	SC	%	SC	%	SC	%	SC	%	SC	%	SC	%	SC	%
Distance Run																												
Skinfolds																												
Sit-ups																												
Sit-and-reach																												
Flexed-arm hang																												
Standing long jump																												
Shuttle run																												
40-yard dash																												
50-yard dash																												
Softball throw																												
Pull-ups																												

and families in an aerobics program before school each morning. The health-education program was supplemented with materials and resource centers that actively involved the child. Recess was changed to a 20-minute fitness session designed to accommodate all students regardless of physical capabilities. In addition, an aerobics fitness program was designed for teachers and conducted after school. This aspect of the program was considered critical to success because of the large extent to which children are influenced by teacher attitudes and behaviors. To stimulate after-school activity (as well as during school), a fitness trail park was installed for use by students and their families. Another similar project, "Super Heart,"[2] which at one time involved approximately 4,000 children, can provide valuable total curriculum materials and teacher training.

[2]For information, contact College of Education, State University of New York, Cortland, N.Y. 13045.

Table 4-4 Individual Fitness Profile

NAME JOHN DOE

CLASS 1-C

AGE 6

YEAR 1983–84

(Space for optional items; skill-related norms from recommended tests may be used, or write raw score above or below 50% line if screening; see Table 4–1.)

	Distance Run			Sit-ups			Sit & Reach			Skinfolds			Broad Jump								
	1	2	X	1	2	X	1	2	X	1	2	X	1	2	X	1	2	X	1	2	X
99																					
95																					
90																					
85																					
80																					
75																					
70																					
65																					
60																					
55																					
50																					
45																					
40																					
35																					
30																					
25																					
20																					
15																					
10																					
5																					

(Use different colored markers for each testing session if both sets of scores are plotted after the second test).

Comments:

Table 4-5 Individual Fitness Profile

NAME __JOHN DOE__

AGE __6__

CLASS __1-C__

YEAR __1983–84__

Items	Test I		Test II	
	Score	Percentile	Score	Percentile
Distance Run	11:20	70		
Skinfolds	12	60		
Sit-ups	34	91		
Sit-and-Reach	30	80		
Standing Long Jump	3'6"	S		
40-yard Dash	8.1	S		

Satisfactory represents a 50th percentile or above; Unsatisfactory, below 50%.

Comments:

A 1982 report by Gilliam and colleagues concerning exercise programs for children presented the following recommendations that support the "total involvement" concept:

1. School systems need to promote vigorous physical education programs and teach the cognitive aspects of exercise and nutrition (it was noted that physical education programs will have only limited success until this is implemented).
2. Schools should set up an exercise trail on the school grounds and encourage children to use it during recess and record their accomplishments on a classroom chart.
3. A large clock with a second hand should be set up on the playground and children encouraged to check their pulse periodically (preferably 160 beats/min for 25 to 30 minutes) to determine if they are achieving high heart rates.
4. Use teachers or physical education students from nearby institutions to conduct fitness activities during recess periods.
5. Encourage all children to run or walk around the school area before participation in recess.

The emergence of such programs is definitely a positive trend toward the improvement of physical fitness in our nation. With evidence that two major causes of heart attacks (and cardiovascular disease) are improper diet and lack of exercise, and that corresponding diseases actually begin in childhood, programs of this nature may be considered a milestone in health education.

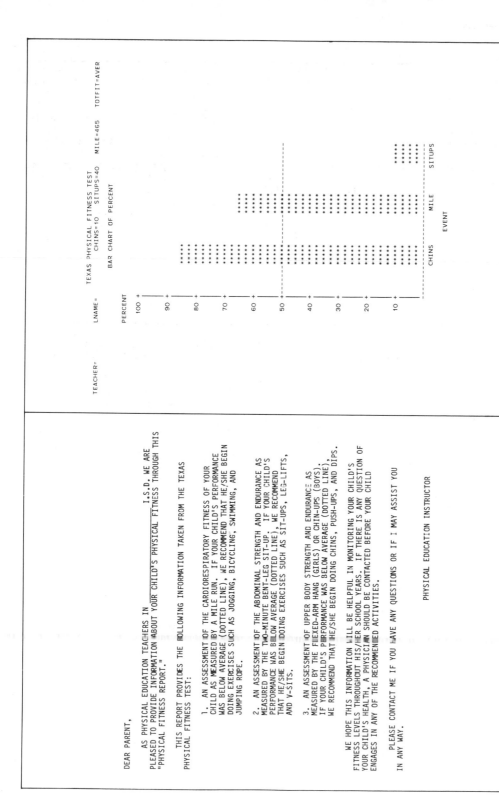

Figure 4-7 Computerized fitness printouts.

REFERENCES

AMERICAN HEART ASSOCIATION COMMITTEE REPORT. (1980). Risk factors and coronary disease: A statement for physicians. *Circulation, 62,* 449A–455A.

ALBINSON, J. G. & ANDREWS, G. M. (1976). *Child in sport and physical activity.* Baltimore: University Park Press.

CORBIN, C. (1973). *A textbook of motor development.* Dubuque, IA: Wm. C. Brown.

EDEN, A. (1975). How to fat-proof your child. *Reader's Digest, 107,* 150–152.

FALLS, H. B. (1980). Modern concepts of physical fitness. *Journal of Health, Physical Education and Recreation, 51,* 25–27.

GILLIAM, T. B., MACCONNIE, S. E., GEENEN, D. L., PELS III, A. E., & FREEDSON, P. S. (1982). Exercise programs for children: A way to prevent. *The Physician and Sportsmedicine, 10,* 96–106.

HEALD, F. P. (1966). Natural history and physiological basis of adolescent obesity. *Federation Proceedings, 25,* 4–7.

KAUFMAN, D. A. (1975). Fundamentals of fat. *The Physical Educator, 32,* 77–79.

PRESIDENT'S COUNCIL ON PHYSICAL FITNESS AND SPORTS. *Newsletter,* March 1980.

ROSE, K. (1973). To keep the people in health. *Journal of the American College Health Association, 22,* 80.

STEIN, E. A. (1981). Coronary risk factors in the young. *Annual Review of Medicine, 52,* 601–613.

WILMORE, J. H. & MCNAMARA, J. J. (1974). Prevalence of coronary heart disease risk factors in boys, 8 to 12 years of age. *Journal of Pediatrics, 84,* 527–533.

SUGGESTED READINGS

AAHPERD: Health-related fitness. (1981). In *Journal of Physical Education and Recreation, 52,* 26–39.

AAHPERD *health-related fitness test manual.* (1980). Washington, DC: American Alliance for Health, Physical Education, Recreation and Dance.

BERG, K. & ERIKSSON, B. (Eds.). (1980). *Children and exercise.* Baltimore: University Park Press.

BOILEAU, R. (Ed.). (1984). *Advances in pediatric sport sciences. Vol. 1.* Champaign, Illinois: Human Kinetics.

CORBIN, C. C. & LINDSEY, R. (1979). *Fitness for life.* Glenview, IL: Scott, Foresman.

CORBIN, C. (1980). *A textbook of motor development.* Dubuque: W. C. Brown.

CUNDIFF, D. E. (Ed.). (1979). *Implementation of aerobic programs.* Washington, DC: American Alliance for Health, Physical Education, Recreation and Dance.

DAVIS, R. (1982, January/February). An Elementary fitness program that works. *Health Education, 54.*

FALLS, H. B., BAYLOR, A. M., & DISHMAN, R. K. (1980). *Essentials of fitness.* Philadelphia: Saunders.

GALLAHUE, D. L. (1982). *Understanding motor development in children.* New York: Wiley.

GETCHELL, L. (1979). Physical fitness: A way of life. New York: Wiley.

SHEPHARD, R. J. (1982). *Physical Activity and Growth.* Chicago: Year Book Medical Publishers.

ZAICHKOWSKY, D. L., et al. (1980). *Growth and development—The child and physical activity.* St. Louis: C. V. Mosby.

5

CURRICULUM
AND PLANNING

INTRODUCTION

As the reader examines the following sections, the use of the terms "Level I, II, III" (the "Foundation") will be noted frequently, as well as periodic reference to more advanced items categorized by "Levels IV–VI." These categories have been utilized to identify (1) general curricular content, (2) estimated levels of motor performance, or (3) as in the case of movement activities, degree of task difficulty. Although *all* children of a specific age or within a school grade should not be automatically identified with a specific level, the following age range/level chart may prove helpful as a comparison to *general* performance.

Level I	4 to 5 years
II	6 to 7 years
III	8 to 9 years
Level IV	9 to 10 years
V	10 to 11 years
VI	11 years and older

Again, the reader is cautioned that while Levels I–III may be associated with preschool to third grade and Levels IV–VI with grades four to six, a child in the first grade may be performing at Level III, just as the 10-year-old may be at Level II.

CURRICULUM: BUILDING THE FOUNDATION OF FITNESS AND MOTOR SKILLS

As with any area of scholarly inquiry in which a new textbook emerges, much of the information and concepts contained therein were developed from and/or inspired by existing materials and knowledgeable individuals. In holding to the promising trends noted in the 1980s, the authors firmly believe that the use primarily of dance, game (and sport), and gymnastic activities is not the best approach to building an acceptable foundation of skill proficiency in children. The philosophy or assumption that fitness and motor-skill proficiency develop merely as a result of participation in fun activities has not been acceptable to the authors for many years, and that belief is even stronger today. One of the primary objectives of this text is to support the developmental-theme approach and to emphasize the health-related fitness concept. A curricular model is presented that is as scientific as practicality permits and at the same time blends the more traditional and contemporary instructional approaches. Figure 5–1 illustrates the general concept of integration and relationship between the contemporary approach and use of traditional activity areas.

"Building the Foundation" (Levels I–III) refers to program emphasis that focuses primarily upon the development of (1) physical fitness, (2) movement awareness, and (3) fundamental movement skills. The basis (that is, elements) for the curricular model was derived from knowledge related to the developmental psychomotor abilities of children as described in the previous chapters. It is with this information, plus years of experimentation and practical implementation, that the following model is presented.

In addition to a predetermined, structured plan for implementing the physical fitness component of the program (discussed in Chapter 13), the use of developmental themes is the cement by which the "foundation" is constructed, refined, and utilized with proficiency. A *developmental theme* is the focus of a lesson or series of lessons upon a specific fundamental movement skill or movement awareness. More than one movement skill or awareness theme (or the combination) can make up a single lesson. Closely related to the theme approach is the concept of "movement variability," which is discussed in the latter part of this chapter.

Table 5–1 presents the fundamental movement skills and movement awarenesses used to plan and implement the theme concept.

The following is a brief review and explanation of each category.

Figure 5-1 Outline of the curricular model.

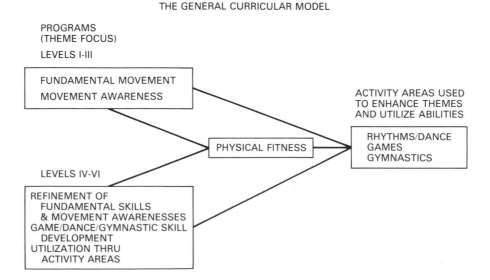

THE GENERAL CURRICULAR MODEL

PROGRAMS
(THEME FOCUS)
LEVELS I-III

FUNDAMENTAL MOVEMENT
MOVEMENT AWARENESS

ACTIVITY AREAS USED
TO ENHANCE THEMES
AND UTILIZE ABILITIES

PHYSICAL FITNESS

RHYTHMS/DANCE
GAMES
GYMNASTICS

LEVELS IV-VI

REFINEMENT OF
   FUNDAMENTAL SKILLS
   & MOVEMENT AWARENESSES
GAME/DANCE/GYMNASTIC SKILL
   DEVELOPMENT
UTILIZATION THRU
   ACTIVITY AREAS

Table 5-1   Fundamental Movement Skills and Movement Awarenesses

MOVEMENT AWARENESSES	FUNDAMENTAL LOCOMOTOR SKILLS	FUNDAMENTAL NONLOCOMOTOR SKILLS	FUNDAMENTAL MANIPULATIVE SKILLS
Body	Walking	Dodging	Propulsive
Spatial	Running	Stretching/bending	Rolling
Directional	Leaping	Turning/twisting	Throwing
Temporal	Jumping (and landing)	Pushing/pulling	Bouncing
Rhythm	Hopping	Swinging/swaying	Striking
Eye-hand	Galloping		Kicking
Eye-foot	Sliding		
Vestibular	Skipping		Receptive
Visual	Body Rolling		Catching
Auditory	Climbing		Trapping
Tactile			

Movement Awareness

Movement awareness refers to a specific aspect (component) of the perceptual-motor system deemed as basic to movement efficiency and the performance of fundamental movement skills. The execution of all motor tasks requires the utilization of various forms of sensory information and perceptual mechanisms. The movement awarenesses are, in essence, the "foundation" (that is, the components) responsible for acceptable motor-skill performance. Figure 5–2 represents an illustrative example of the foundation from which more complex motor tasks can be performed. Following this line of reasoning, one may assume that anything other than a primary emphasis upon the specific components (that is, themes) would not fit the developmental theme concept. Perhaps the major justification for the inclusion of movement awareness themes is the fact that many movement tasks

Figure 5-2   The movement foundation.

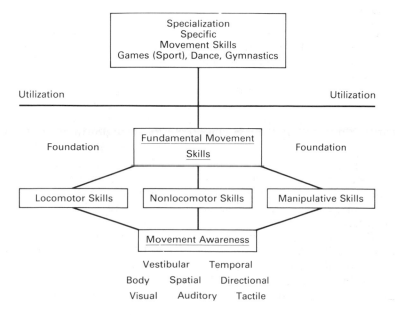

performed by children are not covered under the three fundamental movement categories; therefore, they are not accounted for except as secondary occurrences (as viewed in the "traditional activity approach").

As the reader may recall, one of the major objectives of the developmental-theme approach at the "foundation" level is to provide specific experiences for ensuring the development of specific motor abilities.

Let us consider, for example, two themes under temporal awareness (timing structure), namely eye-hand and eye-foot coordination. Both are undoubtedly the foundation for efficient performance of the fundamental manipulative skills listed in Table 5–1. However, as additional themes, much more emphasis and strengthening of the "foundation" occurs. Activities under an eye-foot theme, for example, are not limited to kicking and trapping, both of which are diverse enough to merit separate emphasis. Eye-foot coordination is a more generalized theme, which may include kicking and trapping activities as well as hopping (for example, hopscotch), jumping, leaping, and walking (on ladders, on lines), to name a few. With an eye-hand coordination theme, the same generalized concept applies. Movement tasks using such gross-motor skills as throwing, catching, bouncing, striking, rolling, and catching are used as fundamental movement themes. The addition of fine-motor activities (for instance, puzzles, building blocks, jacks, marbles) further enhances this component of temporal awareness.

Vestibular awareness (stability) is the most basic form and fundamental foundation of human movement. It is with this awareness that all skills in the fundamental movement categories are executed efficiently. The enhancement of this base generally incorporates using nonlocomotor skill activities and dynamic stability movements.

Without question, all developmental-theme models as well as traditional approaches characteristically provide a great deal of overlapping of movement abilities. This should be perceived as positive and a natural characteristic of human psychomotor behavior. The important point is that the specific psychomotor abilities of children are stimulated through a predetermined program of activities.

Fundamental Movement Skills

Along with an efficient movement awareness base, the acquisition of the fundamental movement skills form the foundation upon which more complex motor tasks (game [sport], dance, gymnastic skills) can be developed and performed. Most research findings have shown that instruction may be a significant factor in the level of proficiency achieved. This information, in addition to the propositions of "schema theory" and "movement variability," strongly suggests the identification and enhancement of individual perceptual-motor elements (that is, awareness and movements) of the desired "motor program." Most complex motor tasks and many individual fundamental movement skills consist of a combination of two or more skill characteristics. Mastery of individual components of the task would appear to provide a better chance for success as well as greater proficiency with individual fundamental skills. For a more detailed discussion of the role and description of the fundamental categories, see Chapters 9 through 12. The following is a brief review of category description.

The three categories of fundamental movement are: (1) locomotor skills, (2) nonlocomotor skills, and (3) manipulative skills. *Locomotor skills* are movements that propel the individual through space from one location to another (run, jump, skip). *Nonlocomotor skills*, sometimes described as skills of stability, are movements executed with minimal or no movement of one's base of support (turn, twist, swing).

The *manipulative* category refers to those skills that focus upon the control of objects primarily with use of the hands and feet. The two classifications of manipulative behavior are *propulsive* (throw, strike, kick) and *receptive* (catch, trap) skills.

Theme Development and Movement Variability

The primary agent for the execution of a theme is the daily lesson plan, which consists of four major parts: (1) Fitness Phase, (2) Skill-Development Phase (movement variability), (3) Enhancement Phase, and (4) Review ("Huddle"). The Skill Development and Enhancement phases will be discussed here because of their significant roles in the curricular model presented. A detailed discussion of planning strategies relevant to each component is presented in a later section of this chapter.

Skill-Development Phase (Movement Variability) is that portion of the daily lesson plan that focuses upon specific theme development and "movement variability" (that is, schema development). This phase of the lesson is the core of the developmental-theme approach. Along with presenting tasks that are developmentally appropriate for the individual child, the concept of "movement variability," as interpreted from Schmidt and others, (see Chapter 3), provides a variety of movement experiences within a specific theme. As a result of movement variability within a specific awareness or movement skill, the child acquires a more diverse, stronger movement schema (that is, the elements of a motor program), thus the chances of performing efficiently in a variety of situations (that is, novel or complex motor tasks) may be greater. The focus is on the acquisition of specific skills and their use in a variety of predictable and unpredictable situations.

Table 5-2 presents the movement dimensions and relationships concept around which specific themes might be varied (that is, movement variability). Although somewhat similar to the movement concepts (that is, movement analysis model) proposed by Laban and modified by others, this model represents a practical interpretation of schema theory with the addition of the authors' preference for the "relationships" concept found in other curricular models. The use of "movement variability" dimensions serves two purposes: (1) enhancement of movement schema as used by the instructor and transmitted to the child through

Table 5-2 Theme Development Movement-Variability Phase (Schema Enhancement)

DIMENSIONS	
SPATIAL (variation in movement pattern)	**FORCE** (amount of muscular exertion)

Basic Patterns
Direction (path of movement)
   up/down   forward/backward
   left/right   zigzag   curved
Levels (height at which movement
   is performed)
   low/medium/high
	light to heavy
	related to: distance/height projected
	          size/weight of objects
	          manipulated

TIME (speed at which movement is performed)	**RELATIONSHIPS** (movement with objects and/or people)

slow motion to fast
sudden/sustained
smooth/jerky (also known as "flow"
   of movement)
	Objects small equipment/large equipment
	            (attached and apart)
	People solo/partner/group/mass

problems and movement experiences, and (2) to provide the child with a movement vocabulary and understanding of "how" and "where" the body moves. Through "movement variability," the two occur simultaneously; however, at times children should be afforded the opportunity to program their own movements using their understanding of the concepts.

Enhancement Phase is considered by the authors as an optional (that is, the skill development phase may continue for the duration of the period) yet complimentary part of the lesson that can add significantly to the development of the theme. It is with this phase that the teacher has the option of integrating developmentally appropriate, and theme specific, dance, game, and gymnastic activities into the lesson; hence, there is a blend of the traditional and more contemporary curricular approaches. Serving as vehicles to enhance movement awareness, and fundamental skills, "activities" play an integral role in movement utilization. They also provide an element of fun, socialization, and motivation. One of the criticisms of the pure-movement education (movement analysis) approach is that children may not acquire many of those traditional and fun activities associated with childhood and societal play preferences. The authors believe that this phase presents an optional and acceptable solution to the enhancement of movement awareness and fundamental skills of elementary-level children. It has been the authors' observation that even if teachers have been trained in the instruction of dance, game, and gymnastics activities, many prefer just one or two of the areas and reflect this in their planning. This approach allows teachers to present appropriate activities within their selected areas of preference. At the end of each movement awareness and fundamental skill chapter is included a list of selected rhythm/dance, game, and gymnastic activities that are developmentally categorized (that is, Levels I–III) and specific to the theme. Suggested activities for Levels IV–VI may be found in Chapters 14 through 16.

PLANNING STRATEGIES

Planning is essential for effective teaching, and effective teachers plan with a purpose in mind. This is true for all educational endeavors of which physical education is no exception. The end result of effective planning is a smooth lesson in which students improve their levels of fitness, motor-skill proficiency, cognitive and affective behaviors, and teachers are free to give individual feedback on skill performance and other behaviors demonstrated by students. Instruction that does not produce minimal change of behaviors over a reasonable period is "wasted" time and the tax-paying public is not keen on paying for experiences that do not positively affect students' behavior. Physical education must be presented as more than supervised recess, and effective planning is one of the major tools used in accomplishing this mission.

Physical educators are accountable for their students' accomplishment of fitness and skill objectives just as the math teacher is responsible for the attainment of stated math-skill objectives by their math students. The physical education class of today is not merely a class period in which students are provided the opportunity to "get rid of excessive energy" (what a negative phrase!), but rather a segment of their educational day in which that wonderful energy is focused on healthful exercise and learning how to become better movers, thereby experiencing more fully the joy of graceful and effective movement.

Crucial to effective planning for physical education is a thorough understanding of the overall goals of the profession. As mentioned previously, the goal of physical education is to promote the development of the total child through the domains of psychomotor, cognitive, and affective behaviors. The authors believe that the physical education environment presents the child and the teacher with unique opportunities for the development of organic fitness, motor skills, and cognitive and affective abilities. The world of play is the child's natural environment for expression and learning, and wise teachers will take advantage of the child's natural instincts to be active and, through appropriate and creative planning, present an environment where learning can be realized by both process and product. Systematic planning is a tool utilized by the teacher to ensure that all of the stated psychomotor, affective, and cognitive objectives of the program are accomplished. Planning responsibilities occur at three levels: *yearly planning, theme development*, and *daily planning*, each of which will be described after a discussion of overall primary planning considerations.

Primary Considerations for Planning

The teacher must consider many variables when planning the year's program, each theme, and daily lessons. Prior to beginning initial plans there is a certain amount of background information the teacher should understand. These data are rather general but are as necessary as the more specific data required later. Prior to initiating the yearly plan the teacher needs to survey the following:

1. Nature of the community as reflected by the known customs and mores;
2. Philosophy of the school district as reflected by the goals and objectives of the school board;
3. Needs and interest of the children as reflected by their behavior (successful teachers are constant "people-watchers");
4. Available facilities and equipment as reflected by the current inventory;
5. Campus "time structure" for physical education as reflected by the school schedule (this may be negotiable with the school administrator);
6. Competencies of the teacher as reflected by past performance and continual updating of professional knowledge.

With this background knowledge the teacher is ready to initiate the first step of effective teaching (that is, purposeful planning).

YEARLY PLANNING

The yearly plan is a "flexible outline" of the general content areas of learning to be presented and the amount of time to be devoted to each area. You might look upon the completed yearly plan as the blueprint for the year's building efforts, and as the end result of a significant amount of preplanning. This scope (what will be presented) and sequence (order of presentation) will be different for each grade level because of maturational and skill-level changes of the students from year to year. The yearly plan in general serves two purposes:

1. Provides a written plan for the accomplishment of stated program goals. Most school districts insist on this evidence of professionalism.
2. Helps the teacher to make certain that all of the content areas are given a realistic proportion of the allotted time.

Primary Considerations When Planning for the Year

The overall goals are reflected in the yearly plan, which provides a graphic representation of the scope and sequence of the program. Certain decisions have to be made when devising the yearly plan.

The teacher must first decide on the content for the year's work for each particular grade. Information gathered about the customs and mores of the community might inform the teacher that there are many opportunities within the community for programs and demonstrations and that historically the elementary physical education teachers and the music teacher have cooperatively prepared the community program for the May Fest. These kinds of data would indicate to the teacher that temporal awareness themes (rhythm, eye-hand, eye-foot) should receive as much time as other themes because anytime you require children to move with synchronization, with or without music, a rhythmic awareness is required. Naturally there will be many implements (balls, streamers, jump ropes, lummi sticks) used in the themes of rhythmic awareness, eye-hand, and eye-foot coordination that will develop useful skills needed by all of the children regardless of any participation in the May Fest! On the other hand, the mores of the community may reflect a dislike for any sort of musically accompanied rhythms ("dance"). This information will also influence the decision-making processes of the teacher, primarily at the theme level, because the yearly plan could still reflect the time allotted for rhythms (though the theme would focus more on the rhythmic use of locomotor skills, streamers, and jump rope than "dance"). The stated philosophy of the school board may suggest a strong interest in physical fitness or the way physical education can assist in the learning of academic skills (reading, math, and so forth), or the students may be very interested in jumping rope, soccer, or softball skills because their community has spawned state and/or nationally recognized teams in these sports.

Decisions regarding the teacher's yearly plan will certainly be influenced by data collected about the following: facilities (especially availability of indoor facilities), length and severity of the seasons, class sizes, and time structure allowed for each class. A yearly plan developed for a school that schedules physical education three times a week (30 to 45 minutes per class) will be quite different from a plan developed for a daily (30 to 45 minutes per class) program. Of course, the teacher's interest and skill background will also influence the scope and sequence of the yearly plan. However, this last item should remain just that in order of importance—last. Well-qualified physical educators should be able to devise a yearly plan that reflects diversity and thoroughness.

The authors believe that the yearly plan in the beginning (Level I) should reflect a balance of time spent with fundamental movement and movement awareness themes. Specific emphasis will be dropped (phased out) as the students gain competence in these two areas from year to year. As some themes are phased out, the time that becomes available is shifted to content areas of greater complexity. Phasing out a theme is simply a shift in focus because there is considerable overlapping of all themes. For example, as the student demonstrates competence in body, spatial, and directional awareness themes, they will be phased out and that knowledge will be used to extend further the competencies to be gained in (for example) rhythmic awareness or a complicated manipulative skill like catching or striking. Separate yearly plans are provided for Levels I, II, and III in which this shifting of theme emphasis can be observed and studied. A word of caution to the reader in regard to these yearly plans: As with any teaching plan, they are meant to be a flexible tool that must be developed in such a way as to be useful to a number of similar yet highly idiosyncratic teaching environments. Naturally, it would be convenient if the teacher could assess the motor, fitness, cognitive, and affective abilities of the students prior to writing the plans; however, this is generally not practical. A reasonable yearly plan can be written based on what is commonly known regarding motor skills of children at various developmental levels. When a teacher has taught on one campus for several years the yearly plan is more easily developed because of the knowledge the teacher has acquired about the student population. The beginning teacher must rely mostly on information from current texts and from questioning the more experienced teachers on that particular campus. A more accurate analysis of each grade level can be accomplished at the beginning of the year through informal (but critical) observations of such key items as the following:

1. Selected fundamental skills of locomotor, nonlocomotor, and manipulative patterns;
2. Movement awareness (for example, body, balance, temporal);
3. Cardiorespiratory endurance;
4. Upper body strength/endurance;
5. Flexibility.

The results of these observations will enable the teacher to revise, if necessary, the amount of time to be devoted to the various content areas of the yearly plans for each grade level. Planning the yearly curriculum for each grade level is no easy task, for it is not an assignment of arbitrary choices. The curriculum of each grade level is based on the developmental readiness and movement-skill needs of the children at that developmental level, which may not be consistent with age or grade and may vary across a wide range.

Planning Procedures

Rather than propose grade-level percentages of time to be alloted for each of the content areas, the authors have attempted to simplify the yearly planning process. The reader will note that the suggested form (Table 5–3), "Yearly Curriculum Outline," is a graphic representation of 180 days divided into six 6-week blocks. This is the time available in the "school year." In order to begin, the teacher needs the school calendar (holidays, in-service days, and so forth) and the curriculum content outline (see Table 5–1). Notice that in Table 5–1, which lists the movement awarenesses and the fundamental skills, a total of 32 themes are listed: 10 awarenesses (Temporal is not a theme), 10 locomotor themes, 5 nonlocomotor themes, and 7 manipulative skills. Because fitness development is within the scope of each daily lesson (that is, during fitness phase) it is not treated as a separate content area for development. However, any of the fitness components can be appropriately and effectively handled as a theme, and "special fitness days" are always motivating to children.

Each yearly curriculum outline will reflect the philosophical beliefs of the teacher, school, and community as well as facility and equipment availability. The partial outlines for Levels I, II, and III that follow reflect the authors' general suggestions and should be viewed as flexible guidelines rather than "the last word." As you look at the yearly curriculum outline begin the following procedure:

1. Mark the names of each month so you will be cognizant of the seasons of the year in regard to weather conditions.
2. Place an X on the in-service days; if you do not have the exact dates but know that your students will only be in class 175 days of the 180 days then simpy place five X's arbitrarily on the outline.

Table 5-3 Yearly Curriculum Outline: "General Format"

GENERAL FORMAT FOR LEVELS I–III

1st

	M	T	W	T	F
1	Introduction		Spat Aware	Body Aware	Direct Aware
2					
3	Loco		Move Aware	Nonloco	
4	Manipu		Move Aware	Testing	
5					
6					

2nd

	M	T	W	T	F
1					
2					X
3					
4					
5					
6					

3rd

	M	T	W	T	F
1					
2					
3					
4	X				
5					
6					

4th

	M	T	W	T	F
1					
2					X
3					
4					
5					
6					

5th

	M	T	W	T	F
1					
2					
3					
4					
5					
6	X				

6th

	M	T	W	T	F
1	X				
2					
3		Testing			
4					
5					
6	—Field/Play Days—				

X = in-service/work days

3. During the first few weeks, lessons will include movement themes as well as time spent acquainting the students with the area, class management routines, and optional testing of perceptual ability, fundamental skills, and physical fitness. The last six weeks of the year should also include time for testing (for example, fitness) and a culminating activity.

4. Beginning with the third week, fundamental movement themes are presented in "two-day" segments in the rotational order of locomotor, nonlocomotor, manipulative, with one day of each week devoted to movement-awareness themes. The single-day lessons (usually movement-awareness theme) may be presented on Monday, Wednesday, or Friday. The "two-day" lessons should be taught on consecutive days. (See Table 5–3 for an example of a "general" format for Levels I–III.)

As you plot in the locomotor, nonlocomotor, manipulative, and awareness days, you need a systematic technique so that you are able to allow a balanced amount of time for all of the themes. The authors suggest simply moving your finger down the columns in Table 5–1.

The following examples (Tables 5–4, 5–5, and 5–6) present partial (that is, three blocks) completion of a six-block yearly plan. Completion is generally repetitive, that is, continuance of the system.

5. The Level I curriculum outline should include all themes somewhat equally (that is, approximately four lessons per theme) except for the auditory, visual, and tactile themes; they are 50 percent less (approximately two lessons each). (See Table 5–4.) Note that certain nonlocomotor themes (stretch/bend, turn/twist) are presented on a consecutive two-day period. The plan also reflects an adjustment due to in-service days.

6. The Level II curriculum will display less time spent on some themes (body, spatial, directional, walking, and so forth). (See Table 5–5.) In this example, the movement-awareness day has been set on Wednesdays. After the initial walking theme is presented, the focus is dropped and, in this plan, more rhythm is added. Keep in mind that if more rhythm is desired, it may be presented through the enhancement selection.

7. The Level III curriculum limits its focus on the body, spatial, and directional-awareness themes (after a review) as well as on visual, auditory, and tactile themes; additional time is allocated to rhythm and manipulative themes (see Table 5–6). Note that throwing/catching and kicking/trapping themes are now placed together and that in this example, two rhythm days are on consecutive Wednesdays (this is optional; there could be more rhythm days in a row or the rotation could continue allowing only one day for each theme).

8. When a theme is dropped from the yearly curriculum outline this means that particular content area is no longer emphasized as a theme topic. However, there is always considerable overlapping of the movement-awarenesses and fundamental skills so those skills that no longer receive emphasis by way of theme focus are still being utilized by the children as they participate in the themes that focus on other skills

Other aspects of yearly planning to consider are:

1. Days set aside for assessment are not the only times that skill assessment occurs. The observant teacher assesses performance on a daily basis.

2. The assessment days scheduled during the second week should provide the teacher with general information about each class (for instance, "the children in the 9:00 first-grade class as a whole demonstrate very good body control" or "most of the second graders seem to have not developed beginning-level rope-jumping skills"). In other words, this assessment period is not a formalized testing period. Rather, the skills are assessed as the children participate in the daily lesson of vigorous fitness activities, skill development, and enhancement activities.

Table 5-4 Yearly Curriculum Outline: Level I

1st

	M	T	W	T	F
1	Introduction		SA	SA	BA
2	BA	DA	DA	Loco Walk	
3	MA Rhythm	Nonloco Dodge		Manip Ball Roll	
4	MA Eye/H	Loco Run		Testing	
5	MA Eye/Ft	Nonloco Stretch/Bend		Manip Throw	
6	MA Vestib	Loco Leap		Nonloco Turn/Twist	

2nd

	M	T	W	T	F
1	MA Vis	Manip Catch		Loco Jump	
2	MA Aud	Nonloco Push/Pull		Manip Bounce	
3	MA Tact	Loco Hop		Swing/ Sway	X
4	MA BA	Manip Strike		Loco Gallop	
5	MA SA	Nonloco Dodge		Manip Kick	
6	MA DA	Loco Slide		Nonloco Stretch/Bend	

3rd

	M	T	W	T	F
1	MA Rhythm	Manip Trap		Loco Skip	
2	MA Eye/H	Nonloco Turn/Twist		Manip Ball Roll	
3	MA Eye/Ft	Loco Body Roll		Nonloco Push/Pull	
4	MA Vestib	Manip Throw		Loco Climb	
5	X	Nonloco Swing/Sway		Manip Catch	
6	MA Vis	Loco Walk		Nonloco Dodge	

SA, Spatial Awareness; BA, Body Awareness; DA, Directional Awareness; MA, Movement Awareness Theme.

Table 5-5 Yearly Curriculum Outline: Level II

1st

	M	T	W	T	F
1	Introduction		SA	BA	DA
2	Loco Walk	MA Rhythm		Nonloco Dodge	
3	Manip Ball Roll	MA Eye/H		Loco Run	
4	Nonloco Stretch/Bend	MA Eye/Ft		Testing	
5	Manip Throw	MA Vestib		Loco Leap	
6	Nonloco Turn/Twist	MA Vis		Manip Catch	

2nd

	M	T	W	T	F
1	Loco Jump	MA Aud		Nonloco Push/Pull	
2	Manip Bounce	MA Tact		Loco Hop	
3	Nonloco Swing/Sway	MA SA		Manip Strike	
4	Loco Gallop	MA BA		Nonloco Dodge	
5	X	MA Rhythm	MA DA	Manip Kick	
6	Loco Slide	MA Rhythm		Nonloco Stretch/Bend	

3rd

	M	T	W	T	F
1	Manip Trap	MA Eye/H	MA Rhythm	X	
2	Loco Skip	MA Eye/Ft		Nonloco Turn/Twist	
3	Manip Ball Roll	MA Vestib		Loco Body Roll	
4	Nonloco Push/Pull	MA Vis		Manip Throw	
5	Loco Climb	MA Aud		Nonloco Swing/Sway	
6	Manip Catch	MA Tact		Loco Run	

Table 5-6 Yearly Curriculum Outline: Level III

1st

	M	T	W	T	F
1	Introduction		SA	BA	DA
2	Loco Walk Run	MA Rhythm		Nonloco Dodge	
3	Manip Ball Roll	MA Eye/H		Loco Leap	
4	Nonloco Stretch/Bend	MA Eye/Ft		Testing	
5	Manip Throw/Catch	MA Vestib		Loco Jump	
6	Nonloco Turn/Twist	MA Rhythm		Manip Bounce	

2nd

	M	T	W	T	F
1	Loco Hop	MA Rhythm		Nonloco Push/Pull	
2	Manip Strike	MA Eye/H		Loco Gallop	
3	Nonloco Swing/Sway	MA Eye/Ft		Manip Kick/Trap	
4	Loco Slide	MA Vestib		Nonloco Dodge	
5	X	MA Rhythm	MA Rhythm	Manip Ball Roll	
6	Loco Skip	MA Rhythm		Nonloco Stretch/Bend	

3rd

	M	T	W	T	F
1	Manip Throw/Catch	MA Eye/H		Loco Body Roll	
2	Nonloco Turn/Twist	MA Eye/Ft		Manip Bounce	
3	Loco Climb	MA Vestib		Nonloco Push/Pull	
4	Manip Strike	MA Rhythm		Loco Run	
5	Nonloco Swing/Sway	MA Rhythm		Manip Kick/Trap	
6	Loco Leap	MA Eye/H		Nonloco Dodge	

3. The multiple plan (that is, a different theme for each day, five themes a week) is appropriate during the first two weeks but after that a modified plan (that is, two consecutive days/theme two or three themes/week) should be utilized.

4. As the students gain a functional knowledge of the movement awarenesses (body, spatial, directional, visual, auditory, tactile), these awarenesses need not be presented as themes; they become the components of practice variability in the skill themes. Temporal and vestibular awareness, however, will continue to be presented as themes.

After completing the yearly plan for each grade level, the teacher is ready to begin planning at the next level—theme development.

THEME DEVELOPMENT

Theme development represents the second level of planning. A developmental theme is a *resource packet* usually focusing on one movement awareness or skill theme (catching, running, rhythms, spatial awareness, and so forth). Each of these skills and awarenesses serves as a very important component of the psychomotor "foundation." The theme packet contains information that is needed by the teacher who wants to develop within each lesson the movement variability that is the core of the developmental-theme approach. The movement-variability experiences facilitate the child's developing schema, which enables the individual to become a more versatile and successful mover. Remember, the more complete the theme packet, the more valuable it becomes for daily lesson planning. Visualize having a file of resource packets on all 32 themes!

Primary Considerations for Theme Development

Some skills and awarenesses seem naturally to pair with another or, as with jumping, cannot be completed without another (landing) skill. For example, the following fundamental-skill themes are easier to develop when paired:

Jumping and landing   Twisting and turning
Swinging and swaying   Stretching and bending
Pushing and pulling

Most teachers will find it more efficient and appropriate to consider these skills in pairs when developing themes (see examples in the curriculum outlines). There are other themes, such as throwing and catching, and kicking and trapping, that are usually performed together, but because of their complexity they are focused upon individually during early learning periods (Levels I and II). Another choice the teacher has is to develop themes around the health-related physical fitness components. Here again it sometimes helps to pair the components. For example, health-related themes could be:

Strength and Flexibility
Flexibility and Cardiorespiratory Endurance
Muscular Strength and Muscular Endurance

In most cases the *skill*-related fitness components will be addressed within the movement-awarenesses and fundamental-skill themes, and development of these components will occur as natural outcomes of progressing health-related fitness, and fundamental-movement skills.

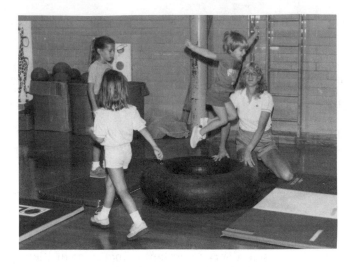

Jumping and landing are a natural pair for a theme.

The teacher is faced with two choices when beginning the composition of a developmental skill or movement-awareness theme. A theme can be developed to include all information necessary for any of the skill levels likely to be performed in grades K–6, or the teacher may choose to develop a theme containing the necessary information for lessons to be taught only at certain grade levels. Because most elementary physical education specialists will teach grades K/1–6, the authors believe the more complete packet to be the most practical. Remember, the theme is an organizational tool for the teacher to use in facilitating the planning of daily lessons. During the development of each theme the teacher keeps in mind that this step in planning is one of the most stable of the three planning levels (yearly, theme, daily), and will *not* have to be repeated each year. Of course, the conscientious teacher will want to update the skill-development and enhancement-activity sections as they discover specific items in these two areas to be less than appropriate for their students. This type of updating should be an ongoing process and will certainly not entail recreating the entire theme packet, because the other elements of the theme are fairly constant. Each theme should reflect all that is needed to enhance the development of that particular skill. The contents of a skill-theme packet are as follows:

CONTENT OF THEMES:

1. Instructional objectives
2. Organizational procedures
3. Safety reminders
4. Equipment (items and quantity)
5. Special contingency plans
6. Evaluation procedures
7. Fitness activities
8. Skill-development–movement-variability activities
9. Enhancement activities
10. Culminating activity
11. References

Instructional objectives are statements that describe the expected performance of students after they have *completed* a unit of instruction. These objectives, although they describe student behavior, are not as specific as the behavioral objectives of daily lesson plans. Objectives are written to describe expected performance in the psychomotor, affective, and cognitive areas as they relate to the theme topic. A more detailed section on writing objectives will be presented later in the chapter.

Organizational procedures are most thoroughly dealt with in the daily lesson plan; however, the following organizational decisions are part of theme development and should be included in the theme packet.

1. Possible teaching style selections.
2. Possible organizational pattern selection.
3. Visual, written, and auditory task stimuli should be prepared and included in the packet. Mini-posters on 8-½-X-11 paper make excellent references for the larger posters, which could be developed later when needed, for the daily lessons.

Safety reminders are both specific to the theme being taught and to general safety rules pertinent to the class at all times. Safety "awareness" is just as relevant to the child as it is to the teacher. Design posters for the class that reflect safety. Verbal reinforcement should be given at the beginning and during class if needed.

Equipment that will be needed for the entire theme is listed as well as the quantities needed for each item based upon the number of students in the class and the available equipment. Posters and other visual aids can also be included in this list.

Special contingency plans are always needed when the children are scheduled to play outside, especially when there is a possibility of foul weather. These plans, which are alternatives, should include activities that will continue to enhance the stated objectives relevant to that theme. With a kicking theme, for example, many eye-foot activities such as jumping rope, hopscotch, and hackey sack would be appropriate in more limited space areas. Sometimes when teaching themes normally taught in the gym, the class will experience interruptions in which the gymnasium is needed for other activities (such as setting up voting booths for local, state, and national elections). This possibility should also be considered during the planning of each theme, and plans should be formulated so that as little disruption as possible will be experienced by the students. For example, during a rhythms theme in which children are learning to use their bodies and small equipment (balls, streamers) while in rhythm to music, an appropriate alternative activity (for use in a small area like a hallway or classroom) might be tapping balloons or lummi sticks in rhythm to chants or music.

Further plans might also include procedures appropriate for larger-than-usual classes in the gym. When the teacher(s) finds it necessary to combine two classes in a space usually reserved for one, it may or may not be possible to continue with instruction that will enhance the objectives of the present theme. During such times, the use of stations are more desirable than mass games for larger groups.

Evaluation procedures for assessing student performance and progress are described in detail and examples of all task sheets and/or skill tests are contained in each theme (see Chapter 8, "Evaluation," for suggestions).

Fitness activities are chosen that may or may not be related to the theme topic. They should, however, enhance the health-related fitness needs of the child.

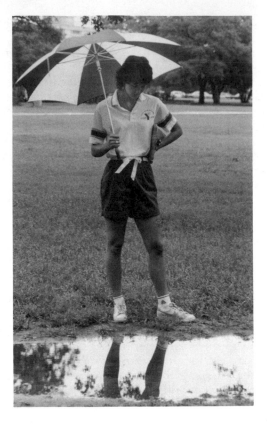

The teacher cannot always count on perfect weather.

These activities are more than calisthenics, although the activities may include some calisthenics. Appropriate activities would include jumping rope, individual tug-of-war, and vigorous movement to music (more examples can be obtained from Chapter 13, "Physical Fitness Activities"). Refer to "Daily Planning" section in this chapter for specific recommendations related to the presentation of fitness components.

The purpose of these initial activities is to stimulate vigorous movement that will enhance the health-related fitness (abdominal strength and endurance, flexibility, muscular strength and endurance, cardiorespiratory endurance, body composition) of the children. Teachers are encouraged to organize the lesson so the child is in an appropriately paced lesson that encourages muscle stimulation, deep breathing, increased heart rate, and perspiration.

Skill-development–movement-variability activities may be stated as problems or challenges (verbal, written, visual, auditory) to children arranged in a variety of organizational patterns. It is best to group these tasks according to levels of skill. In this way the challenges can be taken successively from the prepared theme and used in numerous daily lesson plans. There is no limit to the number of movement-variability tasks one might list in a given theme. Because equipment is used, the manipulative themes will generally contain more opportunities for variability than the other themes.

Enhancement activities are chosen from the areas of games, dance, or gymnastics. Every effort must be made by the teacher to choose enhancement activities that will best serve to help the students to test out and enjoy in a dynamic environment the skills they are acquiring. Enhancement activities are listed at the end of each skill chapter. Each theme should have at least five enhancement activities listed (with references) for each level of skill. Each lesson drawn from the theme utilizes one or more of these enhancement activities.

The culminating activity is planned as the last movement experience for each theme that is taught. This is not the same as an enhancement or final activity of a daily lesson. The culminating activity is much more involved and may take as long as three to four days (a field day or a tournament), an hour (a PTA program) or entire class period (a class contest or creative dance). Only one culminating activity need be planned for each theme. In most cases, the entire class performs as a unit. This activity is normally a creative experience for the younger children (entire class performing a movement rendition of a fairy tale) or it may be a low-keyed contest for older students (entire class involved in an obstacle course relay or a "mini-track meet"). Seasonal programs and PTA programs that involve one or all grade levels of the school offer fine opportunities for a *single culminating activity* to include skills learned during *several themes* that were taught over a period of time. Keep in mind that this single event planned for each theme is an option available to the teacher, who will make the decision to use or not use it on an *individual class* basis. Another point to keep in mind is that one culminating activity containing multiple challenges (like a mini-track meet) could serve all three levels.

References should include specific songs from specific albums, texts, tapes, and other sources.

It should be quite evident that the development of movement-awareness and fundamental-skill themes is a creative task for the teacher. After completing several of these themes, however, the teacher will be accustomed to the format, and the time required to plan such a theme will diminish. The teacher who has a file of well-developed themes possesses an in-depth and task-specific resource library from which effective daily lessons can be planned. Well-developed themes normally can be used year after year with minimal updating being required.

Writing Instructional Objectives

Writing objectives is often viewed by beginning teachers and some seasonal teachers as a futile exercise. The authors value instructional objectives, however, for several reasons:

1. Objectives help to organize the learning material.
2. Developmentally appropriate objectives that identify specific behavioral outcomes provide the teachers with realistic assessment criteria.
3. Specific objectives demonstrate that the teacher believes in teacher accountability.
4. When children are aware of the objectives they are better able to understand the "education" of physical education.
5. Written objectives help to keep the "educational team" (principal, teachers, students) on track.

Each objective states:

1. *Who* (the student)
   will do
2. *What* (the observable skill or behavior; for example, jump)
   under what
3. *Conditions* (rope on the ground)
   and to what
4. *Degree* of competency (eight consecutive) to indicate a minimum (average) level of success.

The following are examples of (1) general (nonmeasurable) objectives and (2) specific (measurable) instructional objectives:

1. The students should know how to jump rope (how is "should know" measured?).
2. At the end of the year, while using a rope stretched out on the ground, kindergarten students will repeatedly jump back and forth over the rope for eight consecutive successful jumps.

Notice that the instructional objective states what the students *will* do, rather than what they should be able to do. By writing this objective the teacher is saying that all of the kindergarten children are expected to develop the skill to enable them to jump back and forth over a rope resting on the ground. Furthermore, each student is expected to be able to jump for eight consecutive jumps without mistakes. The following are examples of affective, cognitive, and fitness objectives.

AFFECTIVE

1. The students should be good sports.
2. The third-grade students will demonstrate good sportsmanship by taking turns while performing jump-rope skills and turning the rope.

COGNITIVE

1. The students will chant while jumping rope.
2. The fourth-grade students will chant (without cues) three of the four jump-rope chants taught.

FITNESS

1. The students will become more physically fit.
2. The fifth-grade students will demonstrate an improvement in their level of cardio-respiratory endurance by jumping continuously (with or without a rope) for one minute longer than performed at the beginning of the semester (pretest).

Specific instructional objectives obviously require more thoughtful preparation than general objectives. However, if the accomplishment of an objective is to be an indicator of success then the objective must be measurable, and in order to be measurable it must be specific. Both teacher and student can measure success or failure when both know the performance expectations. As soon as an objective is conquered, the next objective up the progression is attempted. In some content areas the performance objectives offer a built-in safety mechanism. For example, if students know that prior to attempting a fully extended headstand they must satisfy the objective of " . . . complete 10 tripod lift-ups (knees lifted from elbows) without hesitation . . . ," the teacher has eliminated the opportunity for the famous "crick in my neck" and "fell flat on my back" hazards that suddenly appear. During the tripod lift-ups, the neck, back, and arms are being strengthened and the sense of balance enhanced. At the completion of that objective the students can safely go on to the next, more difficult objective (for example, the fully extended headstand). Another advantage of writing these specific performance objectives is that the teacher is forced to focus on the critical criteria for successful performance and then teach the skills in a safe progression that stimulates healthy practice sessions leading to more rapid success for the individual student. One more comment about objectives: it is beneficial to let students know the objectives of the lesson. This serves several purposes, of which the following are representative:

1. It helps keep students and teacher focused on the goals of the lesson.
2. It promotes the "education" in physical education.
3. It helps students realize that their physical education teacher values the lessons they plan and the children they teach.
4. It encourages the development of "goal awareness" and self-assessment in the children.
5. It provides a yardstick with which to measure the daily progress of the class. A short critique focusing upon which objectives were and were not accomplished offers excellent content for the "huddle" phase of the lesson, and a starting place for ensuing lessons.

The following list of verbs will assist the teacher in writing behavioral objectives for physical education classes.

Behavioral Verbs for Physical Education

PSYCHOMOTOR DOMAIN

bat	pull
bend	punch
bounce	push
catch	roll
chase	run
climb	skip
crawl	slide
dodge	stretch
gallop	strike
grab	sway
grip	swim
hit	swing
hold	throw
hop	toss
jump	trap
kick	turn
leap	twist
	walk

COGNITIVE DOMAIN

check	list
circle	match
copy	measure
define	name
demonstrate	question
describe	show
identify	state
	tell

AFFECTIVE DOMAIN

ask	evaluate
assess	offer
attempt	participate
challenge	praise
choose	share
complete	suggest
cooperate	tolerate
defend	

DAILY PLANNING

The daily lesson plan is a flexible yet highly specific outline of one day's lesson and should include sufficient detail to be appropriate for a substitute teacher to follow. All classes of the same grade level can operate from the same lesson plan, with desired variations for each class being noted on the plan. Some daily plans (especially those involving stations) will have sufficient content material to warrant their use for two days. Moreover, some teachers may prefer to spend one day on fitness activities and skill development (movement variability) and the next day on fitness activities and enhancement experiences.

The daily plan requires several items of information, all of which will be drawn directly from the fundamental-skill and movement-awareness *themes* previously completed.

Daily Lesson Plan Contents

See Table 5-7 for a sample daily lesson plan. The elements within the plan are explained as follows:

Theme Title will come from the areas of movement awareness, fundamental skills, or fitness. All of the awarenesses and skills listed in Table 5-1 are appropriate theme titles (for example, spatial awareness, running, turning/twisting).

Lesson Title will reflect the focus on one day's lesson (for instance, pathways).

Grade Level and Class Number are listed on the lesson plan along with class period (for example, 3rd period—2nd grade—#32).

Equipment Needed indicates not only what equipment is needed for that lesson but also how many of each item. Audio visual teaching aids should be included.

Safety Precautions that are specific to that lesson are listed. General class rules for safety should be posted where they can be seen daily.

Objectives covering all three domains (psychomotor, affective, and cognitive) are stated in *behavioral terms* (remember, *theme* objectives were stated as instructional objectives). Well-stated objectives become tools for assessment at various times during the lessons. An efficient method for stating objectives on lesson plans is to make the initial statement of "The students will" followed by the desired performance, conditions, and criteria for success of each objective (for example, while standing 5 feet apart catch 5 out of 8 beanbags tossed by their partner). Classes with children who have special needs may require additional and/or modified objectives.

References will include all resources used to complete the lesson plan. Good lesson plans can be used year after year with only minimum modifications. Accurate references are valuable timesavers.

Area Layout indicates the spatial organization for the class and the teacher. The diagram should include where the children will be as well as equipment, traffic patterns, positions of stations, and so forth. The teacher's position should be fluid the majority of the time. Beginning teachers will want to note the most advantageous locations for effectiveness of instruction, safety, and other supervisory needs.

In the example of a daily lesson plan format (Table 5-7) it should be noted that approximately one-third of the total time should be devoted to the fitness phase and two-thirds to the remaining phases.

The Four Phases of the Daily Lesson Plan

Fitness Phase

Approximately one-third of each daily lesson is programmed for and devoted to the accomplishment of specific physical fitness objectives; these focus primarily upon the health-related components. In order to ensure somewhat of a balance of fitness activities and objective-oriented program, the following systematic plan is suggested for use during the planning of fitness activities for daily lessons (see Table 5-8).

Examples of activities used to enhance specific fitness components may be found in Chapter 13. The reader will notice that on Mondays, Wednesdays, and Fridays the cardiorespiratory component is given primary focus. This is not to imply that another component such as flexibility may not be incorporated into the

Table 5-7   Physical Education Daily Lesson Plan

THEME _____ LESSON _____ GRADE _____ # _____

EQUIPMENT _____

SAFETY PRECAUTIONS _____

OBJECTIVES _____

_____

_____

_____

_____

_____

REFERENCES _____

_____

_____

Time (min.)   Area Layout

_____ ($^1/_3$) FITNESS:

_____ ($^2/_3$) SKILL DEVELOPMENT/MOVEMENT VARIABILITY:

_____ ENHANCEMENT:

(As skill proficiency is acquired more time should be
allowed for this phase)

_____ HUDDLE:

EVALUATION.

Table 5-8 Recommended Schedule for Planning Fitness Activities

MONDAY	TUESDAY	WEDNESDAY	THURSDAY	FRIDAY
Cardiorespiratory	Upper body strength/endur. Flexibility	Cardiorespiratory	Flexibility Abdominal strength/endur.	Cardiorespiratory
Cardiorespiratory	Flexibility Upper body strength/endur.	Cardiorespiratory	Abdominal strength/endur. Flexibility	Cardiorespiratory

activity. The component listed first on Tuesdays and Thursdays is the component that will receive the *most stress,* either through intensity or duration. Note, too, the different emphasis each week on Tuesdays and Thursdays (that is, flexibility is emphasized more on Thursday of the first week and Tuesday of the second week). The rotation of these two weeks will continue throughout the school year. Based on this system, a typical Level I plan for an entire week may contain the following activities, as listed in Table 5-9.

The following reminders are offered:

1. Fitness activities must be vigorous, with opportunities for individual pacing by the students if needed.
2. Instructions should be brief but clear.
3. Maximum participation is essential; there should be little or no waiting in line or other delays.
4. The use of music can facilitate motivation and smoothness of movement.
5. If games or obstacle courses are used they should already be known or require minimal instructions.
6. Begin with moderately vigorous movement, quickly moving to more vigorous demands for the children.

TEACHER'S ROLE DURING THE FITNESS PHASE OF THE LESSON

1. Be an enthusiastic motivator.
2. Have the area ready when students arrive.
3. Begin quickly (brief but clear directions).
4. Use music at every opportunity.
5. Encourage pacing when needed by individual students.
6. Praise *good effort* as evidenced by accelerated breathing, rosy cheeks, accelerated heart rate, and perspiration.
7. Children should be taught how to locate their "heart beat" (chest, neck, wrist).

Table 5-9 Example of a Week of Fitness Activities

MONDAY	TUESDAY	WEDNESDAY	THURSDAY	FRIDAY
European Running	Streamers Climbing Ropes Horizontal Ladders	Parachute	Movement Stories Floor Exercises	Obstacle Course

Skill-Development Phase (Movement Variability)

The *skill-development phase* is the nucleus of the daily lesson, and the authors believe it is the significant core of the curriculum model presented in this text. According to the latest information available about the motor learning of children, the use of "movement variability" is the best way to strengthen the child's movement schema. It is during the movement-variability phase that students are provided with a variety of opportunities to explore, experiment, and test out the many ways a particular fundamental skill can be performed. During this phase there exists a laboratory-type of attitude wherein the teacher and students are in partnership as they use specific skills in a variety of predictable and unpredictable situations, thereby permitting each child to update his or her functional-movement vocabulary.

Through the variables of space, force, time, and relationships with objects and other people, the students continue to develop their personal schema of concepts and movement patterns that will enable them to respond more efficiently and effectively to both novel and familiar movement challenges. The students receive the challenges or problems verbally or through the use of task sheets (or posters). The predominant teaching methodologies are *guided discovery* and *problem solving*. It is important that the teacher "overplan" this phase of the lesson, for it is better to have too many challenges than to run out of ideas!

The movement-variability challenges and problems are extremely important and should be written with care. The teacher should begin by first recalling all of the performance characteristics that exemplify the mature, proficient movement pattern of that specific skill. The beginning teacher may even want to write down these characteristics. Let us take running, for example. The characteristics described in the skill chapter include:

1. Slight forward lean of the trunk;
2. Arms swing vertically in opposition to the legs;
3. The support foot hits the ground rather flat and close to the center of gravity;
4. The knee of the support leg bends slightly after contact;
5. The driving leg extends at the hip, knee, and ankle;
6. The recovery knee quickly comes forward as, simultaneously, the lower portion of the same leg draws the foot toward the buttocks.

With a clear understanding of what the mature form is supposed to look like, the teacher is ready to begin listing the variability opportunities. At this point it is necessary for the teacher to consider all of the many uses of that skill and how those movement requirements can be reproduced in the physical education class. Then the teacher will consider varying the use of that specific skill (running) through the applications of the variables—time, space, force, and relationships. The list of challenges/problems will represent a rather complete sample of challenges and movement problems appropriate for the various skill levels represented by children. Teachers should consider the children moving along a continuum from simple to complex skill proficiency. In a single class there will be children performing at various stages along that continuum. Each child's progress can be facilitated or hindered by the movement demands made during the movement-variability phase. Therefore the listing of challenges/problems should be from simple to complex and stated in general terms, whereby each child can become a versatile problem-solver at his or her individual level in his or her individual way.

The challenge presented to the children should stimulate them to apply what they know about the skill and use that skill in ways they perhaps have not thought of before (for example, "Can you run faster when your body leans forward or backward?" "What happens to your speed if you hold your arms down at your sides while running?"). The teacher is given many cues in each skill chapter in this text, which can act as stimuli for the development of imaginative and realistic movement-variability challenges.

The following are examples of throwing challenges (and the variability focus) appropriate for Levels I through III.

Level I—How many different ways can you throw the beanbag? Can you throw the beanbag over your head? (space). Can you throw the beanbag behind you? (directions).

Level II—Can you throw the ball to the wall fast, three times? (time). How far can you throw the ball? (force). Can you throw the ball straight while squatting down? (levels). How many times can you and your partner throw the ball to one another without mistakes? (relationships). Can you throw the ball to your partner's knees? (level).

Level III—While running, can you throw the ball and hit the target? (rhythm).

While being guarded, can you throw the ball to your moving partner? (relationships).

The following reminders are offered:

1. Move quickly from the fitness phase to the skill-development phase. Equipment must be ready and instructions should be brief. Difficult transitions should be noted on the lesson plan as this will ensure that the teacher has thought-through the procedure for moving from one phase to the next.
2. Observe critically for possible formation of inefficient skill habits (for example, arms and legs not in opposition when throwing a beanbag) and be ready to employ guided-discovery techniques to facilitate movement toward more efficient skill.
3. Be imaginative when posing variability challenges through the use of force, time, space, and relationships.
4. Refrain from stating the challenges in the same way day after day.
5. Respond to the children's movement with appropriate feedback techniques. Remember, there can be secondary learning by children on the periphery if feedback is given so that several children can hear.
6. Liberal use of equipment facilitates development of movement-variability challenges.

THE TEACHER'S ROLE DURING THE SKILL-DEVELOPMENT PHASE OF THE LESSON

1. To clarify the challenges by those who indicate this need.
2. To motivate all the students to full participation.
3. To encourage unique (rather than only the familiar) movement solutions.
4. To observe critically and give accurate feedback of skill attempts and behavior reactions.
5. To use every "teachable moment" in a positive manner.
6. To avoid being merely a supervisor, clock-watcher, equipment-fetcher.

Refer to Table 5–2 for an outline of the movement dimensions and relationships concept around which themes might be varied.

Enhancement Phase (Games, Gymnastics, Dance)

Although not every lesson will necessarily end with an enhancement activity, (that is, the skill-development phase may continue for the duration of the class period) the enhancement phase is considered by the authors as a very complementary part of the lesson that can add significantly to the development of each skill. When approximately 80 percent of the children are able to perform the skills being practiced with some semblance of accuracy, a carefully chosen enhancement activity can further this development in a fun way. Skills are reinforced as they are used in dynamic games, dance activities, or gymnastics skills. For example, the children have been participating in a balance theme and have become relatively proficient in balancing on low beams while in various static and dynamic positions and can also combine locomotor movements and balance activities. These skills could then be further extended as the students are taught how to use the mini-trampoline. Indeed, they would use many of the same movements while balancing on the trampoline as well as in the air. Likewise, a game such as "Stop and Go" would provide opportunities for extending the developing balance skills. Performing the dance "Seven Jumps" would offer additional opportunities to demonstrate balance skills. Through participation in this organized activity the students are able to use the skill(s) they have been developing in a dynamic way, thereby moving that development to a higher level. Again, it is important for the teacher to "overplan" this segment of the lesson; if one enhancement activity proves to be inappropriate for that particular group of students another can be introduced immediately. Realizing that teachers will often prefer those activities with which they are most familiar, every effort should be made to plan a variety of activities that will draw from all three content areas of games, gymnastics, and dance.

The following reminders are offered:

1. The enhancement is a means to an end (namely, skill development) not an end in itself.
2. Evidence of adequate skill development should be demonstrated by at least 80 percent of the class prior to moving from the movement-variability phase to the enhancement phase.
3. Variety of enhancement activities is very important.
4. Children can develop a repertoire of socially acceptable and developmentally appropriate games and dances that will most likely be utilized during their "away from school" time.
5. Allow for a demonstration or a trial run of relays, tag games, and other similar activities so that all students have a "functional understanding" of what will be required of them. Older students may only need a demonstration, whereas younger students usually require a "practice" prior to the "real" event. Remember, if you allow one of the "teams" to demonstrate a relay or other competitive event, that specific team will have an advantage over the other teams. Hence a trial run for all teams is usually the fairest and often the safest choice for the teacher to make. Children with inadequate skill development should not be expected to participate in competitive events. The teacher's choice is either to schedule competitive and cooperative events simultaneously and let the students choose or to avoid the competitive events until *all* of the children have the appropriate skill development.
6. Children can choose appropriate enhancement activities if they are encouraged and trained to do so.

The teacher's role during this phase of the lesson is to:

1. Have all needed equipment ready and the area marked off appropriately (use of ropes, bases, or cones is most efficient).
2. Divide the class (if necessary) quickly and fairly.
3. Explain the event and safety procedures clearly and quickly (use of visuals can speed up this process).
4. Ask specific questions to evaluate students' understanding of the events. To ask "Are there any questions?" is not nearly as effective as, "Tom, how will you know who is 'it'?"
5. Encourage the students to show their support to the winning team by clapping for the winners, and then teaching the winners to congratulate their opponents for their good effort, fair play, team spirit.
6. Encourage cooperative play among team members by praising this behavior when it is demonstrated by the students.
7. Initiate variations in the event when they are needed to provide opportunities for maximum participation.
8. Be constantly aware of possible safety hazzards.
9. Cease the activity on time, allowing for a one-minute "huddle" before dismissal.
10. Officiate quickly and decisively when necessary.
11. Make changes or simply cease an activity that is not providing opportunities for theme enhancement.

Huddle Phase (Review and Feedback)

The last 30 to 60 seconds of each class period can bring a very special closure to the daily lesson. The teacher calls the children to "huddle" and discuss what went on during that day's lesson. It presents an opportunity for teacher and students to relate to one another on a more personal level. Remarks may focus on a number of items, including skill and affective behaviors. It is best to stress the positive events that occurred; however, it is also appropriate to talk about inappropriate behaviors especially if the students can be led to identify the inappropriate behaviors themselves and then discuss the advantages of appropriate behaviors and possible consequences (relating this to the standing class rules for such behaviors) if the inappropriate behavior continues. The teacher might also want to mention the events planned for tomorrow's lesson.

REMINDERS

1. This is a time for enhancing affective and cognitive skills.
2. All equipment should be placed aside prior to coming to the huddle. When outside this may mean some of the children in the last class of the day will bring the cones and balls with them to the huddle where they will be placed to one side.

The teacher's role during this phase of the lesson is to:

1. Provide an "accepting" atmosphere where the children will feel free to express themselves.
2. See that the lesson ends on a high note even if that psychological high is simply a promise by all to try their best tomorrow! (Remember the "Little Train That Could"?)
3. Let the children know your expectations of them.
4. Insist that the transition from enhancement phase to huddle phase is executed quickly.

Evaluation

At the end of each class period (or, more realistically, for elementary teachers this will be done at the end of the day) the teacher should evaluate the progress of each class in meeting the objectives of the lesson. This evaluation is important not only for making adjustments to the next lesson but also for next year's plan. There is no need to keep making the same mistakes regarding progressions, methodology, or activity selections.

GENERAL SUGGESTIONS FOR THE TEACHER

1. View planning as one of several keys to being an effective teacher. To quote a wise old sage: "Work will win where wishing won't."
2. Most of the educational settings are on a rigid time schedule; therefore, appropriate planning is crucial.
3. Flexibility is a necessity for teacher and students alike. Yearly and daily plans are meant to serve as guidelines—flexible guidelines.
4. By Thursday of each week the plans for the coming week should be completed.
5. A short period of time each day should be spent reviewing what will be taught the following day and checking on the necessary supplies and equipment. Some teachers prefer the time prior to leaving their campus each day, whereas others prefer early-morning planning.
6. Preplanning provides the teacher with more of a trouble-free teaching experience than if plans are left till the last minute when it may be too late to secure the needed equipment, facilities, and so forth.
7. Older students should be given the opportunity to provide feedback to the teacher regarding their likes and dislikes. However, the teacher is responsible for the year's goals and objectives being met through a curriculum that allows these skills to be taught and learned.
8. Teachers who realize their worth to the total educational experience will become excited about planning the yearly curriculum, movement-awareness and fundamental-skill themes, and daily lesson plans that have a purpose and result in academic, motor, fitness, and affective achievements for children.
9. Skeletal outlines are appropriate for initial planning purposes, but these should not be considered sufficient for the daily plans that need considerable detail.
10. Teachers who expect a lot out of students should also be willing to write up creative lesson plans prepared in such a way to cause students to really become excited about participating in a lesson that is different, challenging, exciting, and at times unpredictable. Teachers should not be afraid to risk when planning lessons.
11. Provide for early success experiences.
12. Plan for student leadership opportunities.
13. Be enthusiastic.
14. Observe the children's performance carefully and respond verbally to what you see.
15. Reinforce desired behavior.

THE LEVEL IV–VI PROGRAM: USE OF THE FOUNDATION

"Using the Foundation" (Level IV–VI) refers to program emphasis for children who have acquired proficiency at the "foundation" (Levels I–III) level. This is a curriculum that refines and utilizes those movement awarenesses and fundamental skills acquired during the previously discussed foundation phase. During this period, children are refining specific motor abilities and combining various patterns of movements (locomotor, nonlocomotor, and manipulative) in an attempt to execute more complex dance, game, and gymnastic tasks. It may be assumed that it is the composition (that is, degree of movement dimension variability and proficiency) of the foundation that determines motivation and chances of early success in many of the complex motor tasks. Table 5–10 presents suggested program emphases.

The primary shift from developing the fundamental foundation is to refinement and utilization of the foundation skills in specific task situations. Whereas during the foundation phase, catching and throwing were "generalized" with movement variability, the skills are now utilized in more specific motor-task situations such as fielding and throwing in the game of softball (within these motor-skill areas are several variations and combinations of fundamental skills).

It is at this time that the theme approach and use of teaching units are integrated. In a sport-skill unit (consisting of several lessons and themes) such as softball, for example, base running, sliding, pitching, and batting can all be themes. In this case, movement variability may play a significant role in the development of sport-skill proficiency as used in the ever-changing conditions of dynamic games.

As previously noted, the focus of this text is upon "Building the Foundation" (Levels I–III), and a detailed discussion of its use with more advanced (Levels IV–VI) activities is beyond the scope of the text. However, to place the total curriculum in perspective, general guidelines for planning and selecting activities (see Chapters 14 through 16) for Levels IV–VI have been provided.

The first major step in yearly planning is deciding on content (scope). Before this can be achieved, the teacher must gather and consider the essential background information related to the program. Yearly plan decisions will be significantly influenced by information collected relative to such things as facilities (especially availability of indoor facilities), length and severity of the seasons, class

Table 5-10   Using the Foundation

PROGRAM EMPHASIS LEVELS IV–VI

Fitness (Health and Skill-Related Components)

Refinement of Movement Awarenesses and Fundamental-Movement Skills

Introduction to (and utilization of "foundation" abilities) activities involving greater motor-task complexity:

>   Game (individual, dual, team)

>   Dance (folk, square, creative, aerobic)

>   Gymnastic (stunts/tumbling, apparatus, floor exercise)

Introduction of knowledge concepts, (for example, rules and strategies) and principles related to skill areas and fitness.

---

sizes, and time structure. A yearly plan developed for a school that schedules physical education three times a week (30 to 45 minutes per class) will be quite different from a plan created for a daily (30 to 60 minutes per class) program. Table 5–11 presents suggested content and allotted percentages of time for the Levels IV–VI program. Teacher's selection of specific activities and time allotments may vary, dependent upon a number of factors; however, it is recommended that content areas be presented within the ranges suggested in Table 5–11. In addition to the essential background information gathered (facilities, equipment), variations in the program may also be based upon teacher/community desires. For example, in a community that strongly supports basketball, that instructional unit would demand more than an equal time allotment with other activities. In other situations, football activities may not be desirable in the program; hence the soccer (or alternative) program is given additional emphasis. There are many considerations of this nature; however, the general programming reflected in this model represents a more balanced (that is, within content areas) approach in planning.

After identifying general content, the next step in yearly planning involves "sequence," that is, general placement/order of activities on the school calendar. While this may vary also, certain activities are accepted as being presented at specific times of the year (football in the fall, basketball in the winter, softball in the

Table 5-11 Suggested Content for Levels IV–VI

GAMES (40–70%)

Low Organization	Individual/Partner		Team*	
Relays	Bowling Activities	Frisbee	Basketball	Soccer
Tag	Croquet	Horseshoes	Hockey (Field/Floor)	Softball
Simple Group Games	Deck Tennis	Shuffleboard	Football Activities	Volleyball
	Hackey sack			Track & Field
	Paddleball	Handball	Hocker	Korfball
	Paddle Tennis	Sidewalk Tennis	Speedball	Netball
	Pickleball	Volley Tennis	Team Handball	Pillo Polo
	Badminton		Activities	Flickerball
			Toppleball	

Creative/Cooperative
Games**

RHYTHMS/DANCE (15–30%)	GYMNASTIC ACTIVITIES (15–30%)
Rhythms	Stunts
Folk	Tumbling
Square	Small Equipment (rope jumping, juggling, others)
Creative	Large Equipment
Aerobic	Rhythmic Gymnastics

---

*Team activities emphasize a variety of lead-up games

**May be incorporated with other games or presented as a separate content area

spring). Placement of activities on the calendar necessitates another important general consideration: method of placement. There are two recommended methods of content placement: modified and solid (block).

Modified Method

This plan suggests that a segment of time be shared between two activity areas. For example, during a five-day week (a week is the most frequent unit of planning), soccer skills may be presented three or four days and another activity area the remaining time. This method provides both continuity and variety. In order to provide quality skill development, planning, instruction, and practice are critical. Continuity over a period of days promotes effective instruction and planning. On the other hand, not all children enjoy a specific skill area every day of the week. A "break" can be both refreshing and fulfill program goals. For example, to provide variety, Wednesday (Monday or Friday) may be designated as a "Mod" (modified) or break day. The activities presented should vary enough to provide a change of pace and be simple enough to be completed in a single class period. Some "Mod" day content suggestions include: rhythms, simple dances, simple stunts and small equipment gymnastic activities, individual and partner games, and cooperative and creative game activities.

The modified method is a highly recommended plan. It has continuity, flexibility, emphasis, and variety.

Solid (block) Method

A *solid plan* represents an extended period of instruction (that is, 5 days a week) devoted exclusively to one content area. Its primary asset is that there is no disruption during the presentation of skill-development content. This type of plan requires a highly interested group of children, and while variety is not provided from another content area, an assortment of skill-development activities can provide motivating challenges.

Both methods of content placement provide the teacher with a great degree of planning flexibility. After a feel for general planning and instruction, many teachers find it desirable to combine both methods of content placement. Beginning teachers usually start with a basic skeleton plan and, with experience, refine their outline to meet specific needs and personal preferences.

Table 5-12 (modified plan) and Table 5-13 (solid plan) present two examples of yearly curriculum outlines. The authors have attempted to present a balanced curriculum incorporating all suggested (Table 5-11) general content areas. However, as previously noted, a number of considerations will guide the teacher in determining specific time and placement decisions. The following general planning procedures are suggested: (1) determine areas of content; (2) using a school-year calendar, mark holidays, in-service days, other special days; be sure to designate days not primarily related to content instruction (for example, introduction of class procedures, fitness testing, end-of-school-year events); (3) determine method of content placement, that is, modified, solid, or combination; and (4) decide on order and placement of areas on calendar.

Procedures related to theme development and daily planning generally follow the information for Levels I-III; that is, the skill-development phase is the lesson focus (theme).

Table 5-12 Example of Modified Plan: Yearly Outline Levels IV–VI

	M	T	W	T	F
1	Introduction	Games Low Organization			
2	Rhythms/Dance	Cooperative Games			
3	Football Activities		Testing		Fitness
4	Football Activities	Football Activities	GYMNASTICS		
5	Football Activities			FB	X
6	Individual Games	Individual Games			

	M	T	W	T	F
1	Partner Games				Partner Games
2	Soccer		RHYTHM / DANCE		Soccer
3	Soccer				Soccer
4	Dance*			Dance	X
5	Dance				Dance
6	Partner Games				Partner Games

	M	T	W	T	F
1	Basketball		RHYTHMS / DANCE		Basketball
2	Basketball				Basketball
3	Gymnastics				Gymnastics
4	Tumbling & Stunts				Tumbling & Stunts
5	Volleyball				Volleyball
6	Volleyball				Volleyball

	M	T	W	T	F
1	Gymnastics Tumbling		GAMES / COOPERATIVE		& Stunts
2	Dance			Dance	X
3	Choice**				of
4	Team				Game(s)
5	Floor/Field Hockey				Floor/Field Hockey
6	Floor/Field Hockey				Floor/Field Hockey

	M	T	W	T	F
1	Individual Games		GYMNASTICS / SMALL EQUIPMENT		Partner Games
2	Partner Games				Partner Games
3	Dance				Dance
4	Dance			Dance	X
5	Softball				Softball
6	Softball				Softball

	M	T	W	T	F
1	Gymnastics		DANCE	Gymn.	X
2	Large				Apparatus
3	Track				Field
4	Track/Field			Testing	
5	Track			Fitness	Field
6			-------- Field Days --------		

	Days	Percent
Games	100	61
Dance	30	19
Gymnastics	32	20
	162 days	100%

180 − 18* = 162 days

*Dance (rhythms, folk, square, creative, aerobic).

**Additional Team Games (e.g., team handball, hockey, speedball).

*18 "non-theme" days (introduction, testing, inservice days, field days).

Table 5-13 Example of Block Plan: Yearly Outline Levels IV–VI

Sept./Oct.

	M	T	W	T	F
1	Introduction		Games Low Organization		
2	GYMNASTICS				DANCE
3	Football	Testing		Fitness	
4	Football Activities				
5	Football Activities				✕
6	Individual Games				

Nov.

	M	T	W	T	F
1	Partner Games				
2	S	o	c	c	e r
3	S	o	c	c	e r
4	G Y M N A S T I C S				
5	G Y M N A S T I C S				✕
6	Partner Games				

	M	T	W	T	F
1	G Y M N A S T I C S				✕
2	D	A	N	C	E
3	D	A	N	C	E
4	Field/Floor				
5	Hockey				
6	G Y M N A S T I C S				

Dec. / Jan.

	M	T	W	T	F
1	B	a	s	k	e t b a l l
2	B	a	s	k	e t b a l l
3	D	A	N	C	E
4	D	A	N	C	✕
5	V	o	l	l	e y b a l l
6	V	o	l	l	e y b a l l

March

	M	T	W	T	F
1	Individual/Partner				
2	Games				✕
3	G Y M N A S T I C S				
4	D	A	N	C	E
5	S	o	f	t	b a l l
6	S	o	f	t	b a l l

April / May

	M	T	W	T	F
1	Choice of Team				
2	Game(s)				
3	Track/Field				
4	Track/Field		Testing	Fitness	
5	Track/Field				
6	Field Days				

	Days	Percent
Games	112	70
Dance	25	15
Gymnastics	25	15
180 – 18* =	162 days	100%

*18 "non-theme" days (introduction, testing, inservice days, field days).

SUGGESTED READINGS

DAUER, V. P. & PANGRAZI, R. P. (1986). *Dynamic physical education for elementary school children*, 8th ed. Minneapolis: Burgess.

DAVIS, R. G. & ISAACS, L. D. (1985). *Elementary physical education: Growing through movement*, 2nd ed. Winston-Salem, N.C.: Hunter.

GALLAHUE, D. L. (1982). *Developmental movement experiences for children.* New York: Wiley.

GRAHAM, G., HOLT-HALE, S. A., McEWEN, T., & PARKER, M. (1980). *Children moving: A reflective approach to teaching physical education.* Palo Alto, CA: Mayfield.

KIRCHNER, G. (1985). *Physical education for elementary school children*, 6th ed. Dubuque: William C. Brown.

LOGSDON, B. J., BARRETT, K. R., BROER, M. R., McGEE, R., AMMONS, M., HALVERSON, L. E., & ROBERTSON, M. A. (1984). *Physical education for children: A focus on the teaching process*, 2nd ed. Philadelphia: Lea & Febiger.

MORRIS, G. S. D. (1980). *Elementary physical education: Towards inclusion.* Salt Lake City: Brighton.

NICHOLS, B. (1986). *Moving and learning: The elementary school physical education experience.* St. Louis: Mosby.

6

ORGANIZATION
AND INSTRUCTION

Along with the knowledge of what to teach, the teacher must have the ability to organize the class and select an effective style of subject matter presentation. The fact is, however, there are numerous styles of presentation and organization. Which is best? The topic deserves much consideration before a thorough understanding can be assured, and then a direct answer to the preceding question usually reflects personal preference. A numer of teaching strategies (combination of style, organization, and communication mode) can be used effectively to present the same subject matter; each has advantages and disadvantages, depending upon the specific class situation, content, and desired learning process (Gabbard, 1983). The important criterion in the selection of a strategy is knowledge of the "process," its inherent characteristics, and implications for the development of the child. Although present research indicates that most teachers do not vary their style of teaching, a considerable body of research suggests that the most effective teachers are those who do vary the teaching and learning environment (Dougherty & Bonanno, 1979).

DECISIONS TO BE MADE

Muska Mosston (1981), whose work in physical education has had considerable impact upon the teaching profession, describes teaching as a constant chain of decision-making events. Teachers in all subject areas are engaged in decisions about objectives, organization of the class, subject matter, evaluation, and specifics related to the environment, just to name a few. Every successful lesson is developed from a number of decisions that can be grouped into three categories: preparation (precontact with students), contact, and postcontact (reflection of the lesson). Table 6–1 reveals some of the major decision-making events that occur prior to, during, and after each lesson.

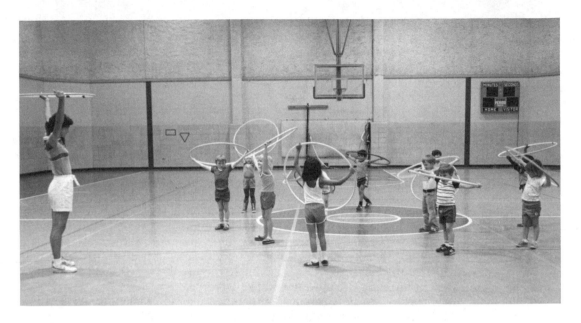

Table 6-1 Chain of Decision-Making Events

DECISION CATEGORIES	COMPONENTS AND DECISIONS

Precontact *(preparation)*	1. General subject area/objectives
	   a. Fitness Activity
	   b. Skill Development
	   c. Enhancement Activity
	   d. Review
	2. Learning/ability level(s)
	3. Number of students
	4. Equipment/material
	5. Facilities/location
	6. Time
	7. General class attitude and anticipated learning climate (how much responsibility is the class ready for?)
	8. Selection of a teaching strategy
	   a. Style
	   b. Organization pattern
	   c. Communication mode (verbal, written, visual, auditory)
	   d. Teacher's role
	   e. Student's role
	   f. Communication
	9. Specific subject matter
	   a. Quantity (desired amount to be accomplished)
	   b. Quality (performance level)
	10. Evaluation of performance (assessment procedures, other)

Contact	1. Adjustment to precontact decisions (weather, mishap, other) 2. Observation of behavior 3. Assessment (against criteria) 4. Feedback (type: gesture, touch, verbal)
Postcontact *(reflection)*	1. Assessment of teaching strategy 2. Assessment of student performance 3. Assessment of teacher performance

Even if accomplished in the subject area, the teacher who does not consider such components as numer of students, amount of time, and resources available, may be allowing a great deal of undesirable events to occur. The selection of a teaching strategy(s) is dependent upon the detailed understanding of numerous precontact factors. If eye-hand coordination (using balls) is the chosen theme, for example, one's selection of a teaching strategy may be severely limited or dependent upon equipment, facilities, and number of students. Are there enough balls so that each child receives one, or are there 12 balls for 35 children? How many vaulting boxes are available for jumping? Are there two for 30 children, or six for the same amount of students? Conditions could vary considerably and, in many instances, class size may vary significantly within the same school setting.

An important point to consider when planning is to be prepared for the unexpected. For example: Your selected location is outside and it rains! Or the ground is wet and the principal (or you) forgot that the fifth graders are scheduled to practice for the school play in the gym! Few if any teachers have not experienced a variation of these unexpected occurrences. Thus, have an alternative set of plans in your lesson-plan book, or at least in your mind. Can you use another large area, classroom(s), or the hallways? Are you going to modify the scheduled lesson (if the situation continues), or use an unrelated activity?

A succcessful lesson is based upon planned decision making that takes into account all phases of the learning and instructional process.

Teaching Strategies

The term *teaching strategy* refers to a process of manipulation of the learning environment. Each strategy is a composite of several possible variables (Fig. 6–1). The essential ingredient in a strategy is the *style* of presentation of subject matter. Along with the style, the instructor may select from a numer of *organizational patterns* and *communication modes* (Gabbard, 1983).

One commonly used method of comparing styles is to place them on a continuum denoting general characteristic qualities (Fig. 6–2).

As one observes the continuum, it is important to keep in mind that no style is superior in every situation. The continuum is not necessarily a "style versus style" representation, but rather something that highlights the relationships. Each style has advantages that are unique to the style itself and that must be effectively matched with the uniqueness of each class (that is, students, equipment available, and other variables), subject matter, and learning outcomes perceived by the teacher. The "master" teacher is one who has the knowledge and experience in matching various conditions and content with an array of teaching styles and organizational patterns to produce the best results.

As noted earlier, the best teachers are those who possess a wide repertoire of teaching strategies. They are not afraid to mix and combine styles.

After experimenting with each style and becoming well versed with its characteristics, learn to modify them to suit your individual needs and desired outcomes. There is nothing as monotonous as a teacher who uses the same style over and over. This procedure stifles both student and teacher.

One last thought, a teaching strategy is only as good as the practitioner. It is hard work to understand the mechanisms involved in the teaching/learning process, but careful preparation and attention to detail are critical for a successful outcome.

TEACHING STRATEGY MODEL

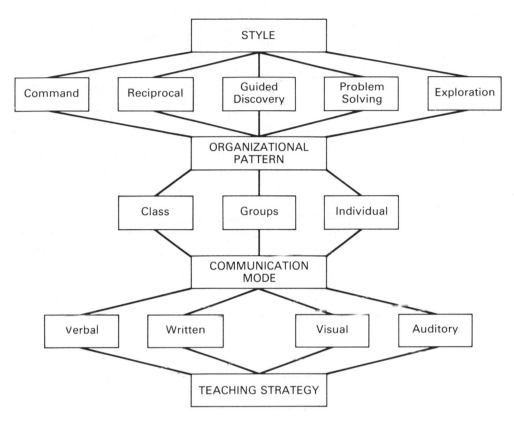

Figure 6-1   The teaching strategy model.

Figure 6-2   Teaching style continuum.

TEACHING STYLE CONTINUUM

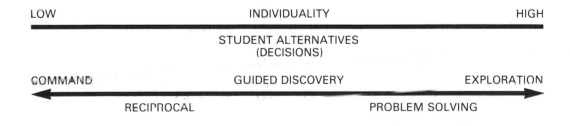

Description of Teaching Styles

Command

The *command* style is considered by many as the most limiting because of the few opportunities for decision making offered the student. The uniqueness and individuality of the student is not acknowledged in a pure command approach. Frequently utilized for "mass instruction," where all students are required to perform the same task at the same pace (relays, mass calisthenics), this style is usually characterized by teacher "demonstration" (and/or explanation) and student "replication." The teacher allows little if any deviation from the presentation. During some lessons involving gymnastics and dance, this tight control is desirable. It is important that the teacher using this style not come across as being rigid and mistrusting, but rather be perceived enthusiastically, desiring that the students learn the skills in an efficient and safe manner.

It is the control characteristic that perhaps influences many new teachers to use this style and seasoned teachers to apply it at the beginning of the school year. When tasks are presented using this style, the teacher usually provides a demonstration and verbal explanation of the task(s), or conveys the material using written "direct" task instructions (task sheets). Examples of direct command statements are:

1. Bounce the ball with your right hand five times; then switch to your left and bounce it five times.
2. Jump up with both feet and land on one. Jump up with both feet and land on both at the same time.
3. Kick the ball with your right foot to the wall, and after it rebounds trap it with the same foot. Switch to the left foot and do the same.

An essential element in this style is the demonstration and/or explanation of the task. If the teacher is going to demand strict adherence to the task criteria, then it is necessary that these criteria be clearly understood by the student. Demonstration is perhaps the most efficient means to make criteria clear. The teacher must be very careful, however, for an incorrect or poorly executed demonstration may confuse the child or lead to inadequate performance of the skill. It should also be noted that the command style of teaching is not as practical for the development of motor schema as other styles because of its emphasis on specific movement outcomes, which excludes the variability needed for schema development. There are, however, several advantages to the command style of subject matter presentation:

1. Clear objectives and specific skill acquisition (the student learns what you have specifically stated). There are skills that can most effectively be presented with the direct style (dance steps, some gymnastic and sport-skill movements, specific exercise movements).
2. Efficiency in terms of time and organization (especially with large classes). Research findings in support of the command style suggest that if the objective is to teach a specific skill within a relatively short period of time, this mode of presentation is superior to problem-solving methods (Toole & Arink, 1982).
3. Some children respond better to the security of knowing what to do, how to do it, and where to go.
4. Class control and safety (such as when teaching gymnastics or swimming).
5. Requires less knowledge of subject matter and dealing with unpredictable questions (as in problem solving). This is perhaps an advantage for the new teacher in a new situation; however, this may also be considered a major shortcoming.

The command style of teaching does have a place in the teaching/learning environment. Situations arise when this style is desirable; however, it should not be used extensively because of the limits it sets on individual creativity, self-discipline, and movement variability—items deemed essential to the total development of young children.

Reciprocal

This method of presentation is characterized by a "grouping" of two or more individuals and is frequently referred to as a "partnership." Although the reciprocal style inherently necessitates that students are grouped (that is, a form of organizational pattern), its unique reciprocal qualities justify its placement as a style in this model.

The reciprocal style is structurally similar to the command style except that interaction and feedback about performance are provided immediately by a peer(s) rather than by the teacher. This style is accomplished by grouping the students into partnerships of at least two (most frequently two or three), with one being the observer that provides feedback (to the performer) based on criteria established by the teacher. After this process, the cycle continues with students switching roles. Although this method can be used with younger children (Levels I–III), a sufficient level of maturity is required for maximum effectiveness. Students must be able to understand and carry out the teacher's criteria; thus they are responsible for a major portion of the instructional process. Secondly, the observer should be able to communicate effectively with the student performing the task. This type of behavior is generally observed with students in the intermediate-grade levels.

Of utmost importance is the teacher's clarity and effectiveness in conveying the established criteria to the partnership. With a clear demonstration and explanation of the task(s), teachers have also found it helpful to provide written task sheets (to be discussed later) outlining the criteria and if possible presenting a visual model of the task. While the teacher should be observant of the environment at all times, direct communication with the partnership, that is, interacting with the feedback process, should take place only through the observer (not the performer) unless safety is a factor.

As mentioned, the advantages of this style, aside from the "grouping" arrangement, provide for a unique learning opportunity. Characteristically, this method provides for a one-to-one teacher/student interaction with immediate feedback of performance, thus enhancing the potential for skill development. Provided that the teacher presents a clear explanation of task criteria (and follows up with supportive materials), additional benefits of this style would be that of mental practice and the potential for overlearning (that is, repetition). Also unique and supportive of this style is the potential for enhancement of self-concept. The image of being an instructor and assisting in the learning process can be a rewarding experience for the student.

Although this style provides many advantages, it can also present problems in the learning process. As previously discussed, a certain level of mental maturity is essential. The potential problem arising when a child is teamed with a partner who is overly critical can be serious. The opposite may also occur, when very little reciprocal communication takes place. The quality of communication and feedback is the essential component in this teaching style. The teacher's explanation of the task criteria and the grouping of students are central to the effectiveness of the reciprocal process.

Further information related to this style may be found in the "Organizational Patterns" section of this chapter.

GUIDED DISCOVERY, PROBLEM SOLVING, AND EXPLORATION

The following styles present a dramatic cognitive shift from the command process. The change is from demonstration/replication (stimulus/response) to a gradual increase in intellectual freedom and opportunity for creativity. With the command approach the student followed a set of guidelines with few if any allowable alternatives. Now the student is presented with the opportunity to think, inquire, and discover; *the process becomes as important as the product!* A demonstration of the "right way," or giving the answer, occurs very seldom if ever when utilizing these styles. At this point, the teacher needs to consider the following: Are *the students* ready for the organizational and intellectual freedom? Can I better serve the needs of the child with one of these processes? Is the presentation of this theme best conveyed using one of these styles? *Am I* ready to present the material effectively using one of these styles?

Communication

Essential to the success of any style is the line of communication between teacher and learner. The teacher presents a stimulus to which the student reacts. The teacher must be a careful and continuous observer in order to respond effectively to the student's performance with appropriate ongoing challenges and feedback. In other words, the student and teacher are communicating through the verbal and motor avenues. In the guided discovery, problem solving, and exploration styles the process becomes as important as the product. A common element that all of the styles exhibit is the presentation of tasks or movement stimuli in problem-solving form. Although the majority of the communication is presented verbally, there is a growing popularity of nonverbal problem-solving communication (for example, task sheets, cards). The characteristic differences between guided discovery, problem solving, and exploration are in the amount of "guidance" and "openness" conveyed through statements; exploration offers the least guidance and greatest "openness," whereas guided discovery conveys the most teacher guidance of the three styles.

The success by which a teacher can get a student to learn is dependent upon the manner in which the student comprehends the information presented. Teachers should phrase tasks or inquiries in an indirect manner through questions and/or challenges without giving away the direct answer, or giving the student a feeling of being commanded.

Teachers should be diverse (as well as challenging) in their presentations. Too often teachers rely on the phrases "Can you . . . ?" "How many ways . . . ?" and "In how many ways can you . . . ?" The following are examples of phrases that may be used to diversify task statements and inquiries:

"Can you dodge this ball with your upper body?"
"Show me. . . . "
"Who can . . . ?"
"How can you . . . ?"
"Try. . . . "
"Could you . . . ?"
"Find a way. . . . "
"What other ways . . . ?"
"How many ways can you . . . ?"

"What different ways are there to . . . ?"
"If you. . . . "
"How else can you . . . ?"
"Is there another way . . . ?"
"Is there a better way . . . ?"

After presenting the problem(s) or stimuli to the class, the teacher's role is far from completed. Communication now extends into reinforcement and providing students with knowledge of their performance (feedback). Feedback can be offered in a variety of ways; however, negative statements very seldom if ever are appropriate. In matters of safety, the teacher may have to be negative if an immediate response is necessary. Praise may be given to a student without verbal statements, and in large classes nonverbal communication may be used frequently. This type of recognition may be in the form of a nod, a smile, or a body gesture. The teacher should, however, try to interact verbally with as many students as possible, giving priority to those who may be "stuck" or who require extra psychological support.

Regardless of teaching style (including *command*), it is essential that the teacher have the attention of all students, especially for initial guidance and delivery of learning information. Voice is both an essential teaching tool and valuable asset. For it is not only what is said but *how* it is delivered that provides understanding and motivation. A teacher's enthusiasm is contagious! Two teachers presenting the same material and using the same script may get far different responses from the same class. It is a common occurrence observed in teacher-education classes that an enthusiastic personality and voice can completely turn around an unassured class of children. Many teachers comment that their afternoon classes (especially the last) do not seem to respond as well as their classes before lunch. The problem, in part, is probably the teacher's delivery. Learn to pace yourself, unless you are an extremely enthusiastic personality and possess a strong voice. Know when to be loud and soft. Be careful not to convey fear by being too loud and direct when a soft, caring voice may be needed.

In order to present an effective delivery, the teacher needs to get the attention of the class. A signal should be established that signifies "stop, look, and listen!" Depending upon the size and personality of the class, this may be done with the voice, a beat on a drum, a clap of the hands, or a whistle. The class needs to understand the importance of this signal, for it is used not only for task delivery but also in an emergency and as an indicator that class time is over.

For delivery, the teacher should be positioned so everyone can see and hear. A scattered or semicircle formation, with students and teacher facing each other, is quite effective. In specific situations it may be best to have the students sit down. This technique controls excessive movement when attention is desired; however, children should not be expected to "sit still" or be too attentive except for short periods of time. Keep verbal statements short, concise, motivating; your job is to get them moving!

Guided Discovery

The *guided discovery* style has been described by Mosston (1981) as the first process that cracks the cognitive barrier and embodies the discovery concept. Guided discovery uses the process of inquiry to "guide" students to the discovery of an end product predetermined by the teacher. Basically, the teacher sets the scene through a series of questions, which brings the students to a point where a common starting point can be assumed. After establishing a foundation, the teacher then guides the students through a carefully planned sequence of steps consisting of questions or clues. Because it is not known how the students will respond, each step is based on the response given by the students in the previous step. If the students are too far "off track," the teacher must guide them back to the target, remembering not to reveal the answer, however. Ideally, each succeeding question narrows in on the target (predetermined objective) until self-discovery is realized by the student. Figure 6–3 illustrates the "ladder effect" of this style.

Essential to the success of this style is the teacher's awareness of the following factors as described by Mosston (1981):

The objective (target)
The direction of the sequence of steps
The "size" of each step
The interrelationship of the steps (general progression)
The speed of the sequence.

Figure 6-3   The "ladder effect" of Guided Discovery.

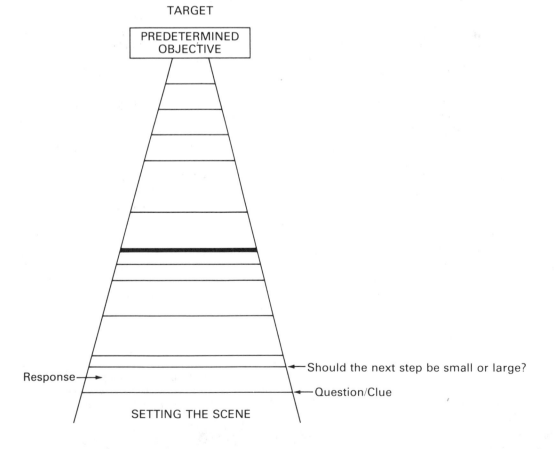

The following suggestions may help to facilitate a smooth development of the guided-discovery process:

1. After stating the challenge, always wait for the student's response; be patient; it takes time to think.
2. Reword the challenge if you must, or state it more simply. If after a reasonable amount of time no response is given, you probably took too big a step. Ask questions to clarify, motivate, or extend.
3. Always reinforce student responses with positive statements (unless safety is in jeopardy); negative ones tend to inhibit student responses.
4. Remember, observe then respond by stating what you have seen; follow this by a question to clarify, motivate, or extend; *observe–reflect–question* (praise when appropriate).

Example
Predetermined objective—Vertical jump for height:

1. proper landing (balls of feet with knees bent)
2. crouch (and toes leaving the floor last)
3. use of arms

Questions to Set the Scene
Today we are going to discover jumping for height. Challenge: pretend that you are jumping up and reaching for an apple that is hanging high above your head. How would you jump to grab it? Try jumping a few times.

Questions: On what part of your feet did you land? How many places on your feet could you land? After trying all three (flatfooted, ball, heel), which is the most comfortable? Did you land with your legs straight or were your knees bent? Select a partner and allow him or her to observe while you jump. Can anyone think of some reasons for landing on the balls of one's feet? Let's talk about the takeoff. Have you discovered any factors that you could share with us that could help us go higher? Good; we have identified the arms and legs as major factors in the takeoff. Let's all practice jumping with our arms in various positions. Try to identify one that lifts you the highest. Share your discoveries with others around you. Would someone like to share some discoveries with us? John says to swing your arms down and then up as your body moves up. Try it! Do you feel a difference? As your body moves up, how do you propel yourself up with your legs? Some of you are crouched deeply and others are just barely squatting down. Does this make a difference? Try different depths. Which depth allows you to go the highest? What part of your foot leaves the floor last? Sally says that she can feel her toes push hard against the floor. What do you feel? Would it help if you extend your hand and fingers to grab the apple? How much higher can you reach if you do? Now let's review the discoveries that we have made. Can we put some of our discoveries together well enough to explain to our friends and parents how to jump the highest and grab something?

Ideal for primary-grade children, this style of presentation allows the teacher to provide intellectual inquiry and at the same time accomplish a designated (specific) objective(s). The concept of "variability in practice" and an understanding of the discovery process by the student are greatly enhanced with this style, especially when compared to the command presentation.

Guided discovery does present possible problems, however. The style has been described as the most difficult for the teacher to master because of the amount of verbalizing and high degree of task competence and knowledge of task sequence required. It may be viewed as time-consuming because of the question-response process. With large groups or groups that possess an extreme range of abilities, this style may also present some problems.

Problem Solving

With *problem solving* emerges individuality, creativity and variability within a general movement area. Where guided discovery is closed-ended (that is, the teacher guides the student to a specific discovery), problem solving is an open-ended process. Each new and different problem leads students to a variety of solutions that, while challenging, are within the student's own unique ability. The teacher still chooses the general subject matter area; however, the student may discover what he or she wishes within that framework. There is room for making new discoveries. Mosston (1981) describes problem solving as a self-perpetuating process. The act of discovery itself becomes a reinforcing, motivating agent that drives the child to continue to seek additional solutions and alternatives.

Problem Design

All problems presented to students must be relevant to subject matter, student readiness, and experience of both the group and the individual. What can be discovered using this style?

Skills/Movement Variability.   This refers to skills that may or may not be designed for specific situations, but ones that enhance the movement schema of a general skill area. Example: In discovering how to roll the body, a number of rolling skills may be acquired. The rolling schema may be greatly enhanced as the child strengthens the dimensions (spatial, time, force) of that skill area, which may help prepare him or her for novel and ever-changing tasks and conditions.

Relationships.   Through problem solving, relationships among parts of the body, equipment, and other bodies are discovered. "Most or perhaps all movements are performed in some relationship to their antecedents and their consequences" (Mosston, 1981).

Concepts.   As a result of the problem-solving process, students discover an understanding of the concepts upon which movement performance is based. An understanding of time, space, force and relationships, and the functions and use of strength, endurance, flexibility, and the cardiorespiratory system (to name a few), may be discovered through problem solving.

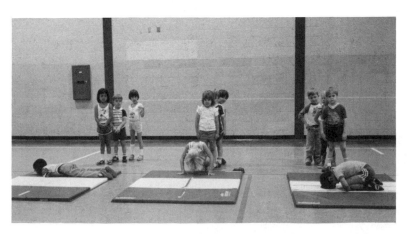

Problem solving provides numerous opportunities to enhance the movement schema.

Preferences. As a result of performing a variety of movements, understanding how the body moves, and judging relationships, the child can make personal judgments as to which movement is the most or the least effective and efficient for specific conditions.

Quantity/Limits. By performing a set of movements in various situations, the child develops an idea of quantitative performance and limitations. How far can I kick the ball using the inside of my foot? How fast can I run backwards? Can I jump higher [vertical jump] by swinging my arms upward? How far can I bend my trunk forward?

Steps in the Problem-Solving Process
1. Identify the skill theme (ball dribbling, jumping, others). Have a clear understanding of the sequence of progression of the skill.
2. Focus upon a specific area (dribbling and moving, jumping for distance, and so forth).
3. Identify a dimension(s) of the skill to focus upon (that is, an element of space, time, force).
4. Design the problems, keeping in mind the desired discovery of skills/variability, relationships, concepts, preference, and quantity/limits.
5. Presentation of problems. Keep in mind that demonstration or disclosing solutions is rarely done! Being an open-ended process, problem-solving questions should be structured in the same manner: allowing solutions, yet stimulating the student to continue inquiring (as opposed to guided discovery of the solution). It will be noted later in this section that the questions can be presented to the class as a whole, in groups, or individually (using problem-solving task sheets).
6. Problem solving. Remember to allow time for students to explore. Refrain from offering additional questions unless children need them for clarification or motivation.
7. Discussion and demonstration of solutions. If possible (class size allowing), all students should have the opportunity to reveal their solutions. Although theoretically there is no "wrong" answer as long as it is appropriate for the problem (yet some answers are recognized as "better"), guidance may provide the student with more meaningful discoveries that result in a broader information base, which may serve further to enhance the schema.
8. Reinforcement. Verbal reinforcement and individual assistance are essential to keeping the process flowing and being motivational for the student. If the student becomes "stuck" (can't think of a solution) on a specific problem, which may occur frequently with younger children, the problem-solving process may be perceived as frustrating, therefore unsuccessful. If such conditions arise it is best to shift over to guided discovery and guide the student away from the frustration and to some solution. Not all children will do well with problem solving.

Example

General subject matter area: Ball Dribbling (Level I)
Specific Theme: Dribbling while moving in various directions
Primary Focus: Body position and ball control; dimensions of space, time, and force.
Background: Children have explored with ball bouncing/dribbling; using two hands and one-hand variations while in their personal space

Questions (General Stimulus)
Let's start out by dribbling with two hands, then one hand (if you can), while staying in your personal space. Can you change hands? Try to change the level of bounce: at your knees, waist, chest. Now, using your preferred hand, move in different directions. Try forward and backward. What other directions can you move to? Is it easier to control the ball

while bouncing it high or low? Are we remembering to not slap at it? Change speeds; moving first slowly then faster. Are you still keeping control of the ball? If you feel ready, try changing hands while moving in various directions.

Problem-solving is not designed to develop a specific skill, nor is it the most efficient style in terms of time or teaching large groups of children. This style is, however, an excellent means for allowing the children the opportunity to understand how their bodies move and to develop schema.

Exploration

The *exploration* style can be utilized quite effectively with elementary-level children. This process takes advantage of the child's intrinsic interests in exploration and experimentation. Compared to guided discovery and problem solving, exploration is more open-ended and offers the least amount of teacher guidance. The teacher designs problems and allows students to explore as they wish, with additional guidance provided only for safety purposes or adjustment owing to lack of communication (for instance, the student did not understand the statement). Generally, exploration is associated with that which is novel. This style is very effective when introducing a new piece of equipment or presenting "old" equipment or movement skills in a new atmosphere of creativity.

This style is also appropriate at the beginning of a lesson when introducing a new theme before a more "guided" style is applied. The uniqueness of the exploration style lies in its flexibility and accommodation to various ages and problem-solving abilities. Exploration instructions from the teacher are generally limited to a few "wide-open" statements such as:

1. Explore handling and bouncing the ball with your hands.
2. Select a ball [various sizes] of your choice and explore ways of balancing it on various parts of your body.
3. What can you and your partner do with a hula hoop?
4. Can you create a new jump-rope routine and chant?

The role of the teacher during exploration is to be aware of safety hazards and to stimulate thought in youngsters who appear "stuck." If needed, it is helpful to inspire children to observe others. This practice, often performed naturally, stimulates thought for movement and creativity. With some children the teacher may need to compensate somewhat by inspiring with pertinent questions that do not "guide" too much, but ask the child to respond to thoughts about his or her movement abilities that are related to the area of exploration.

ORGANIZATIONAL PATTERNS

As previously noted (Fig. 6–1), teaching styles and organizational patterns are independent, yet a teaching strategy must combine elements of both. An *organizational pattern* is utilized to organize students so the desired teaching style may be presented. The basic organizational patterns are: class, groups (two or more), and individual instruction. A number of combinations (styles and patterns) are possible. Some may be more advantageous under ideal conditions (small class size and lots of equipment); however, many teachers find themselves in less than ideal settings. For example, problem solving and guided discovery are very effective if the class size is small and an abundance of equipment is available. Instruction is therefore usually directed to the entire class, and the teacher moves around to interact. But what if there are 60 students in the class and equipment is limited? Can the teacher still provide problem solving? Yes! The alternative is grouping at stations and using written problem-solving techniques (task sheets, cards, other devices). The master teacher is one who can combine style with organization to challenge both the conditions and the student.

Class Instruction. In this pattern, the students are presented information as a whole. Using the desired style, the teacher communicates the same message (command or problem) to the entire class at the same time. Students work as one unit, usually in a scattered formation, responding to the instructions presented.

Group and Individual Instruction. If the teacher wishes to organize the children so that more than one activity can be presented at the same time, dividing the class into units (groups or individual) is excellent.

The use of stations, also known as *learning centers*, has become a very popular and useful technique designed to accommodate group and individual instruction (individual stations). With stations, units are assigned, or allowed the freedom, to perform a task or set of tasks at a number of activity areas that are usually related to a specific theme (Fig. 6–4).

This pattern, one of the most utilized in physical education, is praised by many for its effectiveness in providing sufficient practice of a skill.

A unique quality of stations is that stations may be combined with various styles quite effectively. Among the options are:

1. Dispersing into units (groups) that perform tasks demonstrated or directed by written, auditory, and/or visual materials (task cards, sheets, posters, tape recorders) at each station;
2. Dividing the class into units that perform problem-solving activities as stimulated by written, auditory, and/or visual information.

Figure 6-4 Station work with a theme.

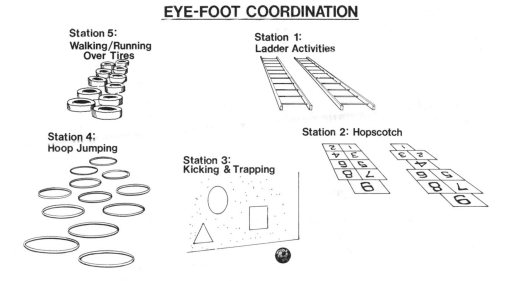

EYE-FOOT COORDINATION

Station 5:
Walking/Running
Over Tires

Station 1:
Ladder Activities

Station 4:
Hoop Jumping

Station 2: Hopscotch

Station 3:
Kicking & Trapping

Basic Station Arrangements

1. Single Task. In this arrangement, each unit (group or individual) is presented a single task at each station. The task could be the same; if so, no rotation (movement to the other stations) is necessary. This arrangement is effective for separating students so maximum utilization of space is obtained. Another option provides a single, yet different task at each station. With this arrangement the units rotate from station to station, thus providing maximum efficiency of equipment use when not enough is available for all to engage in the same activity.
2. Multiple Tasks. Same as the "single task" arrangement, except that at each station more than one task is presented.

With both basic arrangements, the teacher has a number of options in terms of rotation, starting, stopping, and duration between stations.

Among the options are:

1. Setting a specific amount of time for the completion of the task(s) at each station, then giving a signal (whistling, clapping hands, using the voice) for each group to rotate in a designated order (that is, clockwise, station 1 to 2 to 3 . . .).
2. Students (individual) have the choice of pace and location. This is a self-operating design that requires the individual to be in control of his or her own performance and behavior. Students may be given complete freedom or they may be told to complete at least "3 of the 6" stations. A word of caution here: (1) standards must be established by the teacher in regard to number of students allowed at a station at one time, and (2) students need to work up to this freedom with limited decisions.

There are many advantages associated with dividing a class and using stations. One is that stations provide maximum utilization of space and equipment; skills can be practiced without waiting in long lines. Another advantage is that a large number of activities can be conveyed (to large classes) without the direct verbal guidance of the teacher. Stations, in addition to individualizing instruction, can be used to group children by ability (if the task deems necessary) and promote social interaction.

Using Formations to Organize Activity

There are a variety of formations that may be used by the teacher to convey instruction and organize movement activity. Although it is quite common for an entire class (one unit) to be arranged in a single formation, one of the positive characteristics of formations is that they can be used to divide classes into smaller units. When used correctly, formations provide time efficiency and ease in organizing both small and large numbers of children. Whereas some arrangements emphasize uniformity and may be characteristic with teacher-centered (for example, command) teaching styles, others emphasize more freedom with movement space, which is generally more appropriate with child-centered styles (guided discovery, problem solving, and exploration). Table 6–2 presents some of the most commonly used instructional activity formations with children.

Hoffman, Young, and Klesius (1981) have suggested the following additional considerations for organizing students:

1. If in an outside area, face the students away from or at an angle to the sun so they are not looking into the sun.
2. Face the students into or at an angle to the wind so the teacher's voice, when standing in front of the students, is carried toward them by the wind.

Table 6-2   Instruction and Activity Formations

FORMATION	GENERAL DESCRIPTION AND SUGGESTIONS	EXAMPLES OF USE
File 	Position one child for each line desired equidistant apart, then signal the class to line up behind these children, forming single files. Children may also stand side-by-side (line formation). For relay activities, be sure that teams are even and limited to 6 to 8 per line.	Relays, simple games, marching, simple stunts
Circle 	Children form a circle by following the teacher around in a circle. Other methods include all joining hands and forming a circle, or having the class take positions on a circle printed on the floor or play area. The teacher should stand at the edge of the circle when talking, not in the middle. For maximum participation, limit number of children to 8 or 10.	Circle games and dances, parachute activities, marching
Semicircle 	Arrange children in a line facing their leader, then have them join hands and form a half-circle.	Most practical for giving instructions and demonstrations, and skill practice
Scattered 	Children find a spot in the play area. Unless partners or small groups are together, each child should be at least an arm's distance apart. Set geographical boundaries. Be sure to move around the area and interact.	Great for problem-solving and exploratory activities, tag games, stunts, creative dance

3. Keep equipment to be used later in the lesson out of sight, either in a bag, equipment cart, or another area, in order to avoid distracting the students.

4. Choose an activity area that minimizes distractions.

5. Observable boundary markers for movement space are easier for students to respond to than abstract instructions. An area marked off by plastic containers, flags, cones, or painted lines is easier for students to adhere to than instructions such as, "Don't go too far away" or "Stay in line with that tree."

6. The teacher should *circulate* among the students to provide individual teaching points, ask and respond to questions, give reinforcement, or intervene in a potentially hazardous situation.

7. When speaking to the whole class, the teacher should be in a position to view all the children, regardless of the formation used, and to observe the actions of each student.

COMMUNICATION MODES

An additional option in the selection of a teaching strategy is *communication mode*, that is, the mode with which the teacher wishes to convey material. The general options (often combined) are verbal, written, visual, and auditory. The *verbal mode* consists of spoken communication through personal contact, usually between the teacher and student (the most utilized form). An *auditory mode* may be presented using records or tapes that convey the style of presentation selected.

The remainder of this section is devoted to the *written* and *visual* modes of communication; both have been found to be effective and motivating alternatives in the learning process.

The Use of Written and Visual Information

Task cards, task sheets, and posters can be used most effectively with group and individual organizational patterns. Providing written and/or visual information, these techniques promote individualization and convey the instructional style desired by the teacher. Through these media, tasks may be presented directly (command), or be designed to stimulate the problem-solving abilities of children.

Along with promoting general individuality, task materials offer some very functional benefits:

1. Inform about *what* and *how*; especially if a demonstration or explanation was not provided.
2. Help the child remember what was presented in demonstration or explanation.
3. Provide a record (task sheet) for the teacher, student, and parent (optional) of what was expected and to what degree it was accomplished.
4. Provide the flexibility of meeting individual abilities with multiple tasks of varying degrees of difficulty.
5. Release the teacher from the role of direct communicator to the entire class, thus allowing the teacher to interact with individuals.
6. For young children, preschool to first grade, who may not be at a level to comprehend written statements or words adequately, posters with visual information (figures, pictures, other media) provide a means of problem solving without direct teacher communication.

Examples

Poster conveying a direct style of presentation.

Table 6-3   Eye-Foot Coordination

STATION #1—LADDER ACTIVITIES

---

1. Walk forward, stepping on each rung.
2. Walk forward, stepping between the rungs.
3. Walk backward, stepping on each rung.
4. Walk backward, stepping between the rungs.
5. Walk sideways, stepping on each rung.
6. Walk sideways, stepping between each rung.
7. Hop forward between the rungs.
8. Hop sideways between the rungs.

Task card (could be sheet or poster) with problem-solving information.

Table 6-4   Task Card:Eye-Foot Coordination

STATION #1—LADDER ACTIVITIES

Watch where you want your feet to move!

1. Can you walk in different ways from one end to the other without touching the floor?
2. Try walking across by stepping on the rungs only and facing in different directions.
3. Are there other ways to walk across the ladder?
4. Is there a way to cross without stepping on the rungs or spaces between?
5. Have you discovered a direction other than forward in which to cross?
6. If you were a rabbit, how would you move to the other side? Be careful. Be sure to watch where your feet are going to move next.

Poster information conveyed with figures.

Figure 6-5   Poster conveying visual stimuli.

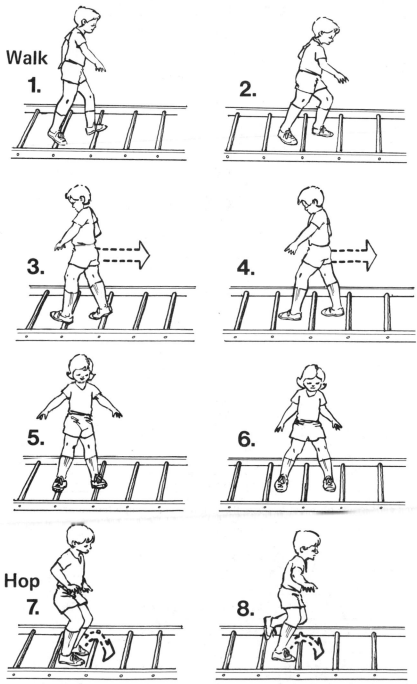

Eye-Foot Coordination
Station 1-Ladder Activities

Table 6-5 Eye-Foot Coordination

LEARNING CENTER TASK SHEET

NAME _____ PERIOD _____

Completed				TASKS
				Ladder
				I can:
				1. Walk forward by stepping on the rungs only
				2. Walk backward by stepping on the rungs only
				3. Walk sideways on the rungs
				4. Hop between the rungs to the end
				Tires
				I can:
				1. Walk across the tires
				2. Run across the tires
				3. Run, stepping in the middle of each tire
				4. Walk across, placing one foot in each tire
				5. Run across in the same way
				6. Hop in the middle of each tire to the end
				Hoops
				I can:
				1. Leap from hoop to hoop
				2. Hop from hoop to hoop
				3. Run across placing one foot in each hoop
				I can:
5	10	15	20	1. Hit the target from 5, 10, 15, and 20 feet away (3 trials)
5	10	15	20	2. Hit the target by kicking with my opposite foot
				3. Trap the ball with my right foot
				4. Trap the ball with my left foot
				Hopscotch
				I can:
				1. Play a successful game of American Hopscotch
				2. French Hopscotch
				3. Italian Hopscotch

Task sheet with checklist; may be completed by student, with partner or teacher.

REFERENCES

GABBARD, C. (1983, fall). A teaching strategy model: The integration of style, organization and communication mode. *Journal of Teaching In Physical Education,* 16–21.

DOUGHERTY, N. J. & BONANNO, D. (1979). *Contemporary approaches to the teaching of physical education.* Minneapolis: Burgess.

MOSSTON, M. (1981). *Teaching physical education* (2nd ed.). Columbus, OH: Chs. E. Merrill.

TOOLE, T. & ARINK, E. A. (1982). Movement education: Its effect on motor skill performance. *Research Quarterly for Exercise and Sport, 53,* 156–162.

SUGGESTED READINGS

ANDERSON, W. G. (1980). *Analysis of teaching physical education.* St. Louis: C. V. Mosby.

GALLAHUE, D. L. (1982). *Developmental movement experiences for children.* New York: Wiley.

GILLIOM, B. C. (1970). *Basic movement education for children: Rationale and teaching units.* Reading, MA: Addison-Wesley.

GRAHAM, G., HOLT/HALE, J. A., McEWEN, T., & PARKER, M. (1980). *Children moving: A reflective approach to teaching physical education.* Polo Alto, CA: Mayfield.

KRUEGER, H., & KRUEGER, J. (1982). *Movement education is physical education: A guide to teaching and planning* (2nd ed.). Dubuque, IA: Wm. C. Brown.

LOGSDON, B. J., BARRET, K. R., BRAER, M. R., McGEE, R., AMMONS, M., HALVERSON, L. E., & ROBERTON, M. A. (1984). *Physical education for children: A focus on the teaching process.* Philadelphia: Lea & Febiger.

MELOGRANO, V. (1979). *Designing curriculum and learning.* Dubuque, IA: Kendall/Hunt.

SCHURR, E. L. (1980). *Movement experiences for children* (3rd ed.). Englewood Cliffs, NJ: Prentice-Hall.

SWEENEY, R. T. (Ed.). (1980). *Selected readings in movement education.* Reading, MA.: Addison-Wesley.

7

CLASS MANAGEMENT AND DISCIPLINE

Although some educators consider class management and discipline to be synonomous, the authors intend for these two topics to be considered as separate. *Class management* is defined in this text as definite procedures used by the teacher in the creation of a positive learning environment that prevent serious disruptions of the learning process. *Discipline*, on the other hand, is defined as technique(s) used by the teacher to interrupt inappropriate behaviors and prevent their recurrence. Basically, class management refers to prevention, whereas disciplinary action occurs "after the fact."

Like the classroom, the gymnasium is meant to be a place of learning. However, it can become the scene of a never-ending battle in which teacher and children struggle to gain the advantage. When this happens, the casualties are usually heavy and most often detrimental to desirable learning.

Many indicators reveal the importance of class management and discipline. The 1979 Gallup Poll on attitudes toward education substantiated what many have expressed for years—lack of discipline is the number-one concern by all who are involved in education, whether they be students, parents, teachers, administrators, or the general public. Student-teachers and first-year teachers report back to their universities that class management and discipline represent the two areas in which they feel the least secure. All have a stake in the positive and negative effects of class-management techniques employed in the classroom, and the gymnasium is no exception.

Students, believe it or not, prefer an orderly environment, one in which they can learn course content and how to relate with others without constant disruption. They become frustrated when lack of structure or proper motivation do not stimulate them to do their best. Parents expect their children to learn both course content and proper behavior in cooperative and competitive efforts with others. Teachers and administrators know that the effectiveness of their class-management strategies will directly influence the quality of learning that occurs in their

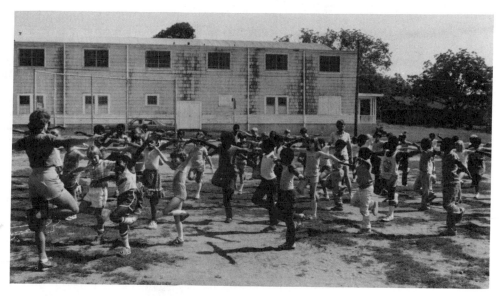

Very large classes require efficient class-management procedures.

classrooms, and affect their emotional health, the evaluation of their success as a teacher-administrator, and even their job tenure. The public fears that students who are allowed to demonstrate hostility, disrespect, and lack of self-control within the structured environment of the schools will eventually manifest this unacceptable behavior to a greater extent on society at large. The authors recognize that the manner in which teachers handle class management and discipline is closely related to their philosophical beliefs. It is beyond the scope of this chapter to examine in detail the complexity and diversity of this topic; however, the reader is encouraged to study the suggested readings at the end of the chapter for a more thorough understanding. The remainder of this chapter focuses on the unique characteristics of a positive learning environment, desirable gymnasium behaviors, communication skills, managerial effectiveness, efficient management of disruption, and discipline strategies.

CREATING A POSITIVE LEARNING ENVIRONMENT

The learning environment can facilitate learning only if the setting is perceived by the students to be psychologically safe, where threats are noticeably absent, expectations are realistic, early success is common, and positive interactions are frequent. In such an environment students feel secure because they are treated as worthwhile individuals.

Of course, the most important variable in a learning environment is the teacher. Teachers who are neatly and appropriately dressed, self-confident, appropriately assertive, consistent, friendly, fair, and competent in their subject matter command a natural respect from the students they teach. Children feel more secure when led by those they respect and like. In other words, the setting is perceived by the children as being psychologically safe, and this perception encourages the children to relax. Such a setting serves as a reminder that the "education" in physical education is a viable, relevant reality. Progressive acquisition of motor, cognitive, and affective skills are diligently planned for with positive expectancy of their attainment. In addition to the teacher's image, there are many teacher tasks that facilitate the development of a positive learning environment (PLE). Children feel more a part of the class when the teacher calls them by name. It is also important for the children to know the names of their peers. Therefore, systems that permit the rapid learning of names must be explored by the teacher. The authors suggest the following:

1. Study the class rolls prior to the first class day. Surnames of former students may be recognized. The wise teacher, however, will refrain from referring to former students as this may be perceived by them as the initial step of a long line of comparisons.
2. Arrange the class in alphabetical squad lines (an even number of squads if possible) prior to the first class meeting. Squad lines should be no longer than six students.
3. On the first day of class, call the roll and make notations beside the names that will help recall faces later. The entire class can become actively involved in this process by having the class say each student's name after the teacher calls it.
4. Play at least one name game on the first day (for example, "Back to Back Tag" with partners having to introduce one another to the entire group).
5. Each evening for the first week go over all squad lists and try to recall faces (now you know the importance of the notations suggested in item 3).
6. Each day have available on an index card a small number of names and diligently try to learn them before the end of the class period.

Perhaps the reader is thinking, "Why spend so much time learning each child's name—I'll know them all by the end of the year." Each of us has a name that signifies *me*. No one likes to be known as "Hey, you" for two to three months. If students perceive that the teacher is making an effort to learn their names, they will help speed up the process. Most teachers also find that students who misbehave find a certain security in anonymity. Thus when children hear their name called they feel more responsible for their behavior.

Teachers who value both their students and the content of what they teach begin each class promptly and with enthusiasm. Remember, even though this may be repetition number six for the teacher, students are experiencing the lesson for the very first time. The teacher's task is to get the children attracted to what has been planned so they will diligently pursue the stated goals of the lesson!

A signal for immediate attention and cessation of activity is important for many reasons, the two most important being safety and efficiency. The stop signal (for example, short blast of the whistle) should be well-known by the students and the accompanying expected behavior should be practiced. Any number of games (for instance, Freeze Tag variation) can be used to help the students learn to listen while moving and to "stop-freeze" on the appropriate stop signal.

BEHAVIOR EXPECTATIONS FOR STUDENTS
IN THE GYMNASIUM

Students should always know what is expected of them, and they should be reasonably sure that these expectations will be assessed within a reasonable amount of time. The students should also perceive the expectations as fair, and that everyone is expected to meet the standards set forth by the teacher. This is not to say that all children will progress at the same rate; however, individualization was never meant to give license to behaviors less than that which the student is determined capable of giving.

Perhaps one of the most difficult decisions a teacher must make is giving priority to student behaviors. It is neither practical nor desirable to react to each and every student behavior whether it is positive or negative. As a general rule, it is best to respond positively to desirable behaviors and to ignore undesirable behaviors. Naturally, there are those undesirable behaviors that require immediate corrective response on the part of the teacher—especially when the inappropriate behavior creates a safety hazard (physical or emotional). Other behavior expectations (no gum chewing, respect for others and equipment, and so forth) should be explained to the students, who should also receive appropriate opportunities for the practice of these behaviors. All rules, rewards, and consequences for misbehavior should be posted. Teachers who relate the consequences in a firm, consistent manner will help students realize that the rules are for their own safety as well as the safety of their fellow classmates. Table 7-1 lists examples of items relating to behavior that may be included on a poster. Items will vary according to school system expectations, teacher philosophies, and maturity of the students.

It is fitting at this time to discuss behavior expectations for minority and handicapped students. The first rule of thumb is to consider all the children as worthy human beings capable of learning (although not always at the same pace). Teachers should help children to understand the many similarities all humans have in common with one another rather than to emphasize differences. Differences can be explained as they occur in overall growth and development of all children (that is, differences in height and weight, hair and eye color). The authors encourage the beginning teacher to realize that children bring to school more than their bodies and lunch pails. Differences in lifestyles and cultural background cannot and should not be ignored. Neither should they be emphasized nor used as an excuse by teachers or students to explain away a lowered expectation of children coming from a different cultural or racial background. Teachers need to make an effort to understand how the children's backgrounds relate to the children's needs and to use that knowledge to guide youngsters to higher achievement. Teachers most clearly demonstrate respect for all people when they facilitate the learning of all students; this positive action helps each student to progress toward becoming fully the person he or she was created to be.

Table 7-1 Grades 1-6

RULES	REWARDS	MISBEHAVIOR CONSEQUENCES
Follow directions Freeze on signal Respect others Take care of equipment No gum chewing Proper footwear required	Class with no marks for 4 days gets to choose fitness activity for Friday Class with no more than 2 marks for 9 consecutive days gets to choose fitness activity for Friday Class with no more than 3 marks for 14 consecutive days gets to choose fitness activity for Friday	1st mark—time out 2nd mark—phone call to parents 3rd mark—loss of play for one entire class period 4th mark—removal from PE—sent to principal

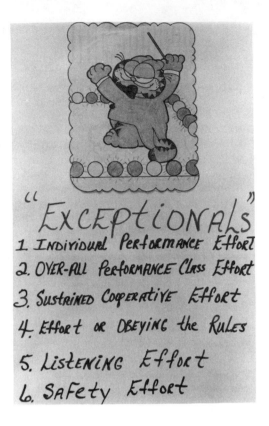

"EXCEPTIONALS"
1. INDIVIDUAL PERFORMANCE Effort
2. OVER-ALL PERFORMANCE Class Effort
3. Sustained Cooperative Effort
4. Effort or Obeying the Rules
5. Listening Effort
6. Safety Effort

Figure 7–1 Behavior expectations.

POSITIVE ATTITUDE DEVELOPMENT

Teachers have excellent opportunities to facilitate the development of positive attitudes within their students. Oftentimes adults take a child's good behavior for granted and find themselves responding to negative behaviors and ignoring appropriate behaviors. Teachers can reinforce, on a daily basis, positive development through the creative use of positive feedback (Fig. 7–1). The attitude of respect for one another (use of self-space principle can be very effective in this regard) and for equipment (for example, when two or four children carry a tumbling mat, "it" does not get a "floor burn" from being dragged!) must be taught, reinforced, and frequently retaught. An attitude of respect for authority will be fostered if the teacher is liked and respected by the students. Attitudes of cooperative play and honorable competition can be fostered through well-chosen games and good officiating. The responsible attitude of safety can be fostered as the children realize they too are responsible for the safety of their play environment.

COMMUNICATION SKILLS

Effective teachers must be able to communicate to the learner the essential information needed. A common mistake of beginning teachers is to present more information than is needed for the initial learning to begin. The following guidelines have been found to be effective by successful teachers when they present a lesson:

1. Students seem to become more involved with the learning process when they are interested in the content.
2. Teacher enthusiasm helps to generate student interest in lesson content.

3. Body language and facial expressions must be congruent with what the teacher is expressing verbally.

4. A detailed lesson plan promotes a more orderly presentation of the lesson.

5. Beginning teachers especially should include on the lesson plan the key points for each skill that is being taught.

6. The class atmosphere should be friendly, but the students should also note a seriousness about the expected accomplishment of the lesson.

7. Objectives for the lesson should be communicated to the students at the beginning of the lesson. This can be accomplished either verbally (for example, "Every time you dribble the ball today, let's see if you can strike the ball at least six times without looking at it") or in writing (chalkboard or posters).

8. The students' attention must be obtained prior to teaching the lesson.

9. If a demonstration is needed, the teacher should allow the students to see the skill from at least two different views (for example, side view and front view).

10. Whenever possible, the skill should be demonstrated simultaneously as the key points are presented. The students also need to see the skill demonstrated both in slow speed and operational speed.

11. Eye contact with as many of the students as possible will help the teacher hold their attention, as will using their names during the instructions.

12. Word pictures help to clarify (for example, "Can you finish off your forward roll in good form, stretched tall as if you are an Olympian?").

13. Questioning techniques can help the teacher evaluate how the students are receiving the direction (for instance, "Mike, what direction are you to rotate when you hear the signal?").

Oftentimes the receiver or the sender will consciously or unconsciously erect *roadblocks* that impede good communication. The following examples show how teacher behaviors can block communication.

Teacher's Messages That Block Communication

1. Threatening
   Blocks: "If you can't keep the ball still during instruction, we simply won't play the game."
   Opens: "Can you hold the ball between your ankles while I give the directions for the game?"

2. Ordering or Commanding
   Blocks: "Keep your mouths shut unless I call on you!"
   Opens: "As I call out the team assignments, I want you to listen carefully so you will know which team you are on."

3. Judging or Criticizing
   Blocks: "John, you are always the main troublemaker."
   Opens: "John, what is the task you are to complete while at this station?"

4. Stereotyping
   Blocks: "Ben, you are as big a talker as your sister was."
   Opens: "After I give the rules for playing the game, I will ask one of you to repeat them to the class."

5. Cross-Examining
   Blocks: "Where was your mind when I explained how we would put away the equipment? Were you talking to your neighbor?"
   Opens: "Kim, I would like for you to tell me the procedure for putting the jump ropes away."

6. Teacher Apathy
   Blocks: "I don't have anything planned for today so why don't we just shoot baskets."
   Opens: "Oh boy, are we going to have fun today. I have a new game for you. It's called flickerball."

MANAGERIAL SKILLS

The effective teacher must be a skilled manager of time. There are many factors to consider such as management of equipment, grouping of students, use of space, and so forth. Research tells us that the smoothness of transitions between phases of the lesson and between activities is of utmost importance to the level of success of the lesson. The *momentum* or *flow* of the lesson is closely related to the transitions because when these factors are efficiently managed the students are provided a maximum amount of quality learning (practice) time. The following managerial techniques have been used by teachers who are considered to be effective managers:

1. Develop lesson plans that include such information as predicted time for each phase of the lesson, kind and amount of equipment, objectives clearly stated.
2. Begin class at a definite time with an established routine.
3. Use task cards (individual or at stations) to impart instructions to the students.
4. Post (usually in a central area) as much class information (team assignments, rotation, procedures, class rules) as is appropriate for the maturity level of the students. Encourage students always to check their "message" center. Issue positive reinforcement to those who look for information upon entering the gym ("Kathy, I was pleased to see you reading the new poster. Can you tell the class what it says?").
5. Shape good self-management skills in the children by frequently reinforcing those who demonstrate good "hustling," cooperation, initiative, and other positive self-management behaviors.
6. Always have the necessary equipment ready before class begins.
7. Teach time-saving routines for equipment issue and retrieval, for reporting scores, for taking skills tests.
8. A specified method for students to secure equipment when additional instruction is needed will eliminate the need for the teacher to demand repeatedly, "Hold the balls, hold the balls!" Students may place the equipment between their feet, or hold equipment overhead, to prevent the distraction of bouncing balls during instruction.

Secured equipment is less of a distraction during instruction.

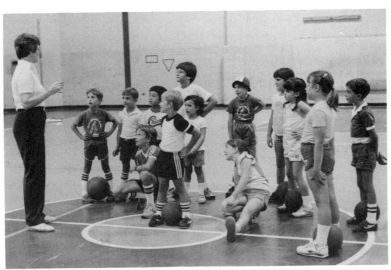

9. Use frequent positive and corrective feedback interactions that have both informative and value content (for example, "Nice work, class, it only took 20 seconds to put the jump ropes back on the hook [information]—now we have time to play with the parachute" [value]). A reasonable goal for a beginning teacher to strive for is two feedback incidents per minute with twice as many positive as corrective interactions. With experience, the feedback frequency should quickly move to three or four incidents per minute.

10. Emphasize the importance of time by challenging classes to complete management-type tasks (organizing groups, handling equipment, and so forth) quickly. Low-keyed competition can also be effective. Classes can compete against each other or against their previous scores.

11. Maintain low percentages of management time (transitions between activities, waiting in line, other).

12. Demonstrate energy, enthusiasm, and "hustle" behavior as you teach the class. This will stimulate the students to become more involved with both the content and the process of the lesson, and therefore remain on task for longer periods of time.

DISRUPTIVE TEACHER BEHAVIORS

Students are not the only initiators of disruption of the learning process. Certain teacher behaviors also contribute to disruption and confusion within the learning environment. Jacob Kounin (1970) provides us with valuable insight into the effect of certain disruptive teacher behaviors upon the momentum of a lesson. Kounin reminds us that *smooth transitions* and *appropriate momentum* are the most important management skills for promotion of work involvement and class control. What follows is a summary of the key points of Kounin's research findings regarding the effect of teaching behaviors on the flow and momentum of a lesson.

"Jerky" transitions are caused by teacher "thrusts," which occur when a teacher suddenly interrupts an activity in progress without regard to the effect of the flow of the lesson. This interrupts the concentration of the students. For example, a group of students playing a game are told abruptly to stop the activity and join another group involved in another activity. It would be more effective to tell the students they had one minute to finish the game. Another cause of jerky transitions can be caused by a teacher behavior that Kounin calls "dangles"—interrupting an activity in progress to initiate a second activity. Later, the teacher may return ("flip-flop") to the first activity (for example, a class working with lummi sticks is stopped while the teacher takes a lunch count [dangle], then lummi activity is resumed ["flip-flop"]). The lunch count should be handled before or after the activity. Obviously, jerky transitions are not desirable teacher behaviors because of the accompanying confusion that encourages student misbehaviors.

Teachers can also interrupt the flow of a lesson if they waste time between activities. The teaching behaviors of "overdwelling" or "fragmentation" are frequent teacher disrupters. Teachers who talk too long experience difficulty in holding the attention of the children. Too much information is boring to children and often a waste of time. A better procedure is to give the bare essentials of directions and proceed with the activity. The teacher can give additional information as it is needed by the students. Overdwelling on misbehavior will be perceived by children as nagging and will be detrimental to the overall learning environment. Fragmentation occurs when group tasks are broken down into too many small steps ("Line up, and one by one, put your rope on the hook, then return to your squad line." After everyone has completed that task—"Now go get a playground ball—one at a time—and come back to your squad line and sit down"—"hold the ball, hold the balls," and so on). A more efficient procedure is to say to a class, "On the signal, take your jump rope to one of the hooks and hang it evenly, then get a playground ball and see how many times you can toss it to yourself and catch it while walking back to your self-space—for every time the ball touches the floor take away one catch."

As the reader can see, the flow of a lesson can be negatively influenced by both student and teacher behaviors. Awareness of the problem is the first step toward eliminating disrupters in the learning process. Videotapes and tape recordings will help teachers determine the frequency of disruptive behaviors.

POSITIVE TEACHER BEHAVIORS

The single most important teacher behavior that teachers want to develop is identified by Kounin as "withitness" (as in "eyes in the back of the head"). Students perceive such a teacher as an alert teacher who is capable of accurately reading the situation (for example, when a discipline problem arises the teacher sees it early and is able to identify the instigators and stop the incident before it grows into a larger problem). In the gymnasium, the teacher must maintain a good position and frequently scan the entire class if this important teacher behavior is to be demonstrated. This means the teacher should move about the periphery of the class rather than maintain a static position in the center.

Discipline Strategies

As mentioned earlier, it is not the intent of this chapter to explore all of the available disciplinary philosophies. Thus, the message contained in the following guidelines for developing discipline strategies is simply that, regardless of the problem a child might have, no student should be allowed to engage in behavior that can cause injury to self or that violates the rights of peers or the teacher.

Guidelines for developing discipline strategies include:

1. List the areas of misbehavior you may encounter (inattentiveness, poor self-control, lack of persistence, off-task, disrespect for others, inappropriate use of equipment).
2. Know what behaviors (by degrees) you will tolerate and what behaviors you will desist; have predetermined methods for discouraging the inappropriate (unwanted) behaviors.
3. Keep class rules short and simple (four to six should suffice).
4. Post rules, rewards, and consequences.
5. Explain rules, rewards, and consequences to students, parents, administrators.
6. Explain students' rights and teacher's rights.
7. Nip misbehaviors in the bud before they become serious.
8. Call the student by name when correcting misbehavior.
9. Be a role model for your students (act and speak in the same manner as you expect them to act).
10. Focus your remarks on the child's behavior rather than on the child ("Tom, what are you supposed to be doing at this station?" rather than, "Tom, why are you not participating?").
11. Be very aware of what is going on in your class areas and let the students know how aware you are by timely responses to both appropriate and inappropriate behaviors.
12. As a goal, strive to correct the child fairly and help guide the child toward self-management.
13. Interact with students on a personal level.

14. Refrain from embarrassing the child. Whenever possible, help with individual difficulties in a manner that does not cause undue attention.

15. Stress choosing good behavior rather than avoiding bad behavior. Help students (with prompts, cues) learn to choose good behavior.

16. For the most part, misbehaviors represent an individual action; hence correction must be directed toward individuals. Group punishment, unless the entire group is at fault, is not regarded as a fair disciplinary technique.

17. Appropriate corrections directed at one individual but heard by several on the periphery will often prevent others from attempting the same misbehavior. This is known as the "ripple effect" (Kounin, 1970).

18. Consistently follow-through with positive and negative feedback.

19. Strive to maintain an appropriate momentum where students are stimulated to remain on task.

20. Choose methods for reinforcement, corrective feedback, and punishment that are developmentally appropriate.

21. Keep expected behaviors posted and call this to students' attention frequently.

22. Teachers, parents, and administrators who work together have higher ratios of success with correcting discipline problems. The teacher is the logical person within this triad to initiate such cooperative behavior.

23. Be firm, consistent, fair, and friendly.

Specific Discipline Strategies

Time-Out

The *time-out* disciplinary technique is used when a disruptive child needs to be temporarily removed from the ongoing activity of the class. To initiate the process the teacher (without anger) removes the child who is not abiding by the stated class rules by saying, "David, you have repeatedly used the equipment in a dangerous way; go to the time-out area and think about the class safety rules, especially the rules for the horizontal ladder. When you think you can obey the rules you may come to me, but the minute hand on the clock [if one is visible] must make

Removal from the activity (time-out) can be an effective disciplining strategy.

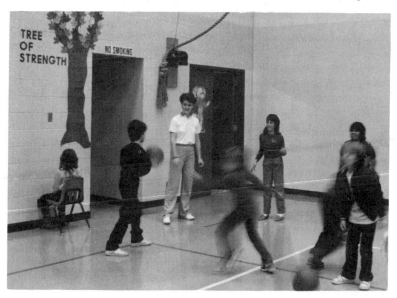

one complete circle." The child may even be told to go and read the safety rules posted on the wall of the gym.

The location of the time-out area (chair, bench, floor) should be on the periphery of the class and in full view of the teacher. The child should have to face away from the class. When the child approaches the teacher at no sooner than one minute later, he or she must state a willingness to obey the rules and what it is that must not occur again ("Teacher, from now on I will obey the safety rules and will not try to shake Joe off the ladder"). This will indicate to the teacher that Tommy did in fact know what he was doing wrong. If a child is sent to the time-out area a second time during the same class period he or she must remain there the rest of the period. Children who can write may be told to copy the safety rule(s) while at the time-out area. Most young children have not developed an aversion to play activity; however, if it becomes apparent that a child is trying to avoid the activity then the time-out technique is obviously not going to be the most appropriate disciplinary technique to use.

Behavior Games

As the name implies, *behavior games*—a disciplinary strategy described by Siedentop (1983)—uses a game format in which the specific goal is the learning of a specific class behavior. The game is played intermittently during the regular lesson for the day. Behavior games are introduced only if the behavior of a class is especially deviant (for example, many of the students are not paying attention to the stop signal, which is supposed to elicit very specific behavior: immediate cessation of activity; control of equipment; look at and listen to the teacher). Specific standards for the class are established, and everyone in the class can earn the rewards. The teacher's goal is for everyone to progress to the point that the desired behavior is demonstrated regularly, therefore signaling that the game is no longer needed. The following is an example of a behavior game suitable for Levels II and III.

CURRENT (UNDESIRABLE) BEHAVIOR:

When the signal sounds, most of the children continue to play, use the equipment and talk to one another.

DESIRED BEHAVIOR:

When signal sounds, the children will stop, be quiet, put equipment down, and listen to the teacher.

GAME STRUCTURE:

1. Entire class plays, all can win.
2. Class is divided into four to six squads; children choose squad names and mascot (optional).
3. Reward will be choice of fitness activities on Friday.
4. Game will be played until 90 percent of students in the class are demonstrating desired behaviors.
5. Game can be played during any lesson being taught. In other words, the game is ongoing.

GAME PROCEDURE

(The following is one example of how a behavioral game might be played.)

1. A timer (out of sight of the children) will be set to go off at a time determined by the teacher.
2. When the timer sounds, all of the children must stop, place equipment on the floor, quickly move to the designated area for their squad, face the teacher, place hands on hips, and not talk. This is to be done within 10 seconds.
3. The teacher will determine quickly which squads are successful and record this on a worksheet.
4. The teacher gives the signal to resume the day's lesson and then resets the timer.
5. Initially, the buzzer should sound four or five times during a 30-minute period. Each behavioral game incident should take no more than one minute (maximum) of time away from the lesson.
6. At the end of the period, the teacher will total the yards (10-yards for each win) for each squad and move the squad marker accordingly on the poster of a football field (this is just an example of one way to record progress in the game).
7. The object is to score a touchdown.
8. Each touchdown will qualify for 10 minutes of "choice of activity" on Friday.
9. The teacher should state that the normal stopping signal (voice, whistle, other) can also signal the beginning of the behavioral game.
10. If one or two students persist in preventing their squad from winning, the teacher should encourage that squad to help their squad members react more quickly. When mainstreamed children are involved, the teacher must determine what level of conformity can be expected from the mainstreamed child.
11. The game should reward positive behaviors but not punish inappropriate behaviors (unless it becomes absolutely necessary; at which time yards can be deducted).

Teacher-Student Conferences

The relationship between teacher and students is most critical to the overall success of the learning environment. Teachers must be viewed by each individual child to be fair, friendly, firm, and consistent. Children normally want to please

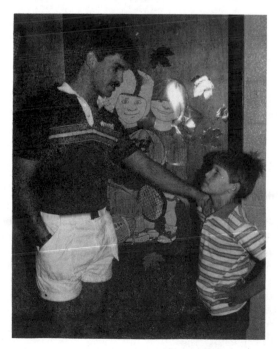

Eye contact is critical when disciplining a student.

adults. This desire to please will usually be prompted either because they are afraid of angering the adult or because they are attracted to the adult. Of course, teachers would much prefer that children obey because they are happy, feel safe, and enjoy what they are learning. When a child does not follow the rules or procedures of the class, the teacher should first look to oneself for the reason. Teachers should ask themselves, "What am I doing or not doing that is causing this child to act this way?" Negative teacher behaviors such as not paying attention to all of the students, giving unclear directions, not being heard, planning inappropriate activities, high frequencies of management time and negative interactions, and low frequencies of positive interactions can adversely affect the behaviors of individual students or even an entire class.

Once the above question has been answered, then it is appropriate for the teacher to consider what deficits the student may be working with (poor hearing or sight, poor nutrition, lack of rest, perceptual motor problems, emotional problems, lack of acceptance by peers, home problems). These questions can only be answered by the teacher making the effort to get to know the student. This can best be accomplished by obtaining data from several sources: the child, permanent records, school counselor, nurse, and other teachers. Sometimes all it takes is for the child to realize that the teacher is interested in him or her as a person and to understand that the teacher's goal is to help the child improve fitness and motor skills and thereby be able to enjoy physical activity.

When a teacher confers with a child privately, several things must occur. First of all, the child must not feel threatened by the thought of a "talk with the teacher." Simply say to the child, "Karen, I'd like to talk to you today after your lunch. I was thinking about asking Miss Jones if you could come to the physical education office when you have finished eating. Would that be okay with you?" This is said in a friendly, nonthreatening manner.

When the child and teacher begin the conference, the teacher should be honest about the reason for the meeting by saying, "Karen, you don't seem to be having much fun when you are in your physical education class. Do you suppose we could talk about this? I really want you to enjoy being in class and participating in the activities, and if there is anything I can do to help you I would like for you to tell me." Then the teacher must be quiet so that the child can ventilate personal feelings about what has been happening.

Occasionally, in the course of the conversation, the wise teacher will ask, "Is there anything I am doing in class that bothers you?" Most likely, the opportunity to "lecture" will arise. This is not the appropriate time to lecture on class rules, behavior, and so forth, and the teacher who succumbs to this natural urge will only destroy the positive interactions that may otherwise occur. Lecturing is merely another act of teacher power and will only serve to destroy communication links between student and teacher.

Teacher-Parent Conferences

Most parents want to help their children to be successful in school, and certainly all parents have the right to know of their child's successes and failures. Just as academic reports of progress are given to parents, so too should behavior reports be issued. At the kindergarten and first-grade level most children respond very well to teacher intervention of their misbehaviors. By the second grade, however, some students have begun to test authority figures and therefore require more sophisticated disciplinary strategies. Children who chronically misbehave are asking for something they need but are not receiving. Oftentimes the child cannot even label what it is that is needed.

The authors believe that parents should be apprised early when misbehavior becomes frequent. Of course, the first step is for the teacher and the child to try to work things out by using some or all of the strategies mentioned earlier. Without a doubt the least effective method for dealing with misbehavior is to send the child to the principal. If the teacher and student reach an impasse then the parents should be called and a parent-teacher visit arranged. During this visit the teacher's job is to communicate concern for the child's apparent unhappiness and state specific incidents where the child has demonstrated inappropriately aggressive behaviors toward self or others. Sometimes rather than aggressive behaviors the child will habitually withdraw from the activity or from the other children. This too is unhealthy and must be addressed. Once the parent believes in the teacher's sincerity then real progress can be made as both teacher and parents strive cooperatively for a better understanding of the child's needs and plan realistically for these needs to be met in developmentally appropriate ways. Whatever reinforcement and corrective strategies are decided upon they should be reinforced both at home and at school. It is important that parents and teacher continue to communicate with one another about the progress that the child demonstrates. The child, knowing that both home and school are working together, should experience the new expectations positively and respond by learning the more appropriate behaviors. This is not to say that correcting behavior is uncomplicated and that change will be rapid and painless. However, a "united front" (if it is realistic, accepting, and fair) is more likely to bring about the desired results.

Some Thoughts On Punishment

Punishment is a contingency brought about by severe, chronic misbehavior. Most children will respond very positively to the disciplinary strategies that we have discussed (time-out, behavior games, teacher-student conferences, and teacher-parent conferences). However, when punishment seems to be inevitable, the authors strongly encourage consideration of the following guidelines:

1. Treat each child with respect and dignity.
2. Refrain from using physical exercise (for example, calisthenics and running) as punishment.
3. If punishment is deemed necessary it must be administered objectively, quickly, and fairly.
4. Once the punishment is completed, the slate is cleared.
5. Refrain from group punishment.

REFERENCES

KOUNIN, J. (1970). *Discipline and group management in classrooms*, New York: Holt, Rinehart & Winston.

SIEDENTOP, D. (1983). *Developing teaching skills in physical education*, Palo Alto, CA: Mayfield.

SUGGESTED READINGS

CHARLES, C. M. (1981). *Building classroom discipline*. New York: Longman.

CORRINGTON, M. V. (1976). *Self-worth and school learning*. New York: Holt, Rinehart & Winston.

CRUICKSHANK, D. R. (1980). *Teaching is tough*. Englewood Cliffs, NJ: Prentice-Hall.

ERNST, K. (1972). *Games students play*. Millbrae, CA: Celestial Arts.

FOSTER, H. L. (1974). *Ribbin', jivin' and playin' the dozens*. Cambridge, MA: Ballinger.

GOOD, T. L. & BROPHY, J. E. (1978). *Looking in classrooms*. New York: Harper & Row.

GREENBERG, H. (1969). *Teaching with feeling*. Indianapolis: Bobbs-Merrill.

HELLISON, D. (1978). *Beyond balls and bats*. Washington, DC: American Alliance for Health and Physical Education, Recreation and Dance.

HOLT, J. (1974). *How children fail*. New York: Dell.

HOLT, J. (1975). *Freedom and beyond*. New York: Dell.

JERSILD, A. T. (1968). *When teachers face themselves*. New York: Teachers College Press.

LONG, J. D. & FRYE, V. H. (1981). *Making it till Friday*. Princeton, NJ: Princeton Book Co.

WOLFGANG, C. H. & GLICKMAN, C. D. (1980). *Solving discipline problems*. Boston: Allyn & Bacon.

8

EVALUATION

By definition, the process of education implies that a change, a modification, or an adjustment of behavior will occur as a result of experience. Changes occur in both student and teacher behaviors. These changes may be minor adjustments in a daily lesson for the teacher, or advancements in skill learning for the student as a result of experiences in the learning environment. Change is a constant in education, and evaluation of changes no matter how small must also be constant. Learning to observe and assess children in activity will enable the teacher (and the student) to locate strengths and weaknesses and make the necessary adjustments toward attaining the established goals of physical education.

This chapter is designed to provide teachers with techniques for evaluating both students and themselves. The first part is devoted to student evaluation, and the second to teacher evaluation. Both are equally important to the success of any program.

OBSERVATION

Observation of change is the first step in the evaluation process. The teacher and student gain important information about progress toward stated goals through skillful observation.

There are several different types of observation that may occur in the physical education environment from a general observation of health habits (grooming, posture, and so forth) or social interactions, to more specific observations of skill performance. From the moment a class arrives, the teacher may begin evaluating the students' health, fitness level, motor skills, attitudes, social, emotional, and cognitive development, all of which are based on observation. Students also gain important information about their performance by observing demonstrations or other students in action. Sometimes both teacher and student will be looking for the same change in behavior. Regardless of who or what is being assessed, the

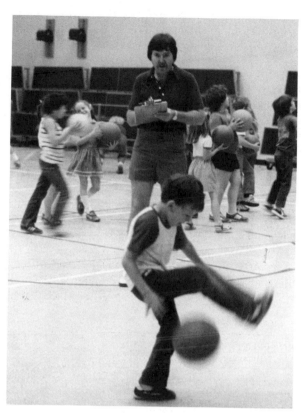

Teachers who make notes about student progress are more effective.

keen observer must know specifically what to expect and only then can it be determined whether or not the movement, social interaction, or knowledge was achieved. For example, if the focus of the lesson is on running, observation of (and focus on) specific movement behaviors, such as the action of the arms, legs, torso, speed, and distance covered, may be used in the assessment process. In order to be accurate in evaluating the child's running form, the teacher should choose only one or two factors to note at each observation until a total picture is drawn. Likewise, the students should be taught to focus on only one or two factors at a time when observing a demonstration.

The key to good observation is pinpointing ahead of time specifically what is to be noticed about the child's movement or behavior.

Student Evaluation

Frequently, the physical education teacher is expected to evaluate the student's physical, motor, social, emotional, and cognitive growth, and to keep records and report on student development. This is a monumental task requiring a great deal of discipline and organization on the part of the teacher. The following section on student evaluation outlines techniques for evaluating and assessing student progress in the above areas.

Health

General health appraisal is a daily responsibility. The teacher looks for signs of illness, neglect, abuse, or emotional strain by scanning the class at the beginning of the period. *Scanning*, as an observation technique, should be done by looking from left to right at the class, noting unusual skin color or markings (such as bruises), unkempt appearances, body odors, unusually fatigued or extremely fidgety children. These children may have problems that will greatly affect their performance and growth.

Should the teacher notice anything unusual about a child's appearance that would indicate possible child abuse or neglect, the proper school authority (usually the principal) should be notified immediately.

Assessment of the child's physical growth and functioning is generally a combined effort with the school nurse. A yearly assessment of height, weight, vision, hearing, and posture should be made. A record of growth is kept either in the nurse's office or frequently with the fitness record, which is the physical education teacher's responsibility (see Chapter 4, "Physical Fitness").

Perceptual Motor Skills

Several good tests exist that may be used to assess the child' perceptual development. Table 8–1 lists selected assessment tools.

When choosing a standardized test the teacher must consider the time available for testing and the ease with which the test can be administered. The teacher may want to screen the students first for potential problems then administer the test only to those children who exhibit obvious weaknesses. The teacher can select

Table 8-1   Summary of Selected Assessment Tools

TITLE	AGE RANGE (YRS.)	ITEMS	COMMENTS
Purdue Perceptual-Motor Survey Charles E. Merrill Publishing Co. 1300 Alum Creek Dr. Columbus, Ohio 43216	6 to 10	balance, posture, body perceptual-motor match, ocular control, form perception	an instrument that allows the examiner to observe a series of psychomotor behaviors and to identify areas that may need attention
Bruininks-Oseretsky Test of Motor Proficiency American Guidance Service Circle Pines, Minnesota 55014	4½ to 14½	gross motor, gross and fine motor and fine motor skills (eight subtests; short form available)	a valid test of motor proficiency as measured by the performance of a child on a given day
Basic Motor Ability Test-Revised In D. Arnheim & A. Sinclair, *The Clumsy Child*, St. Louis: C. V. Mosby	4–12	eleven tests designed to evaluate small- and large-muscle control, static and dynamic balance, eye-hand coordination, flexibility	while validity has not been reported, test-retest reliability was found to be .93. The norming sample was 1,563 children; expressed in percentiles
The Fundamental Movement Pattern Assessment Instrument In B. McClenaghen & D. Gallahue, *Fundamental Movement: A developmental and remedial approach.* Philadelphia: W. B. Saunders.	across ages	five fundamental skills; throwing, catching, kicking, running and jumping	used to classify skill level performance into initial, elementary or mature stage of development changes over time

a simple activity for each of the perceptual-motor areas and scan the class, noting children who are having obvious difficulty with the task. For example, to assess balance, students may be asked to stand on one foot for five seconds; the teacher notes in the scan which students are hopping around unable to maintain a balanced position. To assess directional awareness, students may be asked to place beanbags in different positions in relation to themselves and others. Difficulty in placing to the front, back, side, over, under, or between can be noted as a weakness. A copy of the Dayton Sensory Motor Awareness Survey for Four- and Five-Year-Olds is provided as a simple and easy-to-administer screening device (see Table 8–2). Children with obvious problems should be singled out for further testing and remedial work.

In order to evaluate by means of scanning technique, the teacher must know the students' names. For some this is a monumental task, and teachers often neglect to make an effort. The following technique, which has been used successfully, serves the dual purpose of providing a record of observations and a vehicle for learning children's names.

First, organize the class into squads, rows, circles, or any formation that can be organized quickly. Each child must be assigned a spot within that formation which they take each time the teacher calls for the formation. This may be done alphabetically, by size, or any way the teacher wishes. The teacher then makes a checklist containing each child's name in the spot occupied. While scanning, the teacher glances at this sheet and circles the name of the child who is either having difficulty or who has completed the task assigned. This type of checklist is excellent for screening fundamental-skill performance, especially among large groups.

Fundamental Motor Skills

The assessment of locomotor, nonlocomotor, and manipulative skills should be both objective and subjective. The teacher is concerned with performance outcomes such as the ability to toss and catch a ball consecutively (product-oriented), as well as the form with which the skill is executed (process-oriented); therefore, two different types of evaluation are appropriate.

Objective Evaluation.   The *objective* evaluation of a skill is generally thought of as a "skill test." Because there are no standardized tests for fundamental skills, they must often be devised by the teacher. When devising a skill test the following guidelines should be observed:

1. The test should be designed to measure only one skill.
2. The test should be inexpensive and easy to administer, with time and space factors always considered.
3. The test should accurately reflect the skill it intends to measure. A running test, for example, should reflect the factors of speed and distance.
4. The test should discriminate between high and low levels of skill development. If all children score within two points of each other, for example, it would indicate that the test was either too hard or too easy and the teacher should adjust accordingly (Kirchner, 1985).
5. Scores obtained can be standardized and added to other test battery scores to obtain a total score. A total score can be used to form individual and class profiles, which will in turn enable norms to be established for school or district populations. For example, it may be desirable to group tests in locomotor skills into one test battery; likewise nonlocomotor and manipulative skills for comparison purposes.

Table 8-2   Dayton Sensory Motor Awareness Survey for Four- and Five-Year-Olds

DATE OF TEST _____

NAME _____ SEX _____ BIRTH _____ CENTER _____

Body Image. One-half point for each correct part; nine points possible.

_____ 1. Ask the child to touch the following body parts:

Head _____	Ankles _____	Ears _____	Stomach _____	Elbows _____
Toes _____	Nose _____	Legs _____	Chin _____	Back _____
Eyes _____	Feet _____	Mouth _____	Waist _____	
Wrists _____	Chest _____	Fingers _____	Shoulders _____	

Space and Directions. One-half point for each correct direction; five points possible.

_____ 2. Ask the child to point to the following directions:

Front _____ Back _____ Up _____ Down _____ Beside you _____

Place two blocks on a table about 1 inch apart. Ask the child to point:

Under _____ Over _____ To the top _____ To the bottom _____ Between _____

Balance. Score two points if accomplished.

_____ 3. Have the child stand on tiptoes, on both feet, with eyes open for 8 seconds.

Balance and Laterality. Score two points for each foot; four points possible.

_____ 4. Have the child stand on one foot, eyes closed, for 5 seconds. Alternate feet.

Laterality. Score two points if the child keeps his feet together and does not lead off with one foot.

_____ 5. Have the child jump forward on two feet.

Rhythm and Neuromuscular Control. Score two points for each foot if accomplished six times; four points possible.

_____ 6. Have the child hop on one foot. Hop in place.

Rhythm and neuromuscular Control. Score two points

_____ 7. Have the child skip forward. Child must be able to sustain this motion around the room for approximately 30 feet.

Integration of Right and Left Sides of the Body. Score two points if cross-patterning is evident for each.

_____ 8. Have the child creep forward.

_____ 9. Have the child creep backwards.

Eye-Foot Coordination. Score two points if done the length of tape or mark.

_____ 10. Use an 8 foot tape or chalk mark on the floor. The child walks in a crossover step the length of the tape or mark.

Fine Muscle Control. Score two points if paper is completely crumpled. Score one point if paper is partially crumpled.

Score zero points if child needs assistance or changes hands.

_____ 11. Using a half sheet of newspaper, the child picks up the paper with one hand and puts the other hand behind his back. He then attempts to crumple the paper in his hand. He may not use his other hand, the table, or his body for assistance.

Form Perception. Score one point for each correct match.

_____ 12. Using a piece of paper with 2 inch circles, squares, and triangles, ask the child to point to two objects that are the same.

Form Perception. Score one point if circle is identified correctly. Score two points if the triangle and square are identified correctly.

_____ 13. Ask the child to identify by saying, "Point to the circle." "Point to the square." "Point to the triangle."

Hearing Discrimination. Score one point if the child taps correctly each time.

_____ 14. Ask the child to turn his back to you. Tap the table with a stick three times. Ask the child to turn around and tap the sticks the same way. Ask the child to turn his back to you. Tap the table again with the sticks (two quick taps, pause, then two more quick taps). Have the child turn back to you and tap out the rhythm.

Eye-Hand Coordination. Score one point for each successful completion.

_____ 15. A board is used with three holes in it. The holes are ¾, ⅝, and ½ inch in diameter. The child is asked to put his finger through the holes without touching the sides.

By permission of the Dayton, Ohio, Public Schools, W. T. Braley, consultant.

Table 8-3   Skill Task Sheet

NAME: _____

Dodging

		complete	comments
1	Avoid a ball thrown below the waist from 10 ft. 3 out of 5 times		
2	Avoid a ball thrown above the waist from 15 ft. 3 out of 5 times		
3	Escape partner's tag 3 out of 5 tries		
4	Weave through cones in under 20 sec. 3 out of 5 tries		

The use of objective skill testing is more appropriate for Level III students (and above) whose fundamental skills should be ready for refinement. Objective tests may be necessary to point out those students who have not attained a basic level of skill development. The result of objective tests can be recorded on a master sheet, or students may be allowed to self-test and record the results on task sheets.

Task sheets are often more valuable because they can be used to report to parents, and the children are more intimately involved with their own progress when they are responsible for recording their own performances. Task sheets enhance any program and grading system by individualizing learning in an atmosphere of minimum competition. Task sheets are fun to create and can be very diverse (see Table 8-3). The following guidelines will aid you in formulating a task sheet system:

1. Include at least four separate tasks on each task sheet.
2. Several degrees of difficulty should be developed for each skill. This will provide the children with progressive challenges that will help to individualize the program.
3. Each task should have a criterion for completion (say, 3 out of 5 throws).
4. The teacher should hold the sheets until they are complete and then review them to identify children who are having problems.
5. The teacher should record some of the information for future planning before sending the task sheets home.
6. Sufficient time to complete the tasks should be allotted.

Subjective Evaluation.   Periodic evaluation of a child's movement patterns will provide the teacher with important information about the child's skill development, which should be used in planning future lessons. To be effective, the teacher must aid the child in developing from one stage of motor-skill development to another more advanced stage. To do this the teacher must first determine what stage the child has already achieved. Table 8-1 contains selected assessment instruments for this purpose.

Another choice is a skill-development check sheet. A good skill check sheet is a valuable tool. The teacher should list the positive skill points to be observed and then check them off as they are achieved (Table 8-4). To list the skill points, refer to the individual skill chapters (checklist examples provided with many skills) and study the skill descriptions.

Table 8-4 Skill Development Check Sheet

SKILL THEME: DODGING

Name	Lowers center of gravity in preparation to dodge	Changes direction quickly	Regains balance at the completion of dodging maneuver	Uses feinting-type movements

Social Development

The child's *social development* is many-faceted. The teacher needs to evaluate and foster positive attitudes about physical activity, sportsmanship, and authority. Social development also involves group dynamics such as leadership, sharing, and cooperation. The evaluation of the child's social development is primarily a subjective appraisal. Unfortunately, many teachers wait until report card time to evaluate seriously this area of development, and then they assign a satisfactory or unsatisfactory grade to this complex area of development. The teacher must decide what social skills can be realistically expected of the children and should not try to evaluate behavior that has not specifically been taught.

Cognitive Development

The child's *cognitive development* in the primary grades (and intermediate grades) involves the ability to solve problems, understand physical education concepts, laws of motion, and the vocabulary associated with movement. The teacher can best observe these factors by evaluating the child's ability to listen and move appropriately. Written instruments can be devised by the teacher to facilitate communication of the assessment to the child. These must be kept simple; often pictures are very helpful to the child's understanding. The teacher can use task sheets very effectively to evaluate the child's understanding of movement concepts and vocabulary.

Reporting Progress

Student progress reports are generally required by most school systems in the form of grades. In the primary grades a satisfactory/unsatisfactory system is usually employed, and intermediate grades usually require a percentile or A–B–C-type grade. Both of these grading systems are very difficult for the physical educator for a number of reasons:

1. Diversity of skill levels
2. Number of students
3. Actual contact time.

The need for a more descriptive type of evaluation is apparent.

It is suggested that a task-evaluation-sheet system (see discussion of task sheets in this chapter) be utilized for reporting student progress to parents because task sheets can describe achievement in terms of skill performance and depict what was actually achieved. A further benefit of task sheets for reporting purposes is that they can serve as guidelines for parents who wish to help their children improve. Task-evaluation sheets point out specific areas of performance and skill levels that enable the parents to understand specifically the skills and activities performed in the physical education classroom. This type of system also reduces grade competition among children and enhances individualized learning.

Public relations and parents' understanding are basic to an effective and involved elementary program, and task sheets provide a vehicle for providing information about our programs to the public in understandable terms.

If the teacher is bound by the school system to assign a letter or numerical grade, the most important concern is to establish guidelines or criteria ahead of time and communicate to the children, and if possible their parents, what is necessary to achieve each grade.

Teacher Evaluation

Teacher evaluations are often informal and performed by the school administrator. They are generally viewed by the teacher as a negative experience. The informal assessment based on a five-minute visit provides the teacher with little valuable information about teaching effectiveness. In order to increase effectiveness with children, the teacher must receive relevant feedback about teaching performance. The teacher may employ self-evaluative, student-assisted, or peer-assisted techniques to obtain concrete information about the effectiveness of instructions, interactions with students, management skills, practice opportunities, and teacher movement through the learning environment (Graham, Holt/Hale, McEwen, and Parker, 1980).

Instructions

Giving clear and concise instructions to a group of students from varying backgrounds is challenging for even the most experienced teacher. Teachers usually receive immediate feedback about the effectiveness of their instructions as they observe children begin the activity. Confusion about where to go and what to do will generally look like disruptive behavior as the youngsters try to respond to unclear directions. The teacher can obtain immediate feedback about the quality of instructions by asking questions of the children relating to the instructions that have been given. For example, the teacher might ask Betsy, once Betsy has been given instructions, "What will you do after you get your ball?" Betsy's answer will provide the teacher with the information about the quality of instructions before the students even begin the activity.

Tape-Record.   One of the easiest and most informative techniques for evaluating the ability to give instructions clearly is to tape-record verbal instructions as they are given. The teacher can easily wear a portable recorder, which the students will soon become familiar with, so that all verbal exchanges may be recorded during a lesson. The teacher should tape different classes and at the end of each

Table 8-5 Student Questionnaire: Reaction to Teacher/Student Interaction

DIRECTIONS: CIRCLE THE FACE THAT BEST

DESCRIBES YOUR TEACHER.

	😊	😐	☹️
My teacher gives me good directions.			
My teacher will repeat directions if I misunderstand them.			
My teacher gives me a second chance to learn what I need if I don't the first time.			
My teacher calls me by name.			
My teacher talks to me politely.			
My teacher keeps me working the whole class period.			

class make comments about whether or not the class seemed to run smoothly. When analyzing the tape to improve performance, the teacher should ask these questions:

1. Did I repeat myself frequently?
2. Did the students have a lot of questions before they began the activity?
3. Did I have to shout to be heard?
4. Did my verbal directions take longer than necessary?
5. What evidence did I have that the students understood my directions?

Student Questionnaire. Children can provide valuable information about the effectiveness of instructions and other teaching skills by answering a questionnaire such as the one offered in Table 8-5. The results of such a questionnaire must be interpreted in conjunction with other techniques because this type of instrument will only provide the teacher with information about the children's reactions to teaching.

The written instrument must be simple and the required answers concrete. By using faces on the answer sheet and having the teacher read the questions will increase the effectiveness of the instrument for the primary-grade child.

Interactions

The amount and the quality of interactions a teacher has with students greatly influence teaching effectiveness. The teacher should try to interact either verbally or nonverbally with each child in a class during a lesson. Information about the teacher's interaction patterns with the students can be obtained from the tape-recording technique or the student questionnaire. When using the tape-recording technique, the teacher should calculate (1) the percentage of positive, negative, and neutral comments made during a class; and (2) the percentage of children involved in interaction.

Interaction Checklist. An interaction checklist (Table 8–6) can be used to determine interaction patterns between teacher and student during a lesson.

Table 8-6 Interaction Checklist

CHILD'S NAME	TALKED TO	SMILED AT	TOUCHED	TOTAL
Joan	///	/		4
John	/	//		3
Charles	/			1
Carol	//	/		3
Janice		/		1
Bill	7444 7444 ///	///	////	20
Totals	20	8	4	32

An analysis of the checklist data can provide information about:

1. The sex and race of the children who get the most attention in the class;
2. Whether the skilled or unskilled get more attention;
3. Whether an individual or group of children is being ignored.

A colleague who knows the names of all the children in the class can make a tally in the columns of the checklist. This record can also be derived from a videotape, or even a tape recorder for verbal interactions only. The authors recognize the difficulty of this task; however, the effective teacher will utilize whatever means are available to obtain the information necessary for the development of an optimum learning environment. The tally results can be placed on a graph, which will provide a pictorial representation of the data that have been collected (see Table 8–7).

Table 8-7 Interaction Graph

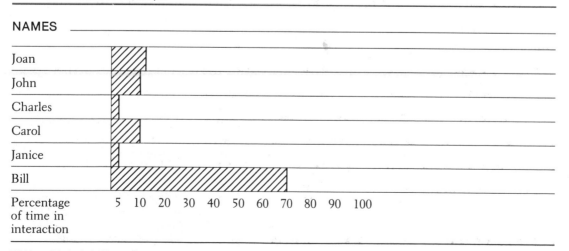

72% = Verbal; 24% = Smiling; 12% = Touching.

Table 8-8 Feedback Checklist

TEACHER _____   DATE _____

OBSERVER _____

THEME _____

	Teacher Feedback			
	Movement Behavior		Social Behavior	
Child's Name	positive	corrective	positive	corrective
George	////		/	
Todd	/	////		卅 //
Susan	卅 卅	/	///	
Ben	卅	/		///
Kristin		////	/	
Total	20	10	5	10

Directions: Mark a slash each time the teacher gives feedback about movement behavior (i.e., "Great catch, John. You really watched the ball all the way"), or social behavior (i.e., "Susan, you put your equipment away very quickly today") occurs. Include both positive and corrective feedback.

Feedback Checklist. A feedback checklist can give the teacher valuable information about the type and quality of the reinforcement provided to the students (see Table 8–8). The teacher should provide feedback about both movement behavior and social behavior.

This type of checklist will be best kept by a colleague enlisted to help the teacher evaluate teaching skills. The colleague chooses several children to observe and codes feedback statements made by the teacher. Using the checklist, positive and negative statements are tallied.

Management Skills

An analysis of management skill utilizes time as a measure of student behavior and involvement. The following techniques involve a time-sampling of behaviors (both teacher and student behaviors) that occur during a lesson, and these techniques will provide the teacher with a better picture of one facet of teaching effectiveness. These instruments can be administered either by a colleague or the teacher can use the tape recorder to gather information during the lesson.

Placheck (Siedentop, 1983). A planned activity check can be conducted to determine the percentage of students involved in meaningful activity during a lesson. The teacher or evaluator scans the class for 10 seconds at five-minute intervals using the left-to-right technique and counts the number of students involved in

either productive or unproductive activity (which is based on the behavioral objectives for the lesson). It is easier to count the number of students in the behavior
category in which the fewest are involved, and then calculate the percentage involved in meaningful movement.

$$\frac{\text{number of students exhibiting productive behavior}}{\text{number of students in class}} \times 100 = \text{percentage of productive behavior}$$

The goal of the teacher should be for 90 percent of the students to be involved
in meaningful activity. Five or more plachecks during a lesson of 30 minutes will
provide the teacher with a good profile of teaching effectiveness.

Duration Recording (Siedentop, 1983). The *duration-recording* system was designed to measure the rate of student participation. It provides the teacher with
indirect feedback about performance. Class time is divided into the categories of
instruction, activity, management, and waiting time. Total times in minutes and
seconds are recorded on a time line for each category. The total minutes and seconds for each category are converted into percentages, which may be compared
to figures from other lessons. A duration-recording system may be either a colleague utilizing the time allotment chart (Table 8–9) or the teacher's analysis of
the recorded lesson. The time line shown in Table 8–9 is divided into 10-second
intervals and the assistant marks with a bar when a change in teacher behavior
has occurred. The duration-recording system may be difficult to use at first, but
with practice it can become an invaluable source of information for the teacher.
The data found in Table 8–9 are derived from the following lesson synopsis.

The second-grade children arrive in the gymnasium where the equipment is
already out and the teacher is ready for them. As soon as the children are seated,
the teacher begins instructions about the fitness activity (30-second instruction)
and students begin activity (5-minute activity). Students gather in center of gym
(20-second management). Teacher explains stations, which are familiar to the students. They number-off and go to stations and begin activity immediately (30-
second management). Each station requires 4 minutes of activity, and 10 seconds
are allotted to change stations (management). The teacher may eliminate the 10
seconds of management time between stations by having children hop to the next
station. Children put equipment down and form a huddle (10-second management). Discussion of the lesson (40 seconds of instruction) follows; children line
up (30-second management).

Practice Opportunities

The more children practice a skill the more likely they are to acquire proficiency in that skill. Therefore, an analysis of teacher effectiveness should include
a calculation of practice opportunities provided by the teacher in the lesson. Recording on a practice opportunities checklist (Table 8–10) can be done by a colleague (Graham and others, 1980). Several children are singled out for observation
and a tally kept of the number of times each child practices a given skill. The
teacher then adds up practice opportunities for each child and utilizes the information to improve the lesson.

Teacher Movement

The teacher who moves well through the learning environment is more likely
to observe and interact with students effectively than one who remains in one

Table 8-9 Time Allotment Chart (Duration Recording)

TEACHER _____   DATE _____

OBSERVER _____   CLASS _____

THEME _____   # OF STUDENTS _____

Time Codes: I = instruction   A = activity
             M = management   W = waiting time

Time Started: _____

I			A		M	I	M

Minutes 1 2 3 4 5 6 7 8 9 10

A	M		A	M	A

11 12 13 14 15 16 17 18 19 20

M	A		M	A	M	I M

21 22 23 24 25 26 27 28 29 30

$$\frac{\text{Activity Time} \quad 1500}{\text{Total Activity Time}} \times 100 = \approx 83 \qquad \text{% Activity}$$
$$\frac{}{\text{Total Lesson Time} \quad 1800} \qquad\qquad\qquad\qquad \text{Time}$$

Activity Time 1500 / Total Activity Time — Total Lesson Time 1800 × 100 = ≈ 83 % Activity Time

Management Time 130 / Total Management Time — Total Lesson Time 1800 × 100 = ≈ 7 % Management Time

Instruction Time 140 / Total Instruction Time — Total Lesson Time 1800 × 100 = ≈ 8 % Instruction Time

Waiting Time / Total Waiting Time — Total Lesson Time × 100 = ≈ 0 % Waiting Time

place throughout a lesson. A student assistant can trace on a diagram of the learning space the pathway the teacher follows during the lesson. The student observer can also make a mark on the pathway where the teacher interacts with a student.

Support Group (Graham and others, 1980)

A systematic evaluation of teacher performance as outlined above can aid the teacher in pinpointing some problems and highlighting some strengths. However, not all teaching skills can be systematically analyzed. Therefore, the teacher

Table 8-10   Practice Opportunities Checklist

DATE _____

TEACHER _____

OBSERVER _____

LESSON TIME _____

Practice Opportunities

Child's Name	Throwing Overhand	Throwing Underhand	Throwing Sidearm				

needs to develop a support group of trusted colleagues with whom questions, problems, and triumphs can be discussed. Often teachers in the same school district can arrange to meet once a month for discussion and sharing as part of a teacher in-service program.

The support group should be used to improve teacher performance by fostering positive feelings and building the self-confidence of its members. Gripe sessions about students, administrators, parents, and other teachers are inappropriate and will be self-defeating to the goal of improved teaching.

PROGRAM EVALUATION

The final area of evaluation to be considered by the teacher is that of the overall program. Specific questions need to be answered about how well the actual execution of the program meets the established objectives. The first step is to review the goals that were established at the beginning of the year.

To determine how effectively these goals have been met, the teacher has several sources available:

1. lesson plan comments
2. student skill- and fitness-assessment records
3. anecdotal notes
4. parental and administrative comments

A formative review (three or four per year) of these sources will provide the most realistic overview as opposed to a summative review (only at the end of the year).

REFERENCES

GRAHAM, G., HOLT/HALE, S., McEWEN, T., & PARKER, M. (1980). *Children moving: A reflective approach to teaching physical education.* Palo Alto, CA: Mayfield.

KIRCHNER, G. (1985). *Physical education for elementary school children* (6th ed.). Dubuque, IA: Wm. C. Brown.

SIEDENTOP, D. (1983). *Developing teaching skills in physical education* (2nd ed.). Palo Alto, CA: Mayfield.

SUGGESTED READINGS

BARRETT, K. R. (1977). Studying teaching: A means for becoming a more effective teacher. In B. J. Logsdon, Barrett, K. R., Broer, M. R., McGee, R., Ammons, M., Halverson, L. E., & Roberton, M. A. *Physical education for children: A focus on the process.* Philadelphia: Lea & Febiger.

GALLAHUE, D. L. (1982). *Understanding motor development in children.* New York: Wiley.

HERKOWITZ, J. Assessing the motor development of children: Presentation and critique of tests. In M. V. Ridenour (Ed.), *Motor development: Issues and applications.* Princeton, NJ: Princeton Book, pp. 175–187.

McGEE, R. (1977). Evaluation of processes and products. In B. J. Logsdon, Barrett, K. R., Broer, M. R., McGee, R., Ammons, M., Halverson, L. E., & Roberton, M. A., *Physical education for children: A focus on the teaching process.* Philadelphia: Lea & Febiger.

SAFRIT, M. J. (1980). *Evaluation in physical education* (2nd ed.). Englewood Cliffs, NJ: Prentice-Hall.

SCHURR, E. L. (1980). *Movement experiences for children* (3rd ed.). Englewood Cliffs, NJ: Prentice-Hall.

9

LOCOMOTOR SKILL THEMES

Movement Description

Walking is the shifting of weight from one foot to the other, with at least one foot contacting the surface at all times. During the movement, each leg alternates between a supporting phase and swinging phase. The heel strikes the surface first as the back leg pushes off, shifting the weight to the leg in front. The body leans forward slightly after the lead foot contacts the surface. The weight is then transferred from the heel to the outside of the foot, the ball of the foot, and the toes. The base of support (with feet parallel to each other, toes straight) should be approximately shoulder-width apart. The arms swing rhythmically in opposition to the legs; the right arm swings forward with the left leg and the left arm moves forward with the right leg (Fig. 9–1).

Movement Observation

The first walking movements can be observed in children aged 9 to 15 months, with most acquiring the skill by 12 months. Walking sideways and backwards occurs approximately 4 to 5 months after walking forward is achieved. Around the age of 4 years, the child has achieved an adult style of walking that is characterized by an easy, rhythmic stride with a smooth transfer of weight.

Figure 9–2 illustrates base of support variations that are related to many problems in walking gait. As previously described, the feet should be close together (shoulder width), with toes pointed straight ahead. "Toeing out" slightly may be all right; however, an exaggeration may cause the child to walk on the inside of the foot rather than shifting weight from the heel to the outside of the foot. Walking "pigeon-toed" (toeing in) may result in a flat-footed step and a knock-kneed condition.

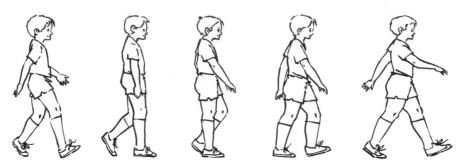

Figure 9-1   Mature walking pattern.

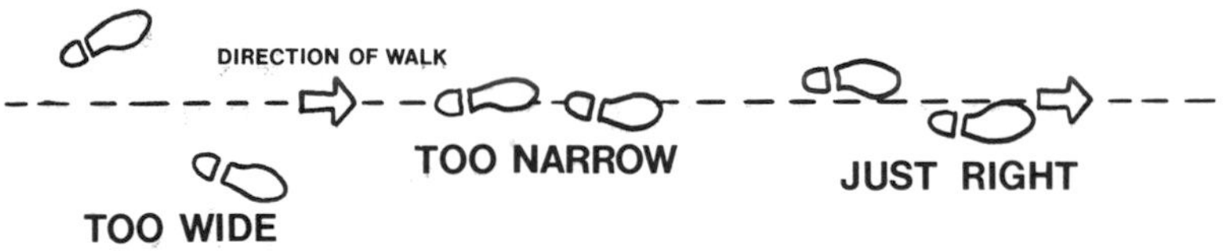

DIRECTION OF WALK

TOO NARROW   **JUST RIGHT**

TOO WIDE

Figure 9-2   Foot placement deviations.

Common Problems

1. Swinging the same side arm and leg forward simultaneously (the arms should swing freely in opposition to the legs);
2. Failure to flex the ankle, knee (stiff), or hip joints, which may cause bouncing or jarring of the body;
3. Incorrect posture as characterized by a forward tilt of the head and body, rounded shoulders, and a titled pelvis (the head and body should be erect);
4. Dragging the heel (push upward and forward from the toe).

Movement Variability

Walking is the most utilized and basic skill that an individual possesses. Used alone or in combination with other movements to form complex skills, walking is the foundation of locomotion.

Spatial

MOVEMENT-PATTERN VARIATIONS

Trunk bent forward, back, or sideward.
Vary base of support (wide to narrow).
Vary length of steps (short to long).
On heels; on toes; shuffle; sides of feet.
Knees stiff.
Vary arm position (straight out, at side, overhead; arms thrusting forward together or alternately; swing arms together from side to side).
Hands on knees; clasped behind back or neck.
Place one foot directly in front or in back of the other.
Sideward (and cross one foot over the other).
Vary foot position (turned out, turned in).
Walk on all fours.
Legs kicking up high in front, back, sideward.

DIRECTIONS/PATHWAYS/LEVELS

In place	Change directions	Over
Forward	Low level (knees bent)	Under
Backward	High level (tiptoe)	Zigzag
Circle	Around	Lower and raise the body

Time

Slow to Fast   Jerky

To musical accompaniment or rhythmic beat

Smooth

Force

Hard	Uphill	Lightly
Soft	Downhill	Knees lifted high

ADDITIONAL MOVEMENT VARIATIONS

Walking in creative ways.

Walk like animals (ostrich, penguin, duck, roadrunner).

Walk (on all fours) like a bear and crab.

Walk "happy" and "sad."

Walk "carrying a heavy load."

Walk on apparatus (benches, balance beams, boards, ropes).

Walk with a partner (side by side, same and opposite direction; back to back, front to front; one behind the other, both facing forward; *all of the variations with variable hand placement*).

Walk as if in a parade.

Walk as if on ice; in mud; on eggs.

Turn, twist, stretch, and bend while walking.

Walk through an obstacle course; forward and backward.

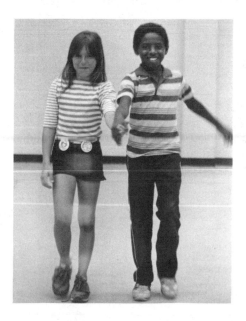

Walk like a tightrope walker in the circus.
Walk like an astronaut in space.
Clap hands under thighs while walking.
Walk like a robot.
Walk with a military goose-step.
Throw and catch an object while walking.
Combine walking with other locomotor skills (walk, run, skip, walk).
Use walking in a gymnastics routine.
Use walking as a movement in dance (see "Movement Enhancement").

Teaching Hints

Provide a visual model of good walking posture.
Provide activities that stress keeping the trunk erect.
Emphasize pushing off from the toes.
Stress walking with the head up and arms swinging freely.

Skill Concepts Communicated to Children

Keep your head up and your trunk straight.
Point toes straight ahead.
Walking is similar to running except one foot is always in contact with the ground.
Your heel is the first part of your foot to contact the ground, and your toes are the last to leave as you walk.
Arms swing opposite the action of your legs in a relaxed, rhythmical manner.
Swing leg from hip.
Swing arms and hands forward easily.

Movement Enhancement

Walking Enhancement Chart

	LEVEL		LEVEL		LEVEL
GAMES		GYMNASTICS		Loobie Loo	
				Mulberry Bush	
Follow the Leader	I–III	Camel Walk	I–III	Farmer in the Dell	
Command Cards		Ankle Walk		The Snail	
		Walking Chair		Sally Go Around the	
Walking Robot	I&II	Bear Walk		Moon	
Cars		Lame Puppy Walk		Did You Ever See a	
Freight Train Relay		Duck Walk		Lassie?	
Kneeling Tag		Elephant Walk		Ten Little Indians	
Marching Ponies		Gorilla Walk		Oats, Peas, Beans,	
Squirrels in the Tree		Inch Worm		and Barley	
Slow Poke				London Bridge	
Red Light		Directional Walk	I&II		
Charlie Over the Water				Jolly is the Miller	II&III
		Crab Walk	II&III	Come Let Us Be Joyful	
Mousetrap	II&III	Knee Walk		Ach Ja	
Old Man/Old Lady				Shoo Fly	
Rescue Relay		DANCE/RHYTHMS/RHYMES		The Wheat	
Fire Engine					
		Sing A Song of Six-	I&II	Glow Worm, Bingo,	III
		pence		Greensleeves	
		Baa, Baa, Black Sheep		Gustaf's Skoal	
		Blue Bird			

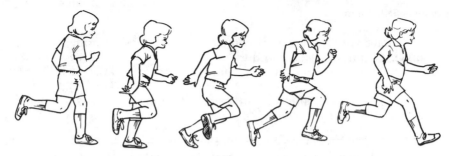

Figure 9-3 Elementary running pattern.

RUNNING

Movement Description

Running is an extension of walking and is primarily characterized by a phase in which the body is propelled with no base of support (flight phase) from either leg. Because of the nonsupport phase, the movement is less stable than walking and demands more bodily control. Jogging, a popular form of running, generally presents a slower pace, more bouncing, and a shorter stride length. As the child propels at greater speeds, more flight time occurs, and there is longer stride length and less bounce. By the age of five, children generally present good running form. They have progressed from the ability to run in a straight line fast to changing directions and dodging.

The majority of children 4 to 8 years of age exhibit running patterns that can be classified as either elementary or mature. McClenaghan and Gallahue (1978) characterize the two stages as follows:

Elementary Stage

In the *elementary* stage, there is an observable but limited flight phase. Although the arms appear to be achieving adequate vertical distance, there is limited horizontal movement. The support leg extends somewhat at takeoff; however, at the height of recovery to the rear, the recovery foot swings across the midline before it is swung forward to the contact position.

Mature Stage

In the *mature* stage, the arms are bent at the elbows in approximate right angles and are swung vertically in a large arc in opposition to the legs. The recovery knee is raised high and is swung forward quickly while the support leg bends slightly

Figure 9-4 Mature running pattern.

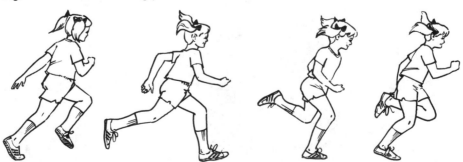

at contact and then extends completely and quickly through the hip, knee, and ankle. Length of stride and duration of flight time are at their maximum. There is very little rotary movement of either the recovery knee or foot as length of the stride increases.

Another description of the mature running pattern as summarized by Wickstrom (1983) suggests that:

1. The trunk maintains a slight forward lean throughout the stride pattern;
2. Both arms swing through a large arc in a vertical plane and in synchronized opposition to the leg action;
3. The support foot contacts the ground approximately flat and nearly under the center of gravity;
4. The knee of the support leg bends slightly after the foot has made contact with the ground;
5. Extension of the support leg at the hip, knee, and ankle propels the body forward and upward into the nonsupport phase;
6. The recovery knee swings forward quickly to a high knee raise and simultaneously there is flexion of the lower leg bringing the heel close to the buttock.

Movement Observation

Most young children acquire an acceptable level of running without formal instruction. This naturally acquired level of proficiency is attributable in part to the amount of experience (time and movement variability) gathered through structured activities and free play. Nevertheless, observation and analysis can both enhance specific phases of the mature runner's form and identify the inexperienced individual.

Common Problems

1. Running in an erect position (slight forward lean should be maintained);
2. Running with the heel touching the surface first (should run on balls of feet during fast, short runs; in long-distance running the heel touches first);

Figure 9-5 Running check-sequence.

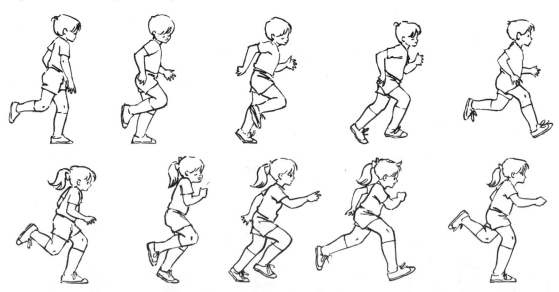

3. Running with feet turned (exaggerated) in or out (feet should be straight);
4. Swinging arms from side to side or allowing to flop at sides (bend elbows at right angles and swing hands and arms forward); motion should resemble putting hands in and out of front pockets);
5. Rearing head far back (head should be positioned straight in direction of run).

When assessing the running pattern, this check-sequence illustration may prove helpful to the instructor and child (Fig. 9–5).

Movement Variability

For pure running efficiency it is important that basic fundamental principles be utilized; however, many movement and game-type activities call upon the child to move in a running fashion using a variety of unorthodox patterns (many being novel to the child). Practice variability allows the child an opportunity to utilize and refine basic patterns as well as experience a variety of situations that call upon bodily adjustment to novel running situations.

Spatial
MOVEMENT PATTERN VARIATIONS

Vary base of support (wide to narrow)
Use short, medium, and long strides
On toes
On heels
Flat-footed
Stiff-legged
Trunk leaning forward, left, right, backward
Toes or knees turned in or out

Standing erect
Arms stiff and down to side
Arms straight out to side; in front; over head; swinging from side to side; folded
Hands on head, waist, shoulders
Knees up high
Crossover step right; left

DIRECTIONS/PATHWAYS/LEVELS

In place
Forward; backward
Sideways (left and right)
Upgrade and downgrade
Over, under, and around objects

Low (squatting down partially)
High (spring into the air)
Changing directions
In circles (clockwise and counterclockwise); zigzag

Time
Slow to fast
Jog
Change speeds while moving

To music accompaniment or rhythmic beat
Running to clapping of hands
Uneven
Even
Jerky motion

Force
Hard   Heavy
Soft   Quiet
Weak   Loud
Light   Shift weight with emphasis

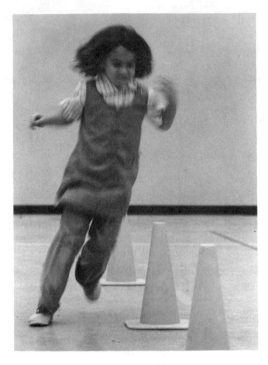

Running through an obstacle course offers the opportunity to enhance agility.

ADDITIONAL MOVEMENT VARIATIONS

Run like various animals.
Run like a character you know.
Pretend you are running in the sand or mud.
Run the pattern of a letter, number, or shape.
Run with a partner (side-by-side holding hands).
Run obstacle-course variations.
Run and stop on a signal.
Run and dodge stationary objects or people.
Combine running with other forms of locomotion (jump, leap, walk, skip, gallop).
Run relays
Run, playing follow the leader.
Run while throwing and catching objects.
Run while shuffling your feet.
Run and touch the ground.
Run while looking over your shoulder.
Run like a rag doll or tin soldier.
Run up and down hills or stairs.
Pretend you are running against a strong wind.
Use running as a movement in dance (see "Movement Enhancement").

Skill Concepts Communicated to Children

Run on the balls of the feet.
Head up, eyes forward.
Bend your knees.
Relax your upper body.

Breathe naturally.
Lean slightly into your run.
Lift your knees.
Bend your elbows and swing the arms freely.
Contact the ground with your heels first.

Movement Enhancement

Running Enhancement Chart

	LEVEL		LEVEL		LEVEL
GAMES		Fire Engine		DANCE/RHYTHMS	
		Beater Goes Round			
Kneeling Tag	I&II	Indian Running		Hickory, Dickory, Dock	I&II
Jet Pilot		Frog in the Pond		Sally Go Round the	
Marching Ponies		Run for Your Supper		Moon	
Command Cards		Flytrap			
Cars		Thread the Needle		Pease Porridge Hot	II&III
Squirrels in the Tree		All Up Relay		Jump Jim Joe	
Red Light		Cat and Rat		Danish Dance of	
Birds and Cats		Count-3-Tag		Greeting	
Charlie Over the Water		Mousetrap		This Old Man	
Catch the Witch		Rescue Relay			
Man from Mars		Race Around the Bases			
		Old Man/Old Lady			
Wild Horse Round-up	II&III	Fire on the Mountain			

JUMPING AND LANDING

Movement Description

Jumping consists of movements that project and suspend the body momentarily in midair with the following basic characteristics: (1) a one- or two-foot takeoff with two-foot landing; (2) two-foot takeoff and one-foot landing. Although classified as a jumping variation, the leap and hop are treated separately in this text because of their extensive use. Wickstrom (1983) describes the following jumping tasks in terms of progressive difficulty:

Jump down from one foot to the other (leap).
Jump up from two feet to two feet.
Jump down from two feet to two feet.
Run and jump from one foot to the other (leap).
Jump forward from two feet to two feet.
Jump down from one foot to two feet.
Run and jump forward from one foot to two feet.
Jump over objects from two feet to two feet.
Jump from one foot to same foot rhythmically (hop).

Fundamental Jumping Variations and Approximate Time of Accomplishment

One-foot takeoff–Opposite-foot landing (jump down; simple leap)	1½ years
One-foot takeoff–Two-feet landing	2–2½ years
Two-feet takeoff–One-foot landing	2½ years

Two-feet takeoff–Landing (broad jump)   4½–5 years

One-foot takeoff–Same-foot landing (hop)   4–6 years

Jumping, regardless of movement variation, is usually attempted with one of two purposes in mind: for height or distance. For either purpose, the hips, knees, and ankles must be bent in order for force to be produced through extension; therefore, takeoff should be from a half-crouched position.

Jumping for Height.   If the primary purpose of the jump is to achieve height, the knees should be bent (crouched position) and the arms lowered with the elbows slightly flexed. As the knees straighten, the arms swing upward. The body stretches and extends as far as possible into the air. The landing should be on the balls of the feet, with the knees flexed to absorb force of impact.

Developmental Progressions of the Vertical Jump and Reach*

Stage 1.   Note the crouching position (illustrated in Fig. 9–6) in which the legs are bent to initiate force. Upward motion is initiated with the arms while the child's head is focused in the direction of the target. After takeoff, the body is fully extended; however, in the upper series, the nonreaching arm is not in an effective position (as shown in Fig. 9–6), where the arm is swung downward as the reaching arm stretches upward.

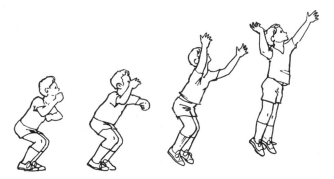

Figure 9-6   Vertical jump: Stage 1.

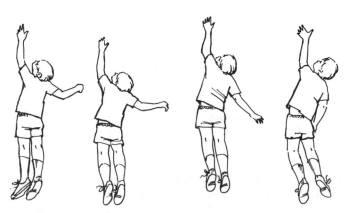

*Material in this section adapted from Wickstrom, 1983.

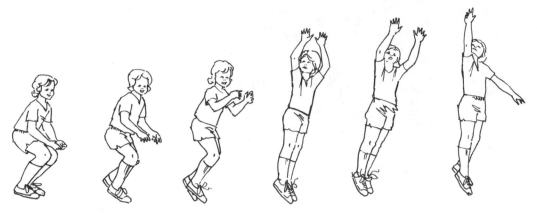

Figure 9-7   Vertical jump: Mature pattern.

Stage 2 (mature).   The preparatory phase is characterized by flexion at the hips, knees, and ankles. A vigorous forward and upward lift by the arms begins the jump; drive is continued by forceful extension at the hips, knees, and ankles. Upon landing, the ankles, knees, and hips flex to absorb the shock (Fig. 9–7).

Jumping for Distance.   To achieve the greatest distance, as in the standing or running long jump, there should be a forward lean, which is counterbalanced by swinging the arms backward and then forcefully forward. The angle of takeoff should be about 45°. The landing should be on the heels first, after which the body's center of gravity shifts forward to maintain balance.

Developmental Progressions of the Standing Long Jump*

Stage 1.   The jumping action of the standing long jump is not initiated effectively by the arms, because of their limited swing. Arms move in a sideward-downward or rearward-upward direction to maintain balance during flight. At take-off, the trunk is propelled in a vertical direction with little emphasis upon the length of the jump. The preparatory crouch is limited and inconsistent with regard to the degree of leg flexion. The extension of the hips, legs, and ankles is incomplete at the takeoff of the jump. Because the child is experiencing difficulty in using both feet simultaneously, one leg may precede the other at takeoff and upon landing (Fig. 9–8).

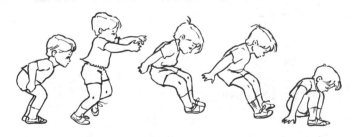

Figure 9-8   Standing long jump: Stage 1.

*Material in the section adapted from McClenaghan and Gallahue (1978), and Wickstrom (1983).

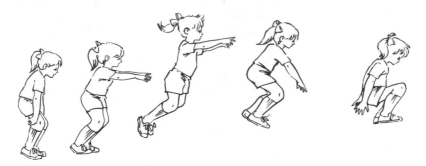

Figure 9-9   Standing long jump: Stage 2.

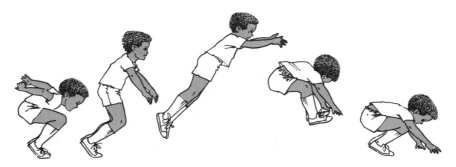

Figure 9-10   Standing long jump: Mature pattern.

Stage 2.   In this stage, the arms are utilized more effectively to initiate the jumping action. They initiate the pattern at takeoff and then move to the side to maintain balance during the jump. There is only a slight change (from Stage 1) in the position of the trunk at takeoff; namely, limited forward lean. The preparatory crouch is deeper and more consistent. At takeoff, the legs, hips, and ankles extend more; however, they remain somewhat bent. During the flight, the thighs are held in a flexed rather than the more effective extended position (Fig. 9–9).

Stage 3 (mature).   In the preparatory phase the crouch is deep and the arms swing backward and upward. At takeoff, the arms swing forward and upward with the thrust being initiated in a horizontal direction (angle of takeoff approximately 45° to 50°). As the body moves forward, the hips, legs, and ankles extend in succession. During flight, the hips flex, bringing the thighs to a position nearly horizontal to the surface. The lower legs extend prior to landing. The knees bend upon impact and body weight continues forward and downward. The arms reach forward to keep the center of gravity moving in the direction of flight (Fig. 9–10).

Movement Observation

Young children begin jumping naturally as soon as they develop the abilities necessary to project their bodies through space with extended "flight." As strength, balance, and coordination levels increase, movement pattern proficiency improves as well as desired height and distance.

In screening for possible weaknesses and determining fundamental jumping ability, the following movement-pattern tasks should be observed:

1. Jumping down from a height of 12 inches using a one-foot takeoff and two-feet landing; two-feet takeoff and two-feet landing.
2. Jump forward using a two-feet takeoff and landing.
3. Jump on to a box (12 inches high) using a two-feet takeoff and landing.
4. Jump up using a one-foot takeoff and two-feet landing.
5. Jump forward from one foot and land on both feet.
6. Run and jump from a one-foot takeoff and two-feet landing.
7. Jump backward using two feet to two feet and one foot to two feet.
8. Jump over, onto, and out of a circle with a diameter of 2 feet.

Common Problems
JUMPING

1. Failure to flex the hip, knee, and ankle joints on takeoff (takeoff should be from a crouched position);
2. Failure to swing arms forward or upward in time with takeoff (if jumping for height, the arms should swing upward as the knees are straightened and the body stretched; when jumping for distance, the arms swing forward and upward explosively);
3. Failure to extend the legs on takeoff;
4. Upper part of body leaning forward in the jump for height (should stretch and reach vertically);
5. Standing too erect when distance is desired (there should be a forward lean and the angle of takeoff approximately 45°)

LANDING

1. Landing flat-footed (should land on balls of feet if jumping for height and on heels if projecting for distance);
2. Landing with feet too close together (width should be same as hips);
3. Knees rigid (knees and ankles should be bent to absorb impact force);
4. Head down (should keep chest and head high, with eyes fixed on direction of movement);
5. Bending forward at the waist (rebound with a small jump into a standing position).

When assessing the standing long jump (two-feet takeoff/two-feet landing), the following check-sequence chart may prove helpful to the instructor and child (Fig. 9–11).

If one is assessing the vertical jump, it is important to provide an overhead target to elicit an effective performance. The target may be an object (bag, ball, balloon) tied to the end of a light rope, horizontal rod, or the tester's hand. For advanced jumpers, chalked fingers, or chalk held in the hand and used to mark the achieved height on a wall, work effectively.

Movement Variability

Jumping and landing are perhaps the most utilized fundamental skills aside from the basic running pattern. A strong schema is necessary if children are to challenge the many and varied jumping and landing tasks that will confront them in almost all movement activities. Aside from the fundamental jumping and landing schema used in performing simple dance, game, and gymnastic activities, jumping variations are an integral part of many advanced movements. Fundamental jumping forms the foundation for such activities as the running long jump, high jump (with variations), and triple jump. Few individual and team-sport activities are performed

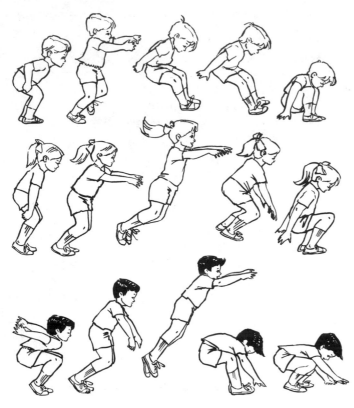

Figure 9-11   Standing long jump: Check sequence.

without some form of jumping. In basketball, for example, players frequently perform a lay-up, jump shot, jump ball, rebound, and jump into the air to retrieve high passes.

In any sport or movement activity in which an object is thrown or hit and must be caught, a jump is frequently utilized (volleyball, baseball, football, lacrosse, racquetball).

Proficiency in dance and gymnastics activities is often based upon one's ability to project through space and land accurately.

Spatial
MOVEMENT-PATTERN VARIATIONS
Jumping

One-foot takeoff–two-feet landing

Two-feet takeoff–one-foot landing (right/left)

Two-feet takeoff–two-feet landing

Jump in a tuck position

Jump in a pike position

Jump in a straddle position

Jump and reach out or up

High jump variations (hurdle, scissors, roll)

Gymnastic vaulting variations

Upright (standing erect)

With knees stiff

Arms in various positions (at sides; swinging forward and backward, or side to side; making circles; folded or extended)

Vary base of support (narrow to wide)

Hands in various positions (on knees, hips, behind head, on head)

Landing

Right foot	With feet apart
Left foot	With feet together
Both feet	Straddle position
With right foot forward	Squat position
With left foot forward	With feet crossed
With arms in various positions	Right foot and right hand
On heels	Right foot and left hand
Flat-footed	Left foot and left hand
With knees bent	Left foot and right hand
With knees stiff	(All of the following are performed on a soft mat or trampoline:)
On toes	On seat
	On knees
	On stomach
	On back
	On hands

DIRECTIONS/PATHWAYS/LEVELS

In place	Off objects (bench, box)
Upward	Unto objects
Forward, backward, sideward	Over objects
Change directions while jumping	Low (knees bent)

Time

	Change speeds while jumping
Slow to Fast	To a rhythmic beat
	To musical accompaniment

Force
JUMP

For distance	For height	For height/distance
Hard	Heavy	
Soft	Smoothly	
Lightly	Loudly	

LAND

Lightly	Hard

ADDITIONAL MOVEMENT VARIATIONS

Jump like a bouncing ball.
Jump into and out of hoops on floor.
Jump with objects on head.
Jump with a partner (side by side, face to face, back to back, face to back; using a variety of hand placements).

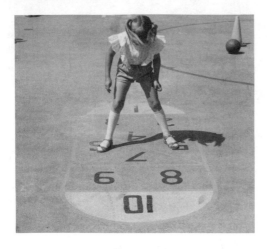

Hopscotch is an excellent and popular
enhancement.

Jump like various animals (rabbit, kangaroo).
Land on designated spots (squares, colors, numbers).
Land on different surfaces (mats, sponge, sand).
Combine jumping with nonlocomotor movements (jump and turn, twist).
Jump while bouncing a ball; while throwing or catching objects.
Combine jumping with other locomotor movements.
Jump onto, on and off of mini-tramp or springboard.
Play hopscotch games.
Try jumping rope and vaulting (discussed in the next two sections of this chapter).

JUMPING ROPE

Movement Description

Traditionally labeled as an activity for young females, *jumping rope* has gained
popularity in recent years due in part to its publicity as a fitness tool and use by
boxers. Sometimes referred to as *rope skipping*, jumping rope can be achieved using a variety of movement variations such as skipping, leaping, hopping, and jumping, all of which require that the performer clear a rope(s) in motion (jump) and
land (rebound).

Equipment and Basic Body Position
Equipment.   There are several kinds of ropes available, ranging from sash cord
to the more expensive Olympic-style mode of plastic links with turning handles.
Homemade ropes can be constructed of inexpensive clothesline and adhesive tape
(tape the cut ends to avoid fraying). An excellent idea is to color-code the ropes
to indicate length.
    The length of the rope can definitely affect the child's performance. To de-
termine the proper rope length, have the child stand in the center of the rope;
the ends should be approximately armpit level (Fig. 9–12). Generally, an assortment
of ropes in 6- , 7- , and 8-foot lengths are appropriate for elementary-school children
(preschool children most often utilize a 6-foot rope). Adults will find that a 9-foot
rope works well. Long jump ropes should be from 15 feet to 20 feet long. Thickness
of the rope may also vary; the authors recommend ⅜-inch to ½-inch thicknesses.

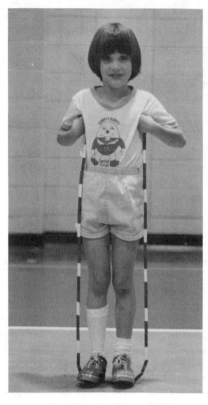

Figure 9-12 Determining proper rope length.

Basic Body Position. The ends of the rope should be held loosely in the fingers with the thumbs positioned on top of the rope and pointing to the sides. The elbows are positioned close to the sides, with hands and forearms pointing slightly forward and away from the body. The rope is started by swinging the arms and shoulders in a circular motion. The wrists and fingers should supply the force necessary to initiate further turning action. The jump is executed with the body erect, a slight push off the toes, and a straightening of the knees, which provides for the lift (approximately one inch). The landing should be made on the balls of the feet with the knees bent slightly to cushion the shock. Specific jumping steps will demand variations in takeoff and landing position; however, the basic principles of posture should apply.

Basic Movement Patterns

It is suggested that rope-jumping patterns and activities be presented in the following order of teaching progression: (1) jumping movements using stationary ropes (or basic jumping, no ropes), (2) long-rope jumping, and (3) jumping using individual ropes.

Because basic jumping and jumping using stationary ropes are discussed in the first section of this chapter, only patterns utilized with long and individual rope jumping will be discussed here.

Jumping with Long Ropes

After the child has been exposed to basic jumping and stationary-rope activities, a confidence in the ability to time one's jumping movements to rhythm is at a level that is appropriate for the introduction of the next rope-jumping category—long-rope jumping. This form of rope jumping is usually performed with one or more children jumping over a rope being turned by at least two others (Fig.

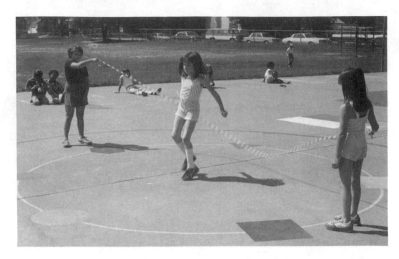

Figure 9-13   Long rope jumping.

9-13). There are two ways that the rope can be turned, which allows the jumper a choice of entries: front door and back door.

Front door means that the child enters from the side where the rope is coming down. The jumper waits until the rope is moving away before entering.

Back door entry is from the side where the rope is coming up. The jumper does not enter until the rope has passed its highest point and is moving downward.

To enhance the rhythmic process, rhymes and chants are very helpful. Children enjoy making up jumping verses, and such a practice is an excellent activity to stimulate creativity (refer to "Movement Enhancement" section for jumping-rope chants and rhymes).

Using the front door (easiest) and then back door entry, the following progression should prove effective in teaching children to jump using long ropes.

1. Run under the rope.
2. Enter, jump once, and exit.
3. Enter, jump several times, and exit.
4. Enter, hop once, and exit (repeat with opposite foot).
5. Enter, hop several times on one foot, and exit (repeat with opposite foot).
6. Enter, hop on alternate feet, and exit.

The child should now be ready for more variations to develop schema (refer to "Movement Variability" section).

Jumping with Individual Ropes

The challenge of turning one's own rope and performing various jumping movements makes this category of rope jumping more difficult than fundamental long-rope jumping (the authors acknowledge that there are some very difficult movements and routines using long ropes).

As with previous rope-jumping activities, music and rhymes/chants can be very helpful in the timing process and stimulation of creativity.

All jumping movements can be varied in speed: slow time, fast time, and double time. An explanation for each of these components is given in the Time dimension, contained within "Movement Variability." Also related to timing is the *rebound*; this is a hop in place as the rope passes overhead. A rebound is used only in slow time with the purpose of carrying the rhythm between steps.

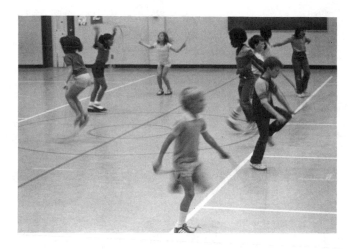

Figure 14 Jumping with individual ropes.

Basic Rope-Jumping Steps

The rope-jumping steps that follow are presented in approximate order of difficulty.

Two-Foot Step.   The two-foot step consists of a two-feet takeoff and two-feet rebound (or landing). The rebound phase is executed while the rope is approximately overhead (Fig. 9–15).

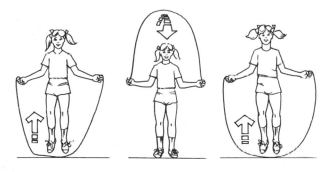

Figure 15 Two-foot step.

Alternate-Foot Step.   The alternate-foot step is characterized by a takeoff and rebound on the same foot (hop), then a switch to the opposite side to continue the same procedure. The rebound step is executed while the rope is passing overhead (Fig. 9–16).

Figure 9–16 Alternate foot step.

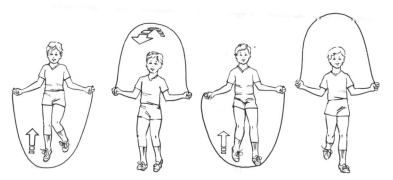

Swing Step.   The swing step is nearly identical to the alternate step, except the *free leg* swings forward, backward, or to the side during the rebound phase (Fig. 9–17).

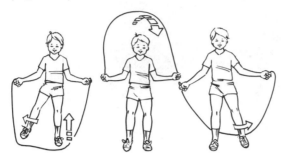

Figure 9-17   Swing step.

One-Foot Hop.   The one-foot hop is similar to the alternate-foot step, except the performer continues hopping on one foot for several rotations of the rope before switching to the opposite foot (Fig. 9–18). This series of movements requires a higher level of balance and general body coordination than does the alternate-foot step.

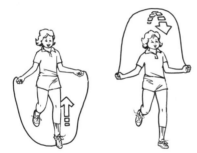

Figure 9-18   One-foot hop.

Rocker Step.   In the rocker step, one leg is always forward and the weight is shifting from the back foot to the forward foot. As the rope passes under the lead (front) foot, the weight is shifted in a forward motion, allowing the back foot to lift and for the rope to pass under. The performer should then rock back, shifting the weight to the back foot (Fig. 9–19).

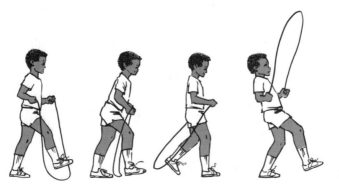

Figure 9-19   Rocker step.

Stride Step.   The stride step starts with the legs in a stride position (one foot forward) with the weight equally distributed on both feet. As the rope passes under the feet, the performer changes foot position and continues (Fig. 9–20).

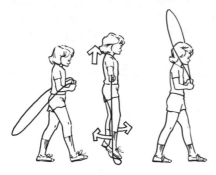

Figure 9-20   Stride step.

Cross-Leg Step.   The cross-leg step begins with one leg crossed in front of the other. As the rope passes under the feet, the legs are crossed in the opposite direction and the pattern continued (Fig. 9–21).

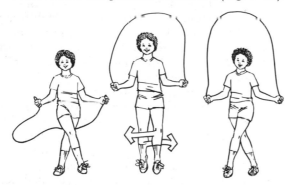

Figure 9-21   Cross-leg step.

Side-Shuffle Step.   As the rope passes under the feet, the performer pushes off with the right (or left) foot and sidesteps to the left, landing with the weight on the left foot (Fig. 9–22). The pattern is then continued in the opposite direction.

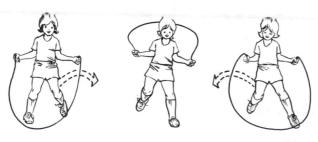

Figure 9-22   Side-shuffle step.

Crossing Arms.   When combined with any selected jumping step, crossing arms while turning the rope provides an interesting challenge for the more advanced jumpers. Once the rope has passed overhead and begins a downward movement, the left (or right) arm crosses over the right and the right hand is brought up and placed under the left armpit (Fig. 9–23). The next jump is executed in this position; the performer now has the option of continuing in the crossed-arm position or alternating positions.

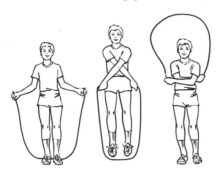

Figure 9-23   Crossing arms.

Movement Observation

Depending upon experience and ability, children will enter programs with a wide variety of rope-jumping proficiency. Generally there will be little difference in skill levels between boys and girls at the primary stage; however, girls seem to extend their interest for the activity over a longer period of time. As previously mentioned, the recent exposure of rope-jumping routines by boxers has helped influence the idea that this activity is not exclusively feminine.

Assessment is essential in determining the entry point of the individual. Corresponding to teaching progression, the following items should also be guidelines for assessment: (1) allow the child an opportunity to jump rhythmically without a rope(s) in motion (jumping in time to a rhythmic beat); (2) allow the child to jump using long ropes turned by others (5 to 10 jumps are considered successful); and (3) allow the child to jump using individual ropes in motion.

Assessment of individual rope-jumping skills can be grouped according to movement pattern and number of turns completed; for example.

NUMBER OF TURNS

Basic two-foot (fast)	_____
Basic two-foot (slow)	_____
Alternate-foot (fast)	_____
Alternate-foot (slow)	_____

The teacher sets a certain criterion to be challenged to meet the requirement for a specific level (that is, Level I, 5 turns; Level II, 10 turns; and so forth).

Common Problems
1. Landing flat-footed (the child should bend slightly at the knees and ankles and land on the balls of the feet);
2. Landing on the rope (in most instances due to incorrect timing; instruct the child to concentrate on movement of rope; offer feedback as to "too soon" or "too late"; slow down rope speed);

3. Not jumping high enough (again, this may be because of incorrect timing or placement of the rope); the rope should hit the surface in front (with individual rope) of the child, thus creating auditory feedback, a cue in the timing process.

Movement Variability

Spatial
MOVEMENT-PATTERN VARIATIONS

I. *Long Ropes*
   A. *Basic Steps*

   one-foot, two-foot variations; leap, hop
   B. *Variations*

   Combine basic steps

   Place hands in various positions (on head, waist, arms crossed)

   Jump with feet in various positions (in, out, close, wide)

   Rope variations

   Double Dutch—two ropes turned alternately, inward (two turners)

   Double Irish—two ropes turned alternately, outward (two turners)

   Egg Beater—two ropes turned at right angles by four turners (more ropes may be added)
II. *Individual Ropes*
   A. *Basic Steps*

   two-foot, alternate foot, swing, one-hop, rocker step, stride, cross-leg, side shuffle, crossing arms
   B. *Variations*

   Combine basic steps

   Toe touch—swing right (or left) foot forward or sideward and land; touch heel with toe of free foot;

   Heel toe—jump with weight landing on right (or left) foot, touch left heel forward; on the next jump, land on same foot, but touch opposite toe to heel; alternate landing foot;

   Heel click—while performing the swing-step sideward (right foot lead), instead of executing a hop (on rebound) when the rope is overhead, raise the left foot to click the heel of the right foot; alternate lead foot;

   Step and tap—this is executed by pushing off with the right (or left) foot and landing on the left. While the rope is overhead, brush the sole of the right foot forward and then backward; alternate push-off foot;

   Create jumping routines from dance steps (Schottische, Bleking);

   Jump with feet in various positions (close, wide, pointed out).

DIRECTIONS/LEVELS/PATHWAYS

I. *Long Ropes*
   Forward body motion or turn of rope
   Backward body motion or turn of rope
   Sideward (shuffle)
   Combinations (change directions while in motion)
   Facing turner; side to turner
   Low level (knees bent)
II. *Individual Ropes*
   Forward body motion or turn of rope
   Backward body motion or turn of rope
   Sideward
   Diagonal
   Combinations
   Low level (knees bent)

Change direction of rope motion (nonstop jumping); forward to backward (as rope starts downward, swing both arms to the left (or right) and make a half-turn facing in the opposite direction. Next, spread the arms and start turning.

Jump with rope turned laterally (rope swung around the body sideways).

Time

Slow Time—slow rope with slow feet movement and a rebound. Rope passes under the feet on every other beat.

Fast Time—fast rope with fast feet movement. Rope turns in time with beat; twice the speed of slow time. Rope speed is approximately 120 to 180 turns per minute.

Double Time—slow rope with fast feet movement. Rope moves in slow time while the performer executes two steps; passing of rope at feet and overhead.

Pepper Time—fast rope with slow feet movement. Two or more turns of the rope while the performer's feet are off the ground.

To a rhythmic beat or musical accompaniment;
Use of rhymes and chants. (see "Movement Enhancement").

Force

Rebound soft; hard
Turn the rope hard; soft
Jump to achieve various heights.

ADDITIONAL MOVEMENT VARIATIONS
Long Ropes

Jumping with partners (start together, or additional jumpers move in while the rope is in motion)

    face to face; back to back; face to back

    alternate role of jumping and turning, with rope in constant motion

    partners attach themselves at various sites and jump (hands on waist, shoulder)

    bounce a ball to a partner or self

    throw a ball to a partner

    jump with more than two

Squat down and touch the surface (one, then two hands)
Create a routine to music.

Individual Ropes

Jumping with partners (start together, or the "extra" jumper moves in while the rope is in motion)

    face to face; back to back; face to back

    the "extra" jumper changes directions

    change role of turning rope

    one jumper holds on to the other at various sites (hands on waist, shoulder, and so forth);

    stand side by side, clasp hands (or arms around waist, shoulders), and turn rope with outside hands;

    side by side, raise inside knees or touch knees;

    the "extra" jumper bounces a ball;

    turning the rope, facing each other, one partner moves in (jumps), then out; partners alternate; another variation is to have one partner move in, followed by the other;

    jump with *three* partners (one in front, one behind the turner);

jump with an individual and long rope (long rope being turned by others in usual fashion).

Create a routine using music.

Jump rope (running) through an obstacle course.

VAULTING

Vaulting, classified as a gymnastic activity, involves a coordination of movements that enable one to bound over an obstacle(s). The obstacles most often used in physical education classes are boxes, benches, and beams. Mini-trampolines, springboards, and beatboards are frequently utilized to aid in the takeoff phase of the vault. Whatever the type of apparatus used in the activity, it is highly desirable that the apparatus be adjustable to accommodate the size and skill level of the participants. There are a number of acceptable models on the commercial market.

Because the use of a springboard or similar apparatus aids in the takeoff phase of some vaulting activities, it is recommended that children be introduced to such apparatus and be allowed adequate practice (with variability) before attempting to vault over obstacles. The control of the body while in flight is an essential prerequisite to this activity. Therefore some forms of vaulting, especially the more complex movements, should be regarded as advanced forms of jumping.

Beginning Vaulting Progression (Nonrunning Approach). Apparatus may be a bench beam, horse, or box; surface approximately knee high to start. (*Note*: Material in this section is adapted from O'Quinn, 1979.)

PUSH OFF

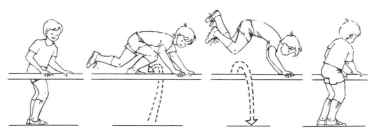

Figure 9–24

Place one foot on the top and push off to the other side.

BOUNCE OFF

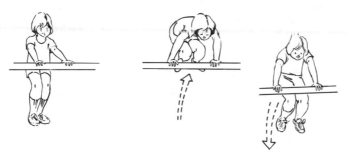

Figure 9–25

With hands on the top, jump up and bend the knees (don't land on the top).

KANGAROO HOP

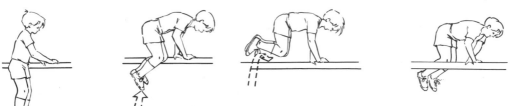

Figure 9-26

Jump up and over.

HIGH PUSH OFF (START AT WAIST LEVEL)

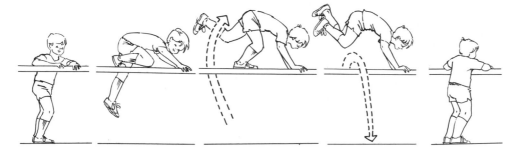

Figure 9-27

HIGH BOUNCE UP

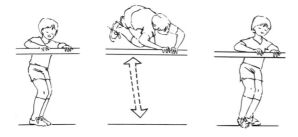

Figure 9-28

HIGH KANGAROO HOP

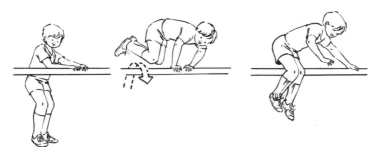

Figure 9-29

TOE TOUCH

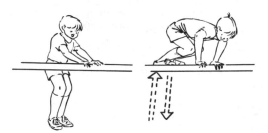

Figure 9-30

Jump up and touch the top with your toes.

ONE FOOT ON

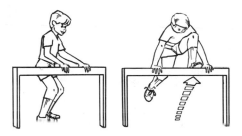

Figure 9-31

Jump up and land on one foot.

TWO FEET ON

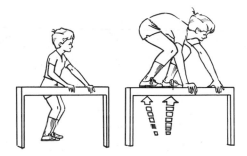

Figure 9-32

Vaulting with Moving Approach

The basic *moving approach* in vaulting consists of a series of running steps and a two-feet takeoff from the floor or bounce apparatus (springboard, beatboard, mini-trampoline). Figure 9-33 illustrates the basic approach and two-feet takeoff. Beginning several yards away from the takeoff point, the child runs into a one-foot liftoff, then brings the legs together for the two-feet takeoff position (which is also the landing on the bounce apparatus or surface). The landing should be on the balls of the feet with the knees slightly bent. The takeoff is performed with a slight forward body lean and hands in place to clear the obstacle.

Figure 9-33 Basic approach and two-feet takeoff.

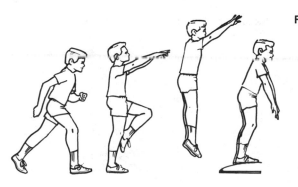

Basic Vaults (Running-Step Approach). Basic jumping skills and bounce apparatus proficiency are a prerequisite when beginning the running-step approach.

The practice-variability method is certainly applicable. However, caution should be taken and spotters utilized as with any potentially hazardous activity. The beginning vaulting movements—bounce off (low and high), kangaroo hop (low and high), toe touch, one foot on, and two feet on—should be the first basic vaults attempted using the running-step approach. *All of the following vaults are performed using a two-feet takeoff:*

SQUAT VALUT

As the child bounds over the obstacle, the hands touch the top as the knees are tucked up close to the chest. The knees should be slightly bent upon landing (Fig. 9–34). The usual landing is on two feet; however, after that is accomplished the child may vary the phase, such as turn, twist (just before landing), or perform a forward roll after landing.

STRADDLE VAULT

The jumping technique is similar to that of a leapfrog. The child reaches forward with extended arms and extends the legs to the side. Maximum height is essential to ensure clearance. The legs are brought together and knees bent slightly upon landing (Fig. 9–35).

FLANK VAULT

With both hands on the top of the apparatus and legs extended toward the right side, the child's right hand is released and motion continued forward until a bent-knee landing is achieved (Fig. 9–36). This vault may be executed from a right or left side takeoff.

HEAD VAULT

The head vault is to be performed only by the highly skilled child. A spotter should be on each side of the apparatus. As the child moves upward, both hands and then the head are placed on the top of the box. When the child becomes overbalanced, the fingertips are used to push off and direct the landing (Fig. 9–37). Caution should be taken by reminding the child not to push off too early and thus fail to clear the apparatus.

Figure 9-34 Squat vault. **Figure 9-35** Straddle vault. **Figure 9-36** Flank vault.

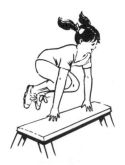 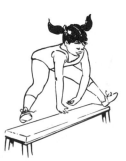 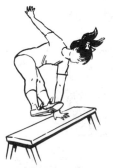

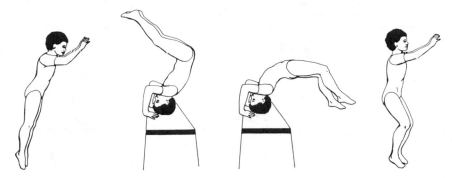

Figure 9-37 Head vault.

Teaching Hints (General Jumping)

Avoid having children jump in socks or in gym shoes that have poor traction.
Use carpet squares to jump to and over.
Emphasize coordinated use of the arms and legs.
Reinforce jumping by measuring individual jumps with a yardstick.
Place a mat on the floor for landing.
Stress proper landing techniques.
Emphasize to the child the need to maintain control while the child is in the air.

Skill Concepts Communicated to Children

Swing your arms forward, bend your knees, and push off with your toes.
Push off equally with both feet.
Your toes leave the ground last.
Lean forward slightly.
Keep your legs shoulder width apart for landing preparation.

Movement Enhancement

Jumping and Landing Enhancement Chart

GAMES	LEVEL	GYMNASTICS	LEVEL	DANCE/RHYTHMS/RHYMES	LEVEL
Hopscotch Games	I–III	Rope Stunts	I–III	Ten Little Indians	I&II
		Lazy Rope			
Train Station	I&II	Snake Rope		Coven Jumps	II&III
Hoop Hop		Circle Rope		Hansel and Gretel	
Toss, Jump, and Pick		Straight Rope		Jump Jim Joe	
		V-Rope		The Popcorn Man	
Eyeglasses	II&III	Rope Rings		Rope-Jump Rhymes	
Weathervane		Frog Jump		Apple, Apple	
Sticky Popcorn				All in Together	
Jump the Clubs Race		Jack in the Box	I&II	Ask Mother	
Stool Hurdle Relay		Missle Man		Be Nimble, Be	
Jump the Shot				Quick	
Over the Brook		Knee Slapper	II&III	Birthday	
Sack Relay		Heel Slap		Blind Man	

(cont.)

Jumping and Landing Enhancement Chart   Continued

GAMES (cont.)		GYMNASTICS (cont.)	LEVEL	DANCE/RHYTHMS/RHYMES (cont.)	LEVEL
Frozen Beanbag		Heel Click		Bobby, Bobby	
Here to There		Human Spring		Bubble Gum	
Slow Poke		Jumping Tubes		Bulldog	
Frog in the Pond		Bouncing Ball		Call the Doctor	
Deep Freeze		Top		Cinderella	
Islands		Up-String		Charlie McCarthy	
Chinese Hurdle		Toe Touch		Chickety Chop	
In the Creek		Tuck Jump		Down in the	
Kangaroo Relay		Rabbit Jump		Meadow	
		Jumping Swan		Down in the Valley	
		Pogo Stick		Fudge, Fudge	
		Kangaroo Jump		Hippity Hop	
		Leap Frog		Hokey Pokey	
		Knee Jump		I Love Coffee	
				Ice Cream Soda	
		Split Jump	III	Lady, Lady	
		Jacknife		Mabel, Mabel	
				Mama, Mama	
				One Two, Buckle	
				My Shoe	
				Teddy Bear, Teddy	
				Bear	
				Tick-Tock	
				Vote, Vote	
				Bleking	III

LEAPING

Movement Description

A *leap* is similar to a run (it may be described as an extension of the run); however, a leap presents more "flight," as well as greater height and distance. A leap is also characterized by a one-foot takeoff and opposite-foot landing (Fig. 9–38).

On the takeoff, the toe of the lead foot leaves last, while the ball of the landing foot contacts the floor first. The movement is usually preceded by several running steps, which add to the momentum needed to produce height and distance. A forward upward motion of the arms also gives added momentum to help carry the body.

Figure 9–38 Leaping.

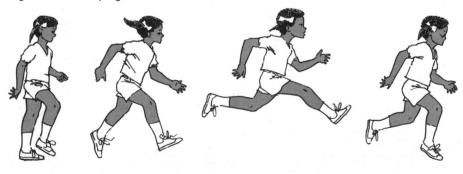

Movement Observation

Without a running start, it is difficult to project the body the necessary height and distance to execute a successful leap. The combination of a run and leap is difficult for many preschool children, although the basic pattern can be achieved. Movement-pattern variations should be held to height and distance during the early learning stages.

Common Problems

1. Not pushing off with enough force to suspend the body in air (push up, stretch, and extend);
2. Failing to swing the arms forward and upward;
3. Landing on heels or flat-footed (land on ball of foot);
4. Landing on both feet (land on opposite foot from takeoff leg);
5. Taking off and landing with stiff knees (knees should be ready to push, lift, extend, and give with the landing).

Movement Variability

While running, children often leap spontaneously when challenged to step over obstacles or space. A leap enables them to hurdle the area (or object) and continue the running pattern; such is the situation in many sport activities. A leap is preferable to a jump while catching an object (basketball, football, baseball) because the running pattern can be continued easily. Leaping can also be observed in such activities as gymnastics, the martial arts, and track (triple jump and hurdling). Except when combined with other movements, the leap is not very easy to use in dancing with others, but it can be frequently observed in solo rhythmic routines.

Spatial

MOVEMENT-PATTERN VARIATIONS

Vary takeoff foot.
Vary arm position (at sides, on head).
Leap with same leg and arm forward; alternate sides.

DIRECTIONS/PATHWAYS/LEVELS

Forward	Various path patterns
Upward	At a low level; high level
To the side (left, right)	Over objects

Time

Slow to fast	To musical accompaniment or rhythmic beat

Force

For height	Land soft; hard
For distance	

ADDITIONAL MOVEMENT VARIATIONS

Leap from a stationary position.
Leap like a deer.
Leap over objects (rope(s), bean bags, blocks, hurdles).

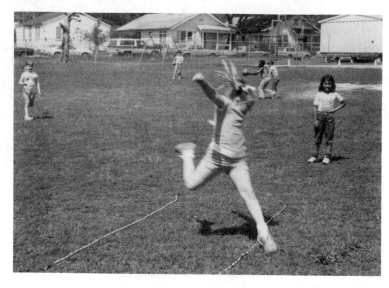

"Leap the Brook" is a traditional and challenging activity.

Leap over a stick or rope in high-jump fashion (gradually increased).
Leap a distance across two lines (gradually widened).
Clap your hands as you leap.
While leaping, catch a ball.
Leap across ropes on the floor at evenly (and unevenly) spaced intervals.
Vary the running pattern before the leap.
Leap, landing on the X's on the floor.
Leap, forming different patterns.
Leap with a partner (side by side holding hands or without attachment).
Change directions.
Combine leaping with other locomotor movements (run, leap, jump).
Use the leap as a movement in dance (see "Movement Enhancement").

Teaching Hints

Combine leaping with two or three running steps.
Provide definite objects or barriers to leap over.
Encourage leaping with either foot.
Suggest imagery-leaping for young children (over mud puddles, or running rivers).
Use devices that "give" if the child comes in contact with an object being leaped over.

Skill Concepts Communicated To Children

Push upward and forward with your rear foot.
Stretch and reach with your forward foot.
Keep your head up.
Lean forward slightly at the trunk as you leap.
Alternate your arm action with your leg action.
Push up, stretch, and reach.
Swing arms up and forward.
Run, run, leap.

Movement Enhancement

Leaping Enhancement Chart

	LEVEL		LEVEL		LEVEL
GAMES		Here to There		DANCE/RHYTHMS	
		Eyeglasses			
Hopscotch Games	I–III	Jump the Clubs Race		La Raspa	II&III
Follow the Leader		Deep Freeze		Fool's Jig	
Over the Brook		Stool Hurdle Relay			
Command Cards		Slow Poke			
Leapfrog Relay		Frog in the Pond			
		Spoke Relay			
Hoop Hop	I&II	In the Creek			
		Chinese Hurdle			
Hurdle Relay	II&III	Islands			

HOPPING

Movement Description

Hopping is characterized by a takeoff from the surface on one foot and landing on the same foot (Fig. 9–39).

Execution is very similar to a jump, but it presents more difficulty in two instances: (1) balance must be maintained across the base of one foot only, and (2) one leg must provide the force necessary to propel the body into space. In hopping, the child should take off and land on the ball of the foot while flexing the hip, knee, and ankle joints to absorb the landing. The free leg is bent under the body so that it makes no contact with the floor.

Movement Observation

Before a child can properly execute a hop, he or she must be able to balance on one foot and have enough strength to propel the entire body using the force of only one leg. A child of 3½ years can usually perform one to three hops, but it is not until approximately 6 years of age that children have mastered the task proficiently. Identification of problems in hopping may be detected easily by directing each child to hop along a straight line (using right and left foot) and over a small object (block, beanbag). Many of the problems associated with hopping are related to lack of balance, leg strength, and experience, which in most instances can be improved upon with proper guidance.

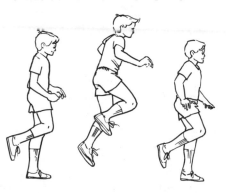

Figure 9-39 Hopping.

Common Problems

1. Landing flat-footed, instead of on the ball of the foot;
2. Inability to propel very far up into space because of being too earthbound (should lift arms up);
3. Taking off on one foot and landing on the other foot or both feet (should take off and land on the same foot);
4. Taking off and landing with stiff knees and ankles (hips, knees, and ankle joints should be flexed slightly to absorb shock of landing);
5. Taking off with the trunk bent too far forward, backward, or sideward (body should lean slightly in the direction of the takeoff leg, with the angle of takeoff close to vertical).

Movement Variability

Hopping is an integral component in many dance, game, and gymnastic activities. It is used in hopscotch, jump rope, skipping, dance steps (step-hop, schottische, polka, mazurka, tinikling), as well as a component in endless movement combinations.

Spatial
MOVEMENT-PATTERN VARIATIONS

Hop on right foot; left foot.   Flat-footed

Hop with trunk tilted forward, backward, or   With body stiff
sideward.

Short, medium, and long hops.

Free leg placed in various positions (extended forward, sideward, backward, or bent up high in front or at side).

Hop with hands in various positions (on head, behind head, on hips, around knee of free leg).

Hop with arms in various positions (at sides, straight out in front, straight out at sides).

Click heel of hopping foot to free leg heel.

DIRECTIONS/PATHWAYS/LEVELS

Upward   Hop in place
Forward; backward; sideward   Hop over
Low (knees bent)   Change directions/levels
High

Time
Slow to fast   To the rhythm of music,
                or a rhythmic beat

Force
For height   Soft, lightly
For distance   Heavily

ADDITIONAL MOVEMENT VARIATIONS

Hop and turn.

Hop, forming a pattern (number, letter, shape).

Hop over objects (ropes, beanbags).

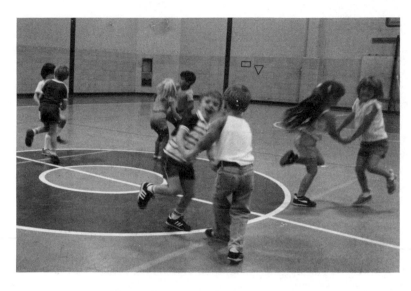

Hopping is used in many
traditional dance steps.

Hop with a partner (side by side, face to face, back to back, front to back; hand placement variable).

Hop like a wooden soldier (short hops with a stiff body).

Hop through an obstacle course; over, around, in and out (tires, ropes, ladders, hoops, cones, tape).

Hop on a trampoline or bouncing board.

Hop while holding the nonhopping leg (foot).

Hop holding the nonhopping leg in various positions.

Hop while blindfolded.

Hop and clap your hands.

Hop using a jump rope.

Hop while dribbling a ball.

Pop a balloon with foot while hopping.

With a partner, try to "mirror" each other.

Combine hopping with other movements (run, jump, skip, step, walk, leap, gallop).

Hop while catching, throwing, or juggling (with a partner).

Hop and kick.

The Hop in Dance.   Hopping is usually combined with other movements for use in partner dancing. The hopping movement is found in the following traditional dance steps:

Skipping—discussed separately in this chapter.

Step-hop—a combination of a walk and hop. The walk is strongly accented and the hop executed in place. The step-hop is performed to the two beats of an accompaniment in ¾ meter time.

Schottische—a combination of three short running steps and a hop. The accent is on the first run and the hop is executed on the foot that takes the third run. The movements are performed in ¼ meter time.

Polka—a combination of a hop and three springy walking steps performed on the balls of the feet. These movements are usually performed in a sideward direction. Preliminary lift for the first walking step is initiated by the hop. The walking step is taken sideward with the outside edge of the lead foot. The feet are brought together into a closed position by the second walk. The third walking step is taken in the same direction as the first, completing the combination in an open position, held for part of the fourth count. The movements are performed to one equally divided and one unequally divided pulse interval in ¾ meter time.

Mazurka—a combination of two springy walking steps and a hop. The two walking steps are taken forward and the hop is performed after the second walking step on the same foot. The movements are performed in ¾ meter time.

Teaching Hints

Avoid letting children perform hopping activities when wearing only socks or gym shoes that have poor traction.

Use marks on the floor to hop to and over.

Emphasize coordinated use of the arms and legs.

Skill Concepts Communicated to Children

Hop up in the air on one foot and down on the same foot.

Stay on the toes while hopping.

Arms should be used for balance.

Reach for the sky.

Crouch halfway down for takeoff.

Movement Enhancement

Hopping Enhancement Chart

GAMES	LEVEL		LEVEL	DANCE/RHYTHMS/RHYMES	LEVEL
		Islands			
		Thread the Needle			
Command Cards	I–III	In the Creek		Ten Little Indians	I&II
		Rescue Relay			
Cars	I&II	Kangaroo Relay		This Old Man	II&III
Slow Poke		Come Along			
Train Station		Jump the Clubs Race		Bleking	III
Charlie Over the Water		Indian Running		Schottische	
Hoop Hop				Crested Hen	
Eyeglasses	II&III				
Chinese Hurdle					
Sticky Popcorn					
Over the Brook					
Stool Hurdle Relay		GYMNASTICS			
Here to There					
Deep Freeze		Rope Stunts	I–III		
Frozen Beanbag					

GALLOPING

Movement Description

Galloping is an advanced extension of walking combined with a leap. It is similar to a slide except the directional progress is forward or backward. Just as the slide, the rhythm is uneven (Fig. 9-40).

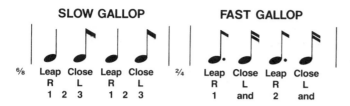

Figure 9-40 Galloping.

The lead leg thrusts forward, supporting the weight, while the rear foot quickly closes behind the lead foot and takes the weight. In a series of gallops, the same foot takes the lead. The takeoff is from the ball of the rear foot and landing is on the ball of the forward foot.

Movement Observation

Galloping (and skipping) is one of the most difficult locomotor skills for young children to master. This may be partly due both to lack of experience with the movement and the complexity of the skill, which is a combination of locomotor movements. Galloping rarely appears before 4 years of age, and children usually do not achieve the mature stage until 6½ years.

Common Problems

1. The rear foot is not brought up quickly to support weight;
2. Lack of a "sliding" movement;
3. Lack of flexibility in lead leg (lead leg should be lifted and bent);
4. Tempo not fast enough;
5. Weight not taken on heel of lead foot (increase stride of leg in front);
6. Failure to stay on toes of foot in rear (take shorter steps on rear leg);
7. Stride of leap too short (should be long-short uneven rhythm);
8. Body too erect (body's center of gravity should be shifted forward).

Movement Variability

Although not utilized extensively in most fundamental and advanced movement programs, galloping is known as one of the traditional dance steps with variations that range from the simple to complex when combined with other locomotor movements.

Spatial
MOVEMENT-PATTERN VARIATIONS

Alternate lead foot

Change arm position (at sides, overhead, in front)

Alternate stride length

Legs stiff; very loose

Base of legs set wide; set close together

DIRECTIONS/PATHWAYS/LEVELS

In place	Low Level	Around
Forward	Change Directions; Levels	Between
Backward	Zigzag (through cones)	Curve
Circle (clockwise, counterclockwise)	Turning gallop (lead foot acts	
High Level	as a pivoting center	

Time

Slow to fast   To a rhythmic beat or
                    musical accompaniment

Force

Heavy   For distance (strong leaps)
Lightly

ADDITIONAL MOVEMENT VARIATIONS

Gallop with a partner (one behind, both facing forward or side by side; hands joined optional).

Combine galloping with other locomotor movements (slide, gallop, run, leap, step, skip).

Gallop through an obstacle course (cones, beanbags, ropes).

Gallop while throwing and/or catching.

Gallop like various animals (race horse, mule).

Gallop like a bouncing ball.

Use a wand and ride a horse.

Be a horse on a merry-go-round.

Be a horse carrying a heavy load.

Gallop over two ropes ("jump the river").

Gallop in different patterns (C, Z, S, 7, 9).

Use the gallop as a movement in dance (see "Movement Enhancement").

Teaching Hints

Begin with exploratory experiences then progress to skill drills.

Stress not crossing the feet.

Stress bending of the knees, trunk leaning forward, and staying on the balls of the feet.

Rhythmical accompaniment aids in galloping.

Skills Concepts Communicated to Children

Keep one foot in front of the other.

Use arms as needed for balance.

Move on the balls of the feet.

Lean forward slightly at the waist.

Movement Enhancement

Galloping Enhancement Chart

GAMES	LEVEL	Man from Mars	LEVEL	DANCE/RHYTHMS/RHYMES	LEVEL
		Gardner and Scamp			
Command Cards	I–III	Come Along	II&III	Sally Go Around the Moon	I&II
Run For Your Supper	I&II	Beater Goes Round		Loobie Loo	
Marching Ponies		Thread the Needle			
Cars		Cat and Rat		Paw Paw Patch	II&III
Charlie Over the Water		Catch the Witch		Pease Porridge Hot	
Flowers Blowing in the Wind		Indian Running		Hobby Horse	
Broomstick Relay		Rescue Relay			
Wild Horse Round-Up		All Up Relay			

SLIDING

Movement Description

Sliding consists of a long-short uneven movement pattern that is executed in a sideward direction (Fig. 9–41).

When sliding to the right, the right foot moves sideward, taking the weight, and the left foot follows quickly. The same foot always leads. The first step is a slow gliding movement and the second a quick closing step. The movement should be performed on the balls of the feet, with the weight shifted from lead to follow-up foot. After the follow-up foot catches the lead foot, a slight hop (with little height) occurs; balance is easily maintained, and the body is ready for a quick change of direction or continuation on the same pathway. The slide is the easiest way to move continuously in a sideward direction.

Movement Observation

By 5 years of age, most children are ready to learn sliding, provided they have had some success with hopping movement. The uneven rhythm that is characteristic of sliding, galloping, and skipping presents a more complex challenge to the child (as compared to running, jumping, and hopping). If a child is having difficulty, the skill should be broken down and practiced at a slow tempo.

Common Problems
1. Sliding on the heels rather than on the balls of the feet;
2. Failure to shift weight from the lead to follow-up foot;
3. Hopping too high and not gaining distance (hop should be slight and provide momentum for next movement);
4. Legs too stiff (both knees should be bent).

Movement Variability

Variations from the basic movement can be seen in many sport and dance activities. Sliding movements are frequently utilized in skating, basketball, badminton, tennis, volleyball, and baseball (also softball). Sliding is also a basic step found in many dances.

Spatial
MOVEMENT-PATTERN VARIATIONS

Change lead foot
Slide with arms in various positions
Change slide lengths

Change feet position (heel to heel, heel to side)

Figure 9–41 Sliding.

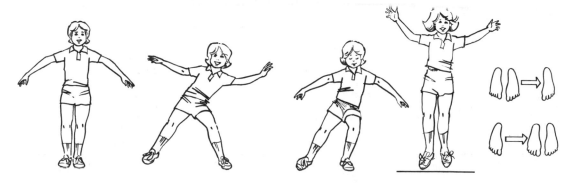

DIRECTIONS/PATHWAYS/LEVELS

Sideward to the right; to the left
Change directions

Low level (knees bent); high level (on toes)
Around objects

Time

Slow to fast   To musical accompaniment or rhythmic beat

Force

For distance (short to long)   Heavily
With a high lift (hop); slight lift   Lightly

ADDITIONAL MOVEMENT VARIATIONS

Sliding with a partner (facing, holding both or one hand; facing, without holding hands; one or two hands on partner's hips, facing or one behind the other; hand(s) on shoulders, facing or one behind; side by side, holding one hand(s) or without holding hands; side by side, skater's style; back to back, holding one hand, both hands, or none).
Slide in a circle with others (hands joined, facing toward or away from center).
While sliding, form various patterns (shape, letter, number).
Slide through an obstacle course.
Catch and throw objects while sliding.
Slide so a hand(s) can touch the floor.
Combine sliding with nonlocomotor movements (slide, turn, slide, bend).
Combine sliding with other locomotor movements (slide, skip, slide, gallop, run).
Use the slide as a movement in dance (see "Movement Enhancement").

Teaching Hints

Rhythmical accompaniment can aid in sliding.
Stress keeping the knees slightly bent, trunk forward, and staying on the balls of the feet.

Skill Concepts Communicated to Children

Step to the side.
Draw foot up toward the other and hop.
Do not bounce.
Slide the feet.

Movement Enhancement

Sliding Enhancement Chart

		LEVEL		LEVEL		LEVEL
GAMES			Old Man/Old Lady		Come Along	
			Cars		Charlie Over the Water	
Command Cards	I–III		Flowers Blowing in the		Indian Running	
			Wind		Rescue Relay	
Slow Poke	I–II		Man From Mars		Beater Goes Round	
Gardner and Scamp					Thread the Needle	
Catch the Witch			Cat and Rat	II&III	All Up Relay	

Sliding Enhancement Chart   Continued

DANCE/RHYTHMS/RHYMES	LEVEL		LEVEL		LEVEL
		Chimes of Dunkirk		Kinder Polka	
				Jump Jim Joe	
Loobie Loo	I&II	A Hunting We Will Go	I&III	Ach Ja	
Sally Go Round the					
Moon		Pease Porridge Hot	II&III	Little Brown Jug	III
Baa, Baa, Black Sheep		Paw Paw Patch		Carousel	

SKIPPING

Movement Description

Skipping is a rhythmic combination of a walking step and hop. It consists of stepping forward on one foot, quickly hopping on the same foot, then duplicating the process on the opposite foot (Fig. 9–42).

To maintain balance and provide the body with upward momentum, the arms should be swung forward and upward in opposition to the legs while hopping. The weight should be on the balls of the feet throughout the movement.

Movement Observation

Skipping may be the most difficult locomotor skill for young children to acquire. Successful performance requires the combination of two fundamental movements—a walking step and hop—that must be executed in an uneven but rhythmic pattern. Skipping is usually the last locomotor skill to be acquired. Research indicates that skipping appears at approximately 5 years of age; however, it is usually not perfected until about age 6½.

Aside from lack of experience, especially among males, young children experiencing difficulty in skipping usually have problems with the hop or coordination of movements. Initial remediation should focus upon the child's ability to hop and then the step-hop combination.

Common Problems

1. Inability to hop (work on the hop, then the combination; step-hop);
2. Landing flat-footed (should land on toes);
3. Stepping on one foot and hopping on the other foot (should step and hop on same foot);

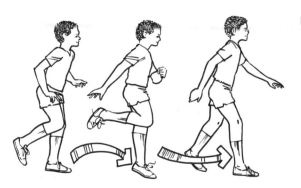

Figure 9-42   Skipping.

4. Failing to swing the arms in opposition to leg movements (arms should swing forward and up in opposition to legs while hopping);
5. Body lean is too far forward or backward (slight lean toward movement direction, with vertical takeoff on hop).

Movement Variability

Although not used in many sport and game-type activities, skipping is a traditional dance step used in many folk dances.

Spatial
MOVEMENT PATTERN VARIATIONS

Vary base of support (feet wide; narrow)

Skip with arms in various positions (folded, straight out, at sides)

Change lead foot (right, left)

Skip with hands in various positions (on head, on hips, behind head)

Trunk bent forward or backward

Skip on tiptoes

Free knee swings out to side, or bent up high in front

DIRECTIONS/PATHWAYS/LEVELS

In place	Low (body crouched)	
Forward	Around	In and out
Backward	Over	
Sideward	Various patterns (circle, square, zigzag)	
High (on toes)		

Time
Slow to fast   Slow motion

To musical accompaniment or rhythmic beat

Force
Lightly   High on the hop

Heavily   Low on the hop

ADDITIONAL MOVEMENT VARIATIONS

Skip with your eyes closed.

While skipping, catch and throw a ball or beanbag.

Skip and clap your hands.

Skip low, touching the ground with the hands.

Skip through an obstacle course.

Skip rope.

Skip with a partner (side by side; face to face; right or left sides together; arm and hand placement variable).

Skip and add other locomotor movements (skip, jump, slide).

Skip and add nonlocomotor movements (skip and turn).

Use skipping as a movement in dance; best performed to music in ⁶⁄₈ meter time (see "Movement Enhancement").

Teaching Hints

Child should be able to gallop with either leg leading before teaching skipping.
Child should be able to hop on either leg before teaching skipping.
Provide a slow-motion demonstration if necessary.
If child has difficulty with the pattern, take his or her hand and skip with the child.

Skill Concepts Communicated to Children

Step forward and hop up!
Swing arms up.
Skip on the balls of the feet.
Keep eyes forward.
Bend the knees.
Relax the upper body.

Movement Enhancement

Skipping Enhancement Chart

GAMES	LEVEL	DANCE/RHYTHMS/RHYMES	LEVEL		LEVEL
Command Cards	I–III	A Hunting We Will Go	I–III	Fool's Jig	
				Maypole Dance	
				Jolly Is the Miller	
Old Man/Old Lady	I&II	Loobie Loo	I&II	Grand March	III
Slow Poke		The Muffin Man		Gustaf's Skoal	
Run for Your Supper		Did You Ever See A		Skip to My Lou	
Cars		Lassie?		Little Brown Jug	
Catch the Witch		Oats, Peas, Beans,			
Gardner and Scamp		and Barley			
Flowers Blowing in the		Baa, Baa, Black Sheep			
Wind					
Man From Mars		Paw Paw Patch	II&III		
Charlie Over the Water		Hansel and Gretel			
		Round and Round the			
Mousetrap	II&III	Village			
Come Along		This Old Man			
All Up Relay		Shoo Fly			
Rescue Relay		Pease Porridge Hot			
Thread the Needle		The Wheat			
Beater Goes Round		The Popcorn Man			
Indian Running		Seven Jumps			

ROLLING

Movement Description

Rolling is one of the earliest locomotor abilities acquired. Before infants crawl or creep they can be observed rolling from stomach to side, stomach to back, back to side, and later back to stomach.

Rolling may be described as: (1) moving along a surface by turning over and over, and (2) forming into a mass revolving over and over. Rocking, which is to move or sway to and fro or from side to side, is often used in the preliminary stages of rolling development, especially as a component in rolling backwards or sideways.

The rolling schema, consisting of a multitude of directional and axis roll patterns, can be developed extensively utilizing a system of progression with practice variability.

Basic Log Roll

The easiest roll to execute is performed with the child lying across one end of a gymnastics mat with arms stretched overhead (Fig. 9–43). The child tries to roll across the mat evenly, keeping the body in a straight line. Initial attempts may be performed without demanding that the child roll across the mat evenly.

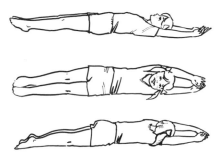

Figure 9–43   Log roll.

Forward Rolling Progression

(*Note*: Material in this section adopted from O'Quinn, 1979.)

Bunny Hop.   Jump out and land with hands first.

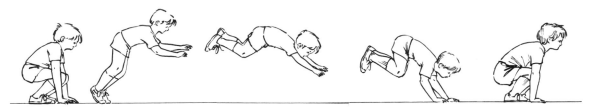

Figure 9–44

Look Behind.   Peek between legs and balance.

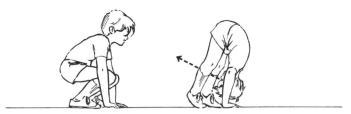

Figure 9–45

Tip Over.   Duck down slowly and tip over.

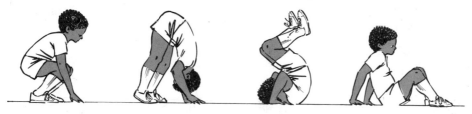

Figure 9-46

Back Rocker.

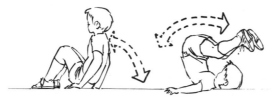

Figure 9-47

Seat Lifter.   Do the back rocker, rock forward, then reach out and lift seat off the floor.

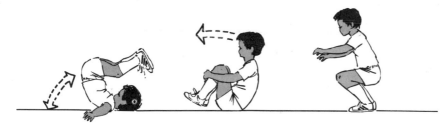

Figure 9-48

Forward Roll.   The *forward roll* is characterized by the child starting in a standing position, then squatting down with the arms extended forward and the fingers pointing straight ahead. There is a push-off from the toes, a rising of the seat, and the chin is tucked to the chest. The arms and hands receive the body weight as the force is transferred to the base of the neck and the top of the shoulders as the roll continues. The arms assist the forward motion by moving forward until first a crouch, then a standing position, is attained (Fig. 9–49).

Figure 9-49   Forward roll.

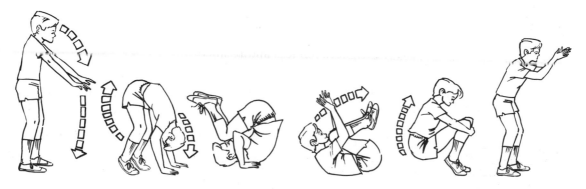

Step-Jump Roll.

Figure 9-50

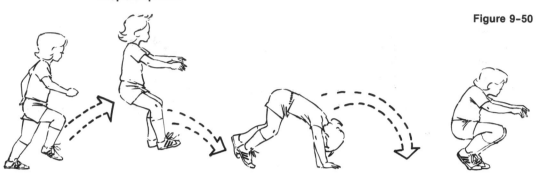

Reach-Over Roll.

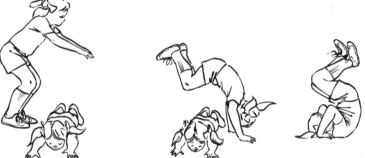

Figure 9-51

Dive Roll.

Figure 9-52

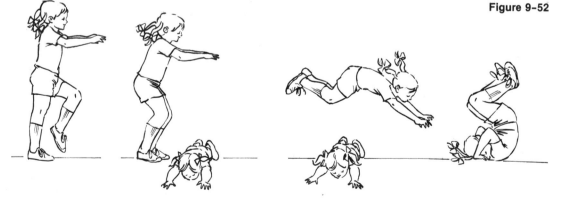

Side Roll. Starting in a back-lying position, with the elbows, knees, and nose tucked in, the performer rolls like a human ball in a sideward direction (Fig. 9–53).

Figure 9-53 Side roll.

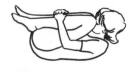
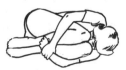
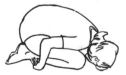

Backward Rolling Progression
Back Rocker.

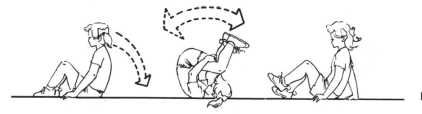

Figure 9-54

Back Balance.   Do the back rocker and hold balance.

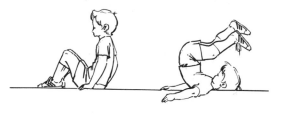

Figure 9-55

Shoulder Balance.   With palms of the hands pointing backward, rock back and balance.

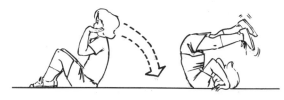

Figure 9-56

Reach and Look.   While performing a "back rocker," look sideways at an extended hand.

Toe Touch.   While performing the "reach and look," one foot is extended over the head to touch the floor.

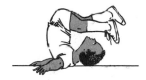

Figure 9-57

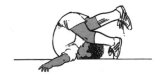

Figure 9-58

Back Shoulder Roll.   Combine a "rock back," "toe toucher," and rollover.

Figure 9-59

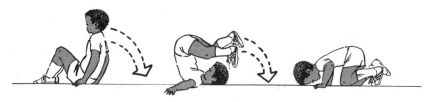

Sit Back. Sit, rock back, balance on shoulder, and return.

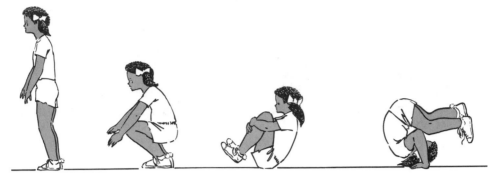

Figure 9-60

Sit Back to Shoulder Roll (diagonal roll).

Figure 9-61

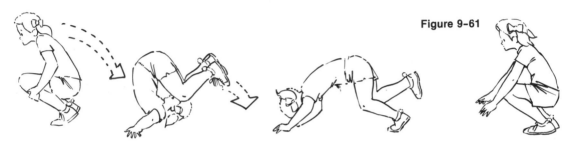

Backward Roll. The *backward roll* is the most difficult basic roll to execute because weight has to be taken on the arms as the body rolls in the backward motion. With the back facing the mat, the child rocks forward slightly, pushing off with the hands, and rolls backward while keeping the knees close to the chest and chin down. The backward motion continues until the weight is well over the shoulders; at that time the hands push off the floor, exerting enough force to lift shoulders off mat and allow head through and then bring the body to a landing position on the knees and toes (Fig. 9-62).

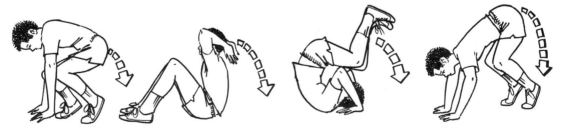

Figure 9-62   Backward roll.

Movement Observation

Aside from focusing on skill performance, the instructor should constantly be aware of possible hazards especially when children are attempting unfamiliar rolls. *Spotting* demands that the instructor understand what the child is going to do next and be ready to assist by giving momentary support (psychological and physical). Figures 9-63—9-65 illustrate proper spotting techniques for the forward and backward rolls.

Forward Roll.   The spotter, positioned on the left side of the child in a kneeling position, places the right hand on the back of the child's left thigh and left hand on the back of the child's head. As the child rolls forward, the right hand pushes forward against the thigh while the left hand lifts (Fig. 9–63).

Backward Diagonal Roll.   Facing in the direction of the backward roll, the spotter takes a kneeling position on the child's left side. The right hand is placed under the child's left shoulder and the left hand on the lower back ready to assist (Fig. 9–64).

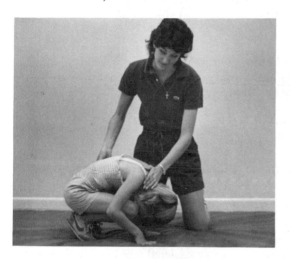

Figure 9-63   Spotting a forward roll.

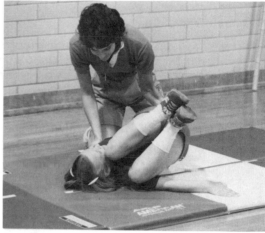

Figure 9-64   Spotting a backward diagonal roll.

Backward Roll.   Positioned in a standing posture on the right side of the child, the spotter places the hands on the child's hips. As the child rolls backward, the spotter gently lifts upward and then backward (Fig. 9–65).

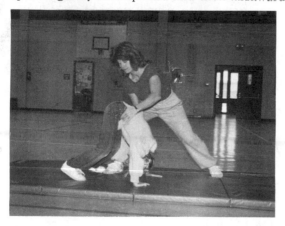

Figure 9-65   Spotting a backward roll.

Common Problems
FORWARD ROLL

1. Body collapses to one side; little use of the arms and hands (arms and hands should take the body weight and push evenly);
2. Too much weight taken onto the head (head should slide through the roll, not be a primary support);

3. The performer does not achieve an ending on the feet (body should be curled with knees tucked in until erect position; arms not coming off the mat as the shoulders touch may also cause lack of momentum).

BACKWARD ROLL

Child cannot roll over backwards:

1. Roundness of back not held during roll (knees should be positioned close to chest);
2. Hands not positioned properly to exert force necessary to accomplish rollover (refer to placement of hands in Fig. 9–62).

Movement Variability

Rolling, a movement youngsters find naturally fascinating, has an extended utility far beyond the basic rolling foundation. Variations of the foundation can be observed in such activities as gymnastics, dance, football, soccer, volleyball, trampolining, wrestling, and judo.

Spatial
MOVEMENT-PATTERN VARIATIONS

ROCKING (forward and backward with hand and leg position variations)

LOG ROLL

Vary arm positions (at sides, crossed, overhead)
Vary leg positions (crossed, wide, close)

SIDE ROLL

Vary arm/hand position (on ankles, shins, knees, chest, behind head)
See Figures 9–89 and 9–90 (Human Ball and Egg Roll)
Vary leg position (crossed)

FORWARD AND/OR BACKWARD ROLL

Walking takeoff
One-foot takeoff
Running takeoff
Diving takeoff
Kneeling takeoff
One-knee takeoff
Squatting takeoff
Standing takeoff
Legs crossed (takeoff and/or landing)
More than two parts (takeoff and/or landing)
Vary arm/hand position (close, wide, grasping feet, ankles, knees, chest)
Vary leg position (crossed, wide, close, one in front of the other)

DIRECTIONS/PATHWAYS/LEVELS

Backward	Down	Low and High level (vary bend of knees)
Sideways	Change directions	Roll in a circle
Forward	Under	
Up	Over	

Time
Slow to Fast   Changing speeds
                To a rhythmic beat
                To musical accompaniment

Force
Smoothly   Roll, diving over objects (mats or markers)
Soft
Hard

ADDITIONAL MOVEMENT VARIATIONS
Forward Rolling Progression Using a Spring Board

(*Note*: Material in this section adapted from O'Quinn, 1979.)

Land and Squat.

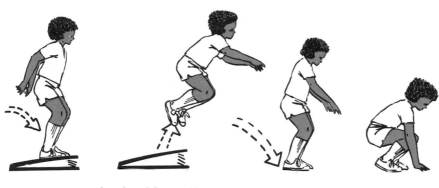

Figure 9-66

Land and Bunny Hop.

Figure 9-67

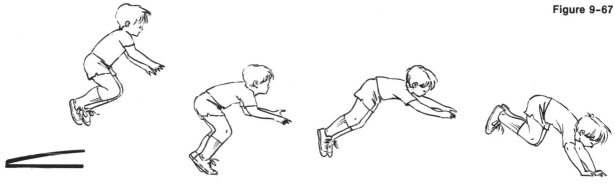

Land, Bunny Hop, and Tip Over.

Figure 9-68

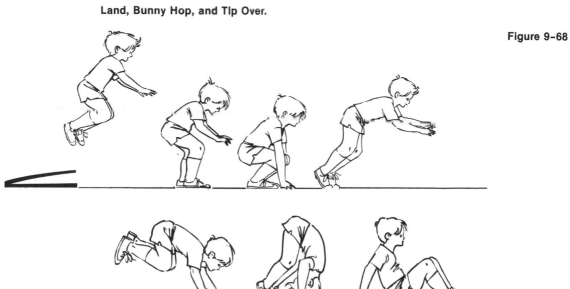

Knee Slapper and Tip Over.

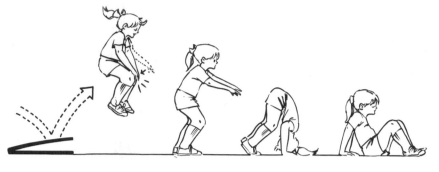

Figure 9-69

Seat Kicker and Tip Over.

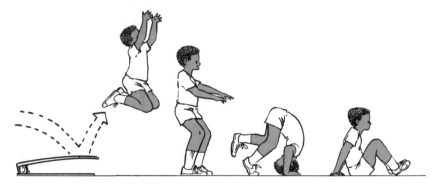

Figure 9-70

Seat Kicker and Forward Roll.

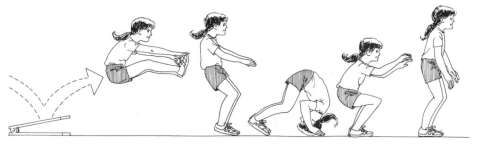

Figure 9-71

Jack Knife and Forward Roll.

Figure 9-72

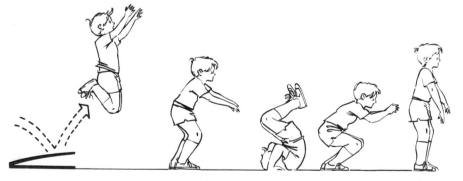

Straddle Bounce and Forward.

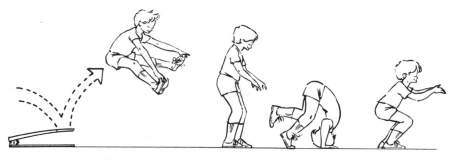

Figure 9-73

Full Twist and Forward Roll.

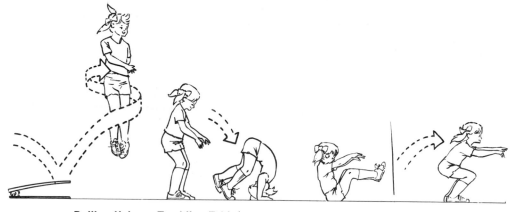

Figure 9-74

Rolling Using a Tumbling Table*
(*Note*: Place well-cushioned mats around the table.)

Log Roll.   Start on the stomach and then the back.

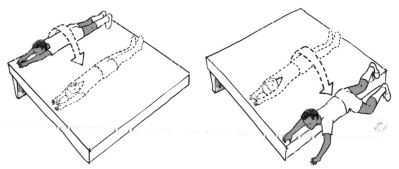

Figure 9-75

Dog Roll.

Figure 9-76

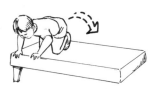
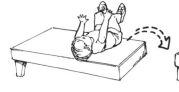
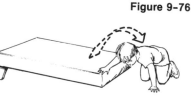

*The tumbling table may be purchased from Physical Fun Products, Inc., Box 4548, Austin, Texas 78765.

FORWARD MOTION ROLLING
Tip Over.

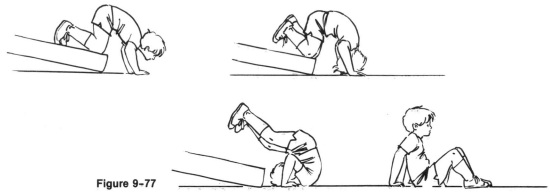

Figure 9-77

Kick Roll Up.

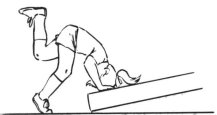

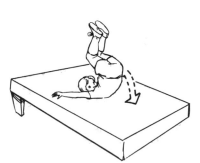

Step Jump Roll.

Figure 9-78

Figure 9-79

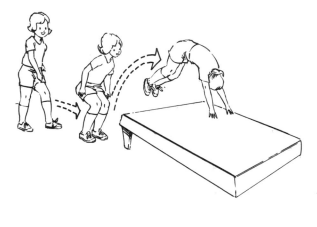

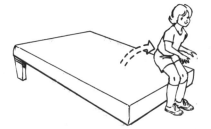

Step Jump, Roll, and Straddle.

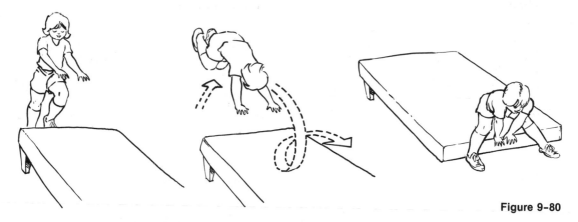

Figure 9-80

Tuck Roll Down.

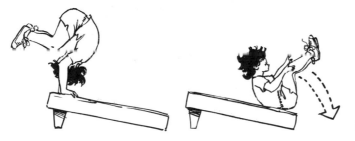

Figure 9-81

Straddle Roll Down.

Figure 9-82

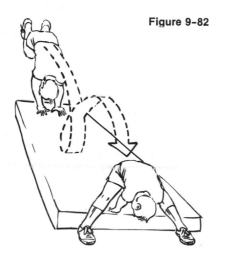

Pike Roll Down. Keep legs straight. Backward motion.

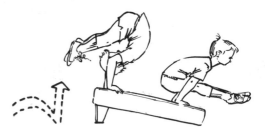

Figure 9-83

BACKWARD MOTION ROLLING

Tip Over.

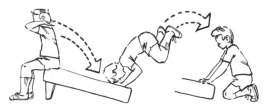

Figure 9-84

Roll Back to Feet.

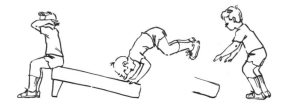

Figure 9-85

Roll Back and Straddle.

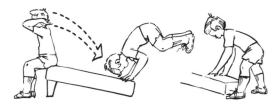

Figure 9-86

Roll Back and Leap.

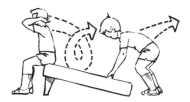

Figure 9-87

Straddle Roll Back and Tuck Roll Back.

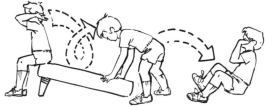

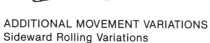

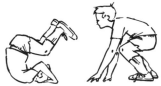

Figure 9-88

ADDITIONAL MOVEMENT VARIATIONS
Sideward Rolling Variations

Human Ball.   Beginning in a sitting position with feet flat on the mat, knees bent, and held close to the chest, the hands are locked together around the lower legs. The child rolls first to one side, then the other, on the shoulder (Fig. 9-89).

Figure 9-89   Human ball.

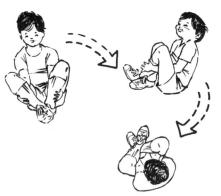

Egg Roll.   From a sitting position, the arms are stretched down the inside of the knees and the hands are wrapped around the lower legs to overlap the ankles. The child rolls as in the Human Ball movement (Fig. 9–90). How many other arm and leg variations can you create?

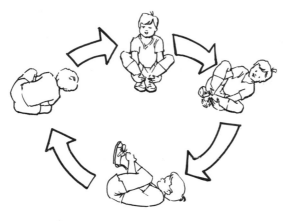

Figure 9-90   Egg roll.

MISCELLANEOUS VARIATIONS

Dive and roll (over and under objects).
Roll with something in hand(s).
Combine rolling with other locomotor movements (jump and roll).
Combine rolling with nonlocomotor movements (balance and roll).
Roll onto, along, and off apparatus (balance beam, bench, plank).
Roll after catching an object.
Roll and stop on signal.
Roll up in a blanket and unroll.
Roll down an incline (hill, ramp).
Roll in a cardboard box.
Play "Follow the Leader"; use various rolls.
Roll with a partner.
Roll with a hoop.
Toss a ball against a wall, then roll and catch.
Allow children to create "rolling routines" (with and without musical accompaniment).

Teaching Hints

See Chapter 16, "Gymnastics."

Skill Concepts Communicated to Children

Stay tucked in a small ball throughout the forward roll on back.
The head should touch the floor as little as possible, so push off on the hands to compensate.
Keep the chin against the chest.
Push evenly with both hands.
Focus the eyes on an object in front to help roll in a straight line (forward roll).

Movement Enhancement

Rolling Enhancement Chart

	LEVEL
GAMES	
Round Stones Command Cards	I–III
Wagon Wheels	II&III

CLIMBING

Movement Description

Climbing is moving upward or downward (ascending and descending) by using hands and feet, with the upper limbs usually initiating primary control. Climbing, an outgrowth of creeping, is often performed before walking, especially if the opportunity to practice is made available. Shortly after the child learns to move in an upright position, the child then attempts to ascend and descend obstacles (usually stairs and steps). This form of climbing is performed without the use of the upper limbs, and although it is prevalent among older children, it will not be discussed in this chapter.

Depending upon the climbing condition (stairs, ladders, frames, nets, ropes), a number of movement patterns may be utilized by the child.

During the initial stages of stair and ladder climbing, the child moves in a "marking-time" pattern, that is, stepping up or down on the level with the same foot each time followed by the trailing foot to the same level. This type of behavior is frequently observed in children 2 years of age. (See Fig. 9–91a, b.)

Figure 9–91 (a) Start of marking-time pattern; (b) completion.

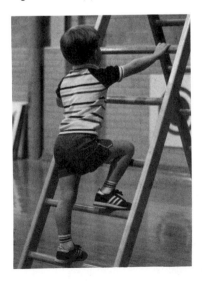 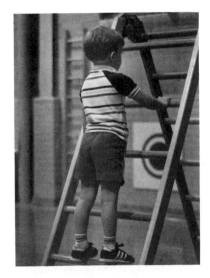

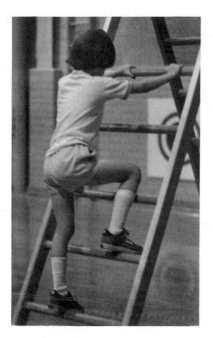 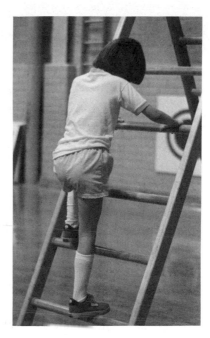

Figure 9-92 (a) Start of cross-lateral pattern; (b) completion.

It is after this stage that the child demonstrates the alternate-foot ascent and descent characterized by a cross-lateral pattern, that is, alternating sides, right-left, or vice versa, with only one foot on each level. (See Fig. 9–92a, b.)

Children are usually capable of descending ladders by 5 years, and at 6 years of age they are proficient climbers in general. Espenschade and Eckert (1980) summarize the studies in stair-climbing ability as follows:

1. Ascending is achieved prior to descending at the same level of achievement.
2. An activity is accomplished with help before it is performed alone.
3. The child will negotiate a shorter flight of stairs before a longer flight.
4. Stairs with lower risers are mastered prior to those of adult size.

Rope Climbing

Movement-pattern variations performed on vertical climbing ropes vary with the "hands only" technique usually not observed among primary-grade children because of upper body strength and endurance limitations.

ROPE-CLIMBING PROGRESSIONS

Lying to Sitting. In the lying position, the child pulls up the upper body into a sitting position. This is executed by placing one hand over the other, moving up the rope. To return to the lying position, the child places one hand under the other, moving the hand on top first (Fig. 9–93).

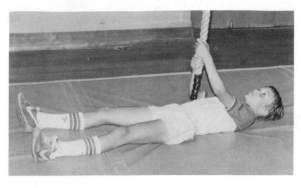
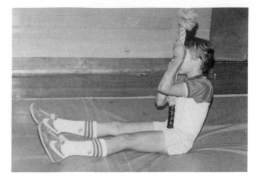

Figure 9-93 Lying to sitting.

Lying to Standing Position. While keeping the knees straight as possible, the child pulls, using the hand-over-hand technique until in the standing position. Again, the child moves hand under hand to lower the body down to the lying position (Fig. 9–94).

Hanging. While standing close to the rope, the child grasps it as high as possible with both hands and pulls, bringing the feet up off the floor. This position is held for progressively longer periods of time (Fig. 9–95).

Climbing. Positioned close to the rope, the child grasps it firmly as high as possible with elbows straight and hands close together. The knees should be bent and feet crossed over the rope. As the child attempts to move up the rope, the knees are straightened and elbows bent. To initiate the pull, the hands move up as high as possible (one hand at a time; hand over hand during initial stages), followed by an upward pull of the knees (Fig. 9–96).

To descend, the foot grip is released as the hands move, using the "hand-under-hand" technique. The body should always be positioned close to the rope. The child should be instructed not to slide down the rope because of possible body burns, loss of control, and orthopedic damage.

Figure 9-94 Lying to standing position.

Figure 9-95 Hanging.

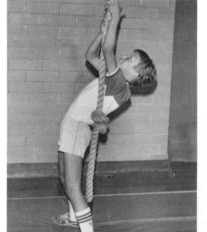
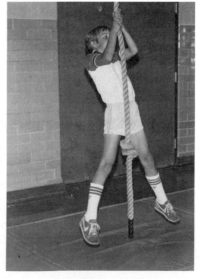

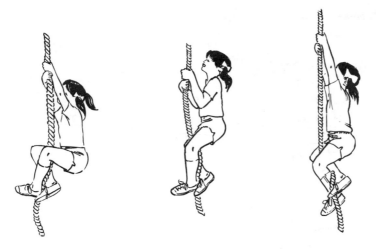

Figure 9-96 Climbing.

Swinging. The child grasps the rope firmly and backs up before running forward. While moving forward, the child slides the hands up and jumps onto the rope. The feet are crossed around the rope and squeezed firmly (Fig. 9-97).

Climbing, aside from being a primary mode of early-stage locomotion, is an excellent means of developing young bodies. Research indicates that children who participate in regular programs utilizing climbing apparatus (overhead ladders) should reveal significantly increased upper body muscular strength/endurance levels as a result of the experience. This is compared to children who have limited opportunities on climbing-type apparatus during the day. Unfortunately, many of our pre- and elementary-level schools today do not provide adequate outdoor play environments, and as a result those children may be deprived of a very essential benefit to their motor development. The overall contributions of general play activities on muscular strength and endurance—often weaknesses in children—should not be underestimated.

Climbing apparatus offer children a wide variety of opportunities to enhance a great number of developmental components.

Figure 9-97 Swinging.

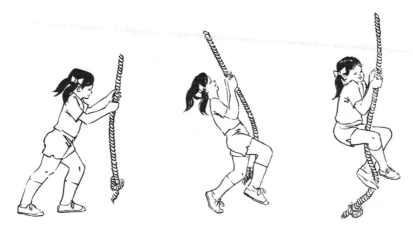

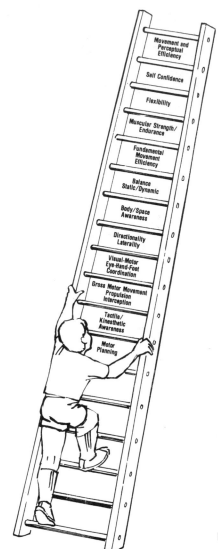

Movement and Perceptual Efficiency

Self Confidence

Flexibility

Muscular Strength/ Endurance

Fundamental Movement Efficiency

Balance Static/Dynamic

Body/Space Awareness

Directionality Laterality

Visual-Motor Eye-Hand-Foot Coordination

Gross Motor Movement Propulsion Interception

Tactile/ Kinesthetic Awareness

Motor Planning

Figure 9-98   Contributions of climbing apparatus to child development.

Movement Observation

A point of observation that the instructor should always be concerned with is safety, especially among those children who are learning control of their bodies in early developmental stages. The instructor should consider such factors as apparatus height, depth, distance between rungs and surface, as well as the child's strength and endurance limitations and perceptual-motor capabilities. When observing the climber, points of periodic focus should be on foot placement, hand grip, eye focus, and general body coordination. Remembering that children are children, and sometimes their confidence borders on the reckless, one should always be alert for possible trouble.

Common Problems
1. Inability to use alternating hand and/or foot placement.
2. Failure to grip the grasping object efficiently.

Movement Variability

Considering the wide variety of climbing challenges that children may encounter, opportunity and variability of practice should be regarded as prime factors to enhance proficiency. Climbing behavior among children depends to a large degree on whether or not they have been exposed to specific challenges. As previously mentioned, climbing apparatus vary widely in dimension and type. Equipment variability, an asset to the development of movement schema, certainly can be experienced in the climbing program.

Spatial

MOVEMENT-PATTERN VARIATIONS
Step-Type Apparatus (alternate lead side)

Unilateral—Same side leg and then arm movement; opposite leg and then arm follow to same level (marking time).

Simultaneous Unilateral—Movement from same side leg and arm simultaneously followed by opposite-side movements to same level.

Cross-pattern—One side leg moves then opposite side arm, alternating sides.

Simultaneous Cross-pattern—One side leg and opposite arm move simultaneously, alternating sides:

Dragging legs
Replacing feet position with knees
Without using hands
Using one hand (alternate)
With knees together/wide
Arms together/wide
Using various grips (thumbs under bar, thumbs over bar)
Changing forearm positions (pronated, supinated)
With the back facing the obstacle.

Rope- and Pole-Climbing Patterns

Refer to "Rope-Climbing Progressions" in earlier section.

DIRECTIONS/PATHWAYS/LEVELS

Ascending (upward)

Descending (downward)

Sideways (moving across; ascending or descending)

Varying levels (degree of incline/decline
Backwards (head first or reverse)

Time
Slow to fast   To musical accompaniment
To a rhythmic beat

Force

Force requirements related to: (1) degree of incline and decline, and (2) amount of weight carried during movement.

ADDITIONAL MOVEMENT VARIATIONS
Climbing

Mountains or hills on hands and feet.
While carrying a pack on the back.
With a partner (holding hands or attached by a rope).

Climbing Apparatus

Stairs.

Boxes.

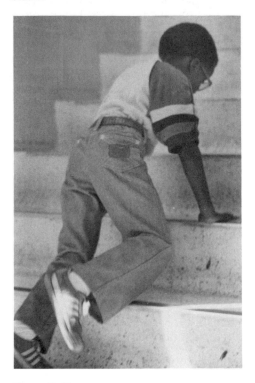

Figure 9-99

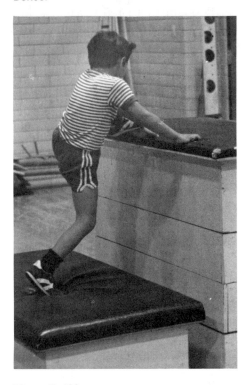

Figure 9-100

Cargo Nets.

Frames.

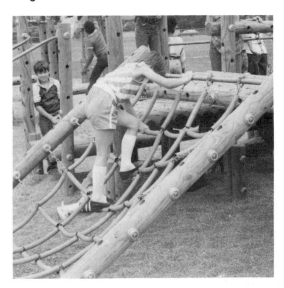

Figure 9-101

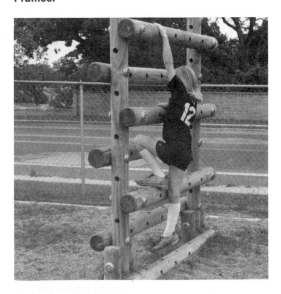

Figure 9-102

Laddors.

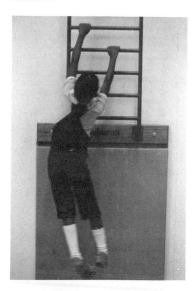

Figure 9-103

Ropes.

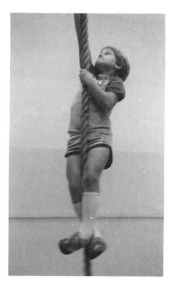

Figure 9-104

Poles.

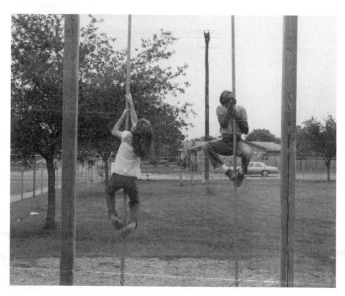

Figure 9-105

Teaching Hints

Spot carefully.

Instruct children to wrap thumbs around the object (rope, pole) when climbing with the use of the hands.

Place a mat under the climbing apparatus.

Stress alternating hand-and foot action.

Skill Concepts Communicated to Children

Place thumbs around the bar.
Use the arms to pull and the legs to push.
Move one hand and the opposite leg at the same time.
Use a follow step and/or a follow grasp.

Movement Enhancement

Climbing Enhancement Chart

	LEVEL
GAMES	
Bridges	I–III
DANCE/RHYTHMS/RHYMES	
Jack the Giant Killer Let's Pretend	I&II

REFERENCES

ESPENSCHADE, A. S. & ECKERT, H. D. (1980). *Motor development* (2nd ed.). Columbus: Charles E. Merrill.

McCLENAGHAN, B. A. & CALLAHUE, D. L. (1978). *Fundamental movement: A developmental and remedial approach*. Philadelphia: W. B. Saunders.

O'QUINN, Jr., G. (1979). *Developmental gymnastics: Building physical skills for children*. Austin: University of Texas Press.

WICKSTROM, R. L, (1983). *Fundamental motor patterns* (3rd ed.). Philadelphia: Lea & Febiger.

10

NONLOCOMOTOR SKILL THEMES

DODGING

Movement Description

Dodging is any sharp change of direction away from an original line of movement. Dodging skills are required to avoid physical contact with one or more objects or individuals that may be either stationary or moving.

Dodging may only require the movement of a portion of the body away from the object or person to be avoided. For example, only the upper portion of the body need be moved to elude a tagger with outstretched arms, whereas the lower portion of the body must be moved to avoid a stationary object or a tagger attempting a tag on the leg.

The dodge is executed by lowering the center of gravity by bending the knees and then shifting all or part of the weight away from the object or pursuer, and then regaining balance by taking a step in the direction of the shift or in the original line of motion. Effective dodging movements include a variety of locomotor and nonlocomotor skills such as jumping, running at different speeds, twisting, bending, falling, and rolling.

Movement Observation

Young children develop rudimentary dodging skills at an early age. As they learn to walk they must also learn to avoid stationary objects in their path. However, the more dynamic situations encountered in games and crowded conditions require a very efficient and mature dodging pattern that must be developed through practice in a variety of situations.

Common Problems

1. Failure to lower the center of gravity (bend the knees and sometimes bend at the waist in preparation to dodge);

2. Failure to stop forward momentum to shift the weight effectively away from pursuer or object (stop forward movement first, then shift the weight or lean away);
3. Maintaining one position too long (push off quickly in new direction);
4. Failure to use deceptive movements (practice feinting to each side and using different body parts).

Movement Variability

The ability to dodge people or objects effectively in gamelike situations is dependent on one's experiences in avoiding moving objects and people. The various conditions that demand dodging movements are rarely the same, so it is very important to practice dodging in as many different and novel situations as possible to enhance the refinement of this skill.

Dodging, probably best known for its use in dodgeball, is also extensively utilized in such sports as football, basketball, hockey, and soccer.

Spatial
MOVEMENT-PATTERN VARIATIONS

Vary base of support (narrow to wide)
Knees bent
Legs straight
Flat-footed
On toes
Movement of:
  head
  shoulders
  abdominals
  hips
  knees
  legs
  feet
  combinations of body parts

Arms held high
Arms held low
Legs in stride position
Legs in parallel position
Upper body stiff
Upper body relaxed
Base stationary
Base moving
Body shapes:
  twist away
  curl away
  stretch away

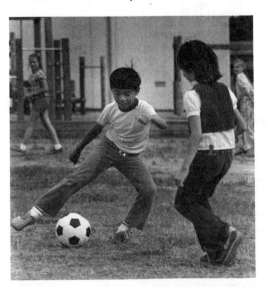

Dodging is a skill used in more advanced games like soccer.

DIRECTIONS/PATHWAYS/LEVELS

Forward; backward; sideways (left and right).
Move to a low level (knees bent, squat), high, middle level.
Change directions on a signal while moving.
Avoid stationary objects in space by changing direction as one encounters them.
Run and dodge in a zigzag or circular path.

Time

Slow to fast	Accelerate forward movement
Combinations	Decelerate forward movement
	Even movement
	Jerky movement
	Dodge on a drum beat

Change direction quickly without stopping movement.

Force

Hard	Weak
Soft	Shift weight quickly

Dodge stationary objects by jumping over them.

ADDITIONAL MOVEMENT VARIATIONS

Dodge balls thrown from different distances.
Dodge various size playground balls (size 5, 6, 7, 8, 10).
Dodge yarnballs.
Dodge a rolling hula hoop.
Use feinting movements before dodging.
Combine different locomotor skills while dodging stationary objects or people.
Dodge objects thrown at varying speeds.
Dodge thrown objects by jumping over them or by ducking from them.
Change running speed while moving forward to avoid a tagger.
Dodge while dribbling a ball (around cones, chairs, people).
Run and dodge through an obstacle course.
Dodge objects or people with a partner (hands joined).

Teacher Hints

Use activities that first demand changing direction on a verbal command, then add stationary objects, and finally moving objects to avoid.
Emphasize bending the knees.
Practice dodging in all directions and use different levels to avoid becoming one-sided.
Practice deceptive-type movements utilizing head, shoulders, eyes, and trunk.
Stay away from dodgeball activities until the child reaches a mature stage of development.

Skill Concepts Communicated to Children

Stop one's movement before dodging one way or the other.

Bend the knees and stay low.

Use different body parts to fake movements; use head, shoulders, and hips.

Change one's speed to fake opponent before dodging.

Movement Enhancement

Dodging Enhancement Chart

	LEVEL		LEVEL		LEVEL
GAMES					
Buffalo Bill	I & II	Fire Engine	II & III	Mousetrap	III
Gardner and Scamp		Wild Horse Round-up		Exchange Dodgeball	
Cut the Pie		Hop Tag		Roll Dodgeball	
Partner Tag		In and Out		Balance Dodgeball	
Birds and Cats		Crossover Dodgeball		Goal Tag	
Scarecrows and Crows		Poison Circle		Snake Catcher	
Seven Dwarfs		Come Along		Snowball	
		Back to Back		Blue and Gold	
		Guard the Toys		Freeze Ball	
		Octopus		Stealing Sticks	
				Chain Tag	
				Chase the Bulldog	
				Man from Mars	

STRETCHING AND BENDING

Movement Description

Stretching is extending or hyperextending any of the joints of the body to make the body parts as long or as straight as possible. Stretching movements are generally done either to increase flexibility or the range of motion of the joints; therefore, they should be done in a controlled manner. Good balance should be required before a maximum stretch is attempted. Children need to understand that stretching involves some minor discomfort and that gradual and static stretching should precede maximum efforts.

Bending, or curling, the body is accomplished by flexing any or all parts of the body at the joints. The structure of the individual joints will determine the range of motion each joint is capable of producing. Bending motions are used both as preparatory actions, as in bending knees before jumping, and ending actions, as in catching a ball by bending the elbows.

Bending is often a preparatory movement for stretching, and both bending and stretching aid in the achievement of maximum force, speed, and distance in combined movements.

The flexibility of the joints can be increased by gradually exerting more force as joints are flexed or extended. If increased flexibility is to be obtained, then bouncing or bobbing movements should be avoided when bending and stretching.

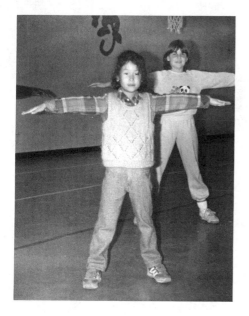

A wide stretch.

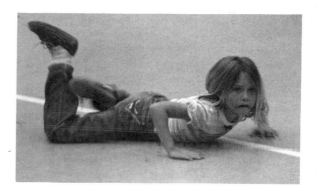

Bending different body parts at a low level.

Movement Observation

A stable base of support is necessary for all bending and stretching movements; consequently, the analysis of a child's pattern should start at the base. Observation should focus on the physical appearance of the child. A heavy or very tall child, for example, may have trouble fully bending the trunk.

Common Problems
1. Stretching and bending movements that are jerky (stress smooth continuous movement, use flowing type music!);
2. Being unable to stretch or bend through the full range of motion (gradually increase flexibility through slow, smooth stretching and bending movements);
3. Loss of balance while bending or stretching (strengthen supporting muscle groups).

Movement Variability

Complete bending and stretching movements greatly enhance the aesthetic beauty of dance and gymnastic activities and increase the child's ability to succeed in the performance of more refined dance and gymnastic skills. A very tight tuck (bent) position, for example, is essential to successful performance of a forward roll. Likewise, a good stretched position is important to the performance of pirouette turns (turning on one foot in dance).

Bending and stretching movements are effective dodging maneuvers for tag and dodgeball games; therefore practice for these skills needs to be dynamic.

Spatial
MOVEMENT-PATTERN VARIATIONS

Bend and stretch with different supports

legs together	on heels	on side
legs apart	on one leg	on back
legs crossed	on seat	on arms
on toes	on stomach	on head and arms

Bend and stretch different body parts

neck	waist
shoulders	hips
elbows	knees
wrists	ankles
fingers	toes

Bend and stretch different combinations of parts with different supports.

DIRECTIONS/PATHWAYS/LEVELS

Bend and stretch
   at high, medium, and low levels
   forward, backward, and side to side
   to trace pathways in the air with different body parts
   curved, straight, and zigzag
Bend one body part in one direction and stretch another the opposite direction.

Time
Bend or stretch

slowly	on a drum beat
continuously	evenly
quickly	unevenly
to music	

Force
Bend or stretch

farther than before	close to the ground
hard	smoothly
soft	roughly
in the air	

ADDITIONAL MOVEMENT VARIATIONS

Hang from a chinning bar-bend and straighten the knees, hips, elbows, neck.

Imitate animals or plants that bend or stretch.

Bend and stretch different body parts while balanced on a box, balance beam, or balance board; use different supports.

With a partner, stretch by gently pushing the partner to stretch farther; bend around the partner in different ways.

Grasping a wand with two hands, bend and stretch to reach the toes from different positions: standing, lying down on back, on front, others.

Stretch and bend while holding different sized and weighted objects in the hands or feet.

Move across the floor by bending, then stretching, the entire body.

Form the letters of one's name by alternately bending and stretching different body parts; use a partner or a group.

Curl or bend around or inside a ball, cone, hoop, rope, or wand, then extend or stretch out over these objects.

Bend to grasp objects on the floor, then stretch to reach objects placed out of reach.

Teaching Hints

Stress smooth continuous movement; use flowing-type music.

Increase flexibility gradually by using slow, smooth stretching and bending movements.

Strengthen supporting muscle groups to aid in balance.

Practice bending and stretching in many positions and utilizing many body parts.

Skill Concepts Communicated to Children

Stretch far enough that it hurts a little.

Stretch slowly and smoothly—do not jerk and bounce.

Alternate stretching and bending to obtain maximum effort.

Try to stretch or bend a little farther each time.

Movement Enhancement

Stretching and Bending Enhancement Chart

GAMES	LEVEL	GYMNASTICS	LEVEL	RHYTHMS AND DANCE	LEVEL
Command Cards Follow the Leader Skin the Snake Octopus	I – III	Giraffe Walk Row Your Boat Long Stretch	I–III	Hokey Pokey	I & II
Partner Tag	I & II	Lame Dog Walk Blow Up the Balloon Over the Head Sky Scraper Pick the Grass Bear Walk Inch Worm Egg Roll Log Roll	I & II	Limbo	II & III
Popcorn	II				
Hop Tag Parachute Play Crossover Dodgeball In and Out Guard the Toys Back to Back	II & III				
Balance Dodgeball Snake Catcher Fly Trap Exchange Dodgeball Chain Tag Goal Tag Roll Dodgeball	III	Egg Sit Ankle Walk Double Roll Bridge Straddle Seat Rocking Horse Corkscrew Thread the Needle V-Sit	II & III		
		Rhythmic Ball Gymnastics Rhythmic Wand Gymnastics Rhythmic Hoop Gymnastics Rhythmic Ribbon Gymnastics	III		

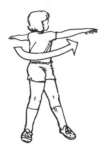

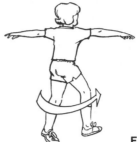

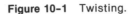

Figure 10-1   Twisting.

Figure 10-2   Turning.

TWISTING AND TURNING

Movement Description

Twisting is the rotation of the body or any of its parts around an axis with a stationary base. Children often call these movements *turning*. For example, one can turn or twist one's head and those movements would look the same.

Turning is a circular movement of the entire body through space, releasing the base of support. Movement of individual body parts without the whole body moving is referred to as *twisting* and not turning.

In twisting and turning movements the base of support should be broadened, and the center of gravity should be lowered to provide a stable position for the next movement and to maintain balance. To twist effectively, the body parts on which the movement is based should be fixed or stable. A slight twist in the opposite direction will add momentum to a turn. The turn from a standing position can be executed by jumping, hopping, or shuffling with the feet and should be made in multiples of quarter turns.

In both twisting and turning, the body should remain relaxed through the range of movements. The speed of these movements can be increased by shortening the length of the moving parts, as a basketball player does when pivoting; he or she draws the ball in close to the body.

Movement Observation

Maintaining balance is a key factor in twisting and turning movements. An analysis of a child's form should be focused on the base of support both at the beginning of the movement and at the conclusion.

Common Problems

1. Losing balance in either twist or turn (widen base of support and lower the center of gravity at start and finish of movement in turn; maintain body alignment throughout movement; don't bend over);
2. Being able to turn one way and not the other (initiate turn by moving one part in the desired direction first—usually the head works best—then combine body forces as skill increases);
3. Landing from a turn stiff-legged (bend the knees when landing and relax);
4. Moving too fast to control the body (perform slow movements until control is achieved);
5. Losing balance or sliding while twisting (hold supporting limbs or parts firm).

Movement Variability

Twisting and turning movements are most commonly used in gymnastic and dance activities. A varied schema is crucial in order to transform these simple movements into the more complicated movement patterns required in such activities as tumbling and apparatus work. An advanced concept of twisting is essential, for example, to execute a round-off on the floor. Turning and twisting movements are present in most dance forms, and their uses in creative movement are numerous. Twisting and turning maneuvers are also a part of dynamic game skills where dodging or quick changes of direction are required. Twisting skill is especially important in manipulating rackets and long-handled implements for striking objects.

Spatial
MOVEMENT-PATTERN VARIATIONS

Twist or turn
    vary base of support (narrow to wide)   with arms in close
    on toes   on one foot
    on heels   knees
    stiff-legged   seat
    knees bent   hips
    arms high   shoulders
      low   head turning only (advanced)
    with arms extended in front
      in back
      to the side
    Twist arms   shoulders
      legs   hips
      head   upper body
          lower body
Twist using different supports and above-body parts
    arms around legs
      around head
      around waist
      around tummy
      around hips
      around knees

DIRECTIONS/PATHWAYS/LEVELS

Twist or turn   Turn while moving in
    right or left   straight
    up or down   curved
    high level   zigzag paths
    low level
Twist body parts on opposite direction.

Time

Twist or turn

to music	evenly
on a drum beat	unevenly
continuously	
slow to fast	

Force

Hard

Soft

Turn while high in the air or close to the ground

Smoothly

Roughly

ADDITIONAL MOVEMENT VARIATIONS

Throw a ball into the air and turn or twist to catch it at different levels.

Twist and turn on balance beam, boxes, ladders, benches.

Twist body around hanging rope or double ropes; on rings.

Twist and turn at the same time.

Twist with or around a partner.

Turn a partner as many different ways as possible.

Mirror a partner's twist-and-turn movements.

Twist in different ways while passing an object back and forth to a partner.

Twist one body part around another.

Using a rope on the floor, turn in different ways while crossing it.

Make shapes with a jump rope and the body.

Twist as if swinging a wand, racket, bat, or other implement around the body.

Twist or turn while carrying various sized and weighted balls.

Turn and twist while moving under and through obstacles.

Teaching Hints

Stress a wide base of support and lower center of gravity at the start and finish of the movement.

When children are turning, stress maintaining body alignment throughout the movement.

To initiate a turn, first move one body part in the desired direction—usually the head works best—then combine forces as skill progresses.

Practice turns and twists to both sides.

Stress bending the knees and relaxing at the landing from a turn.

Have the children slow their movement until control is achieved.

When children are twisting, stress holding the supporting limbs firm as they twist.

Children should start with quarter turns and progress to half turns and then full turns as mastery occurs.

Skill Concepts Communicated to Children

Twisting means keeping one or several body parts on the ground while moving other parts around them.

Turning means to lift one's whole body off the ground and move it around.

Land from a turn with knees bent and body relaxed.

Twist slightly first before turning.

When twisting, place one or more body parts firmly on the ground.

Movement Enhancement

Twisting and Turning Enhancement Chart

GAMES	*LEVEL*	GYMNASTICS	*LEVEL*	RHYTHMS & DANCE	*LEVEL*
Command Cards Follow the Leader	I–III	Human Ball	I–III	Turn the Glasses Over	I & II
Partner Tag	I & II	Top Wring the Washrag Twist Away	II & III	Pease Porridge Hot Hansel and Gretel	II & III
Shoe Twister Human Tangles Crossover Dodgeball Poison Circle Hop Tag Back to Back In and Out Guard the Toys Leap the Brook Skin the Snake	II & III	Floor Touch Thread the Needle Back Scratcher Twist Under Slave Twist Crazy Walk Corkscrew Churn the Butter Crane Twist Greet the Toe Forward Turnover		Klapptanz	III

Exchange Dodgeball
Roll Dodgeball
Balance Dodgeball
Goal Tag
Snake Catcher
	III	Rhythmic Wand Gymnas-
		  tics
		Rhythmic Ball Gymnastics
		Rhythmic Hoop Gymnas-
		  tics
		Rhythmic Ribbon Gym-
		  nastics
			III		

SWINGING AND SWAYING

Movement Description

Swinging movements are pendular or circular movements of the arms, legs, trunk, head, or whole body that occur when the moving part is below the axis. The axis can be another body part, usually a joint (shoulder, hip, knee, elbow), or a fixed object like a bar, which a child can grasp and swing underneath.

Swaying is the same circular type of movement except that the moving part is above the axis. A complete circle of the arms, for example, would involve both swinging and swaying movements.

The pendular motion used in swinging is greatly aided by the force of gravity, whereas swaying movements demand more muscular force to overcome the gravitational pull. For example, for the arms to complete a full circular motion starting above the head, little force need be applied as the arms swing downward below the shoulders, but the arms will stop as speed decreases in the upward portion of the swing unless force is applied to continue the motion back over the head.

In both swinging and swaying motions, when the body is in contact with a supporting surface, momentum of the swinging or swaying part (arm, leg, head)

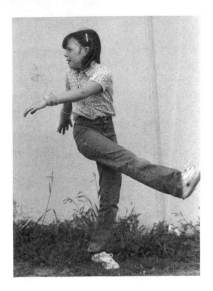

Child swinging a leg.

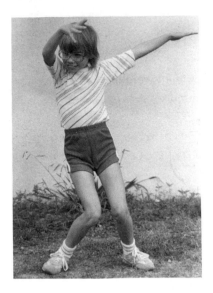

Child swaying arms.

can be transferred to the rest of the body, thus causing movement in the same direction. Also, the speed of the moving part can be increased if the elbow, knee, or entire body is kept straight or extended.

Movement Observation

Swinging and swaying both involve controlling the force of gravity to effect a continuous and graceful movement pattern. Particular attention needs to be focused on the use of gravity in the downward portion of swinging movements, and the exertion of force in the upward portion of swaying movements for the smoothest and most rhythmic action.

Common Problems
1. Loss of body control when swinging or swaying too hard (reduce or eliminate force on downward portion of swing, and allow the weight of the body part swinging to be the force);
2. Movements stiff and jerky (relax body parts, use music to suggest more graceful and continuous movement);
3. Being unable to swing or sway through the full range of movement (increase flexibility of the joints and muscles);
4. Being afraid to swing on high objects like bars and rings (teach proper landing techniques; that is, drop off or dismount at the back of the swing when momentum is briefly slowed).

Movement Variability

Swinging and swaying movements are most commonly associated with dance and gymnastic activities; however, these fundamental movements are also the basis for the manipulative game skills of throwing, striking, and kicking. Therefore, a great variety of experiences in swinging and swaying movements will greatly enhance a child's movement proficiency as he or she progresses through the elementary grades.

Spatial

MOVEMENT-PATTERN VARIATIONS

Supports
Swing or sway arms and upper body with a wide base of support
  narrow base
on toes, on heels
  legs stiff
  knees bent
on one foot
  knees
  seat
Swing or sway legs and/or lower body standing on one foot
  on knees
  on seat
  on stomach
  on back
  on shoulders
Using different supports, vary the extension of swinging or swaying
  body parts
  elbows or knees bent or extended
  ankles or wrists bent or extended
Swing or sway different parts to the front, back, or side of the supporting body.

DIRECTIONS/PATHWAYS/LEVELS

Swing or sway
at high, medium, and low levels
  right or left
  up or down
trace straight
  curved or
  zigzag paths with arms, legs, head.
two body parts in opposite directions.

Time
Swing or sway different body parts
  slowly   to different musical rhythms
  quickly   to a drum beat
  evenly
  unevenly
  continuously

Force
  Hard
  Soft
  Evenly
  Unevenly
  Swing using only force of gravity
  Use individual parts then add whole-body movements.

ADDITIONAL MOVEMENT VARIATIONS

Swing or sway several body parts at the same time.

With a partner, mimic swinging or swaying motions, then do the opposite: One swings the other sways.

Using ribbons or streamers, swing and sway at different levels, speeds, directions, alone and with partners.

Join with a partner and swing or sway together as one.

Swing or sway hoops or wands alone or with a partner.

Swing and sway poi-pois with one hand, then two at the same time; add a body sway to the routine.

Swing and sway holding onto different sized and weighted balls; use one hand or two.

Swing a jump rope doubled up, then extended; continue around to a sway.

Swing various implements around the body using one hand or two; use wands, rackets, ropes, or bats.

Create images for swinging and swaying movements: sway like a stalk of corn, a willow tree, or a flag in a brisk wind.

Holding onto a bar

1. With the body underneath:
   a. Swing one foot up and touch the bar (Fig. 10–3).
   b. Pull one knee up between elbows, then two.
   c. Lift one foot and hook the toe around the bar, then hook one toe, pull the other leg through, and turn over backward (Skin the Cat; Fig. 10–4).
   d. Pull through and balance with legs straight (The Basket; Fig. 10–5).
   e. Swing with the body in different positions: straight, curled, or twisted.
   f. Swing slow, then fast.
   g. Grasp the bar with knees or hands.
   h. Drop off at different points in a slow swing.

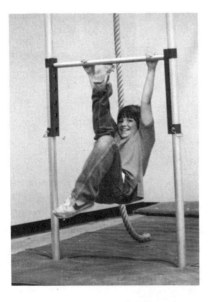

Figure 10–3 Swinging one foot up to touch the bar.

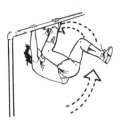
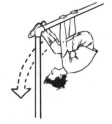
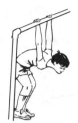

Figure 10–4 Skin the cat.

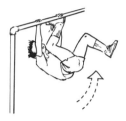
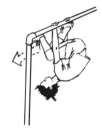
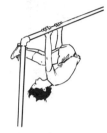

Figure 10–5 Basket.

2. With the body on top of the bar:
   a. Place one knee over the bar and grasp with hands—swing back (Fig. 10–6).
   b. Place both knees over the bar, swing back, and catch on knees or drop back to a basket (Fig. 10–7).

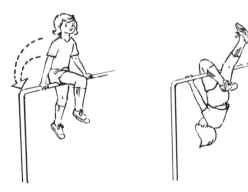

Figure 10–7 Child sits on top of bar, both legs over, and drops back to a basket.

Figure 10–6 Child hooks one knee over bar and swings back under the bar.

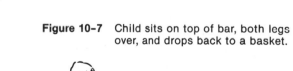
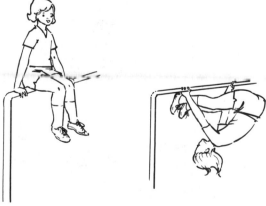

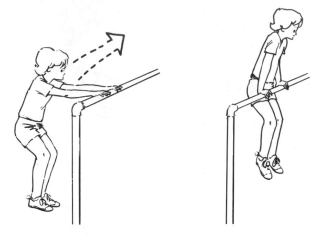

Figure 10-8   Front support position.

3. In a front support, arms straight, bar at hips (Fig. 10–8):
   a. Swing legs forward and back underneath bar.
   b. Sway head, shoulders, and upper body.
   c. Bend arms and support weight at hips.
   d. Lean forward and roll over.
4. Pulling to a support:
   a. Perform flexed arm hang with chin above bar, then pull knees up into a ball (Fig. 10–9).
   b. Curl knees above the bar (Fig. 10–10).
   c. With someone helping, child swings legs over the bar while pulling toward it (Fig. 10–11).
   d. Unassisted—pull with arms while kicking over the bar (Fig. 10–12).

Figure 10-10   Flexed-hang knees over the bar.

Figure 10-9   Flexed-hang knees in tuck.

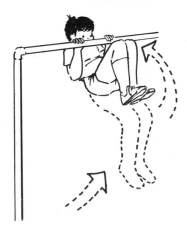

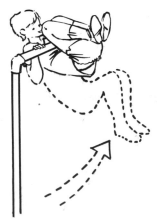

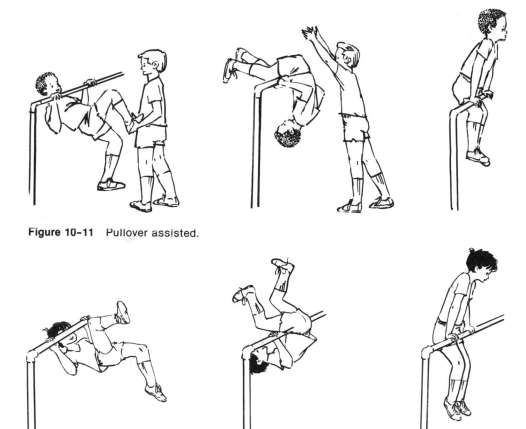

Figure 10-11 Pullover assisted.

Figure 10-12 Pullover unassisted.

Teaching Hints

Use music to relax children and encourage graceful and creative movements.

Stress dismounting apparatus at the back of the swinging movement, and the need to bend knees upon landing.

Stress swinging through the full range of motions.

Skill Concepts Communicated to Children

Allow the weight of one's body parts to pull into a swinging motion.

Relax the muscles when swinging different body parts.

Hold muscles firm when swaying.

When swinging on bars or rings, let go at the back of the swing and land with knees bent.

By adding more force by pumping, one will swing faster and may go all the way around.

Movement Enhancement

Swinging and Swaying Enhancement Chart

	LEVEL		LEVEL		LEVEL
GAMES		GYMNASTICS		RHYTHMS AND DANCE	
Command Cards Follow the Leader	I – III	Elephant Walk	I – III	Hickory Dickory Dock	I & II
				Shoo Fly	II & III
Crossover Dodgeball Poison Circle Guard the Toys Octopus	II & III	Skin the Cat One Knee Swing-up	II & III	Skip to My Lou	III

		Underswing
		Pull Over
		Rhythmic Gymnastics:
		    Ball
		    Hoop
		    Ribbon
		    Wand
			III		

Exchange Dodgeball Roll Dodgeball Balance Dodgeball Snake Catcher	III				

PUSHING AND PULLING

Movement Description

Pushing is exerting force against an object or person either to move the object or person away from the body or to move the body away from the object or person. For example, pushing a small box will cause it to move away from the body, whereas pushing on a wall will cause the body to be moved and not the wall!

Pulling is the application of force that causes objects or people to move toward the body. If the body moves, then pulling will cause the object to follow, as in pulling a wagon; however, if the body remains stationary because of the weight of the object, then pulling will trigger an isometric contraction of one or more muscle groups.

Child pushing.

Child pulling.

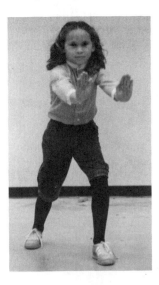

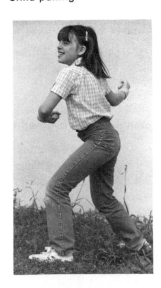

For both pushing and pulling, the body's center of gravity must be lowered and the base of support broadened. All body forces used in pushing or pulling must be directed either toward (in pushing) or away (in pulling) from the center of the weight of the object to be moved. Both pushing and pulling movements should be smooth and controlled, especially when used to move heavy objects. Further, when maximum force is to be exerted, care should be taken to keep the back in a straight position to avoid using the weaker back muscles to impart force.

Movement Observation

Poorly executed pushing and pulling movements can and frequently do cause injuries to the back. Therefore it is imperative that careful observation and analysis of pushing and pulling skills be conducted in order to identify potentially inefficient movement patterns and also to enhance the development of mature patterns.

Common Problems

1. Inability to maintain balance for the duration of the action (widen base of support);
2. Inability to impart maximum force (lower the body and get in line with the direction of the force);
3. Using jerky and inflexible movements (gather body forces and push or pull steadily and evenly);
4. Using an improper body position to lift or pull objects (bend at the knees and keep the back in reasonable alignment).

Movement Variability

Pushing and pulling actions are required in a large variety of game, dance, and gymnastic activities as well as in daily activities not normally associated with physical education. Therefore a variety of practice situations are important to enable the child to adjust to the changing requirements of pushing and pulling movements.

Pushing and pulling movements are most commonly associated with combative games like wrestling and tug-of-war, but they are also used in the games of football and shuffleboard.

Spatial

MOVEMENT-PATTERN VARIATIONS

Vary base of support (narrow to wide)
On toes
On heels
Flat-footed
Stiff-legged
Knees bent
Using different body parts
    feet, legs, hips
    shoulders, back, arms, hands, wrists
    legs in stride position
    legs in parallel position
    standing on one foot
    upper body stiff
    upper body relaxed

arms high, low, in front, in back
stationary base
base moving

DIRECTIONS/PATHWAYS/LEVELS

Forward	Near
Back	Far
Right, left side	Over
Upward	Around
Downward	Under
In	In between
Out	Different angles
High	Circular motion
Low	Figure-8 motion

Time

Slow to fast	To drum beat
Continuously	To beat of music
Even or uneven	To clap of hands
Accelerating, decelerating	

Force

Hard	Evenly
Soft	Steadily
Lightly	
Smoothly	
Roughly	

ADDITIONAL MOVEMENT VARIATIONS

In pairs:
Push finger to finger
  two hands on head
  shoulders together
  side by side
  feet to feet
  back to back
  seat to seat
  knee to knee

PULL

reaching between legs
locking wrists
hand to hand from standing
sitting and prone positions.

Use tug-o-ropes alone to pull on different body parts, and in pairs to pull a partner in different positions and with different body parts.

Use rhythm wands to push and pull against alone and in pairs.

Push or pull a partner on a scooter in open space or through obstacles.

Use objects of various sizes and weights to push or pull through space (balls, beanbags, boxes, cones, hoops, others).

Use a giant tug-of-war rope in a group to pull. Pull in a group in circle formation holding hands.

Push or pull objects with implements (wands to push beanbags or ropes to pull cones).

Teaching Hints

Use lightweight objects at first and gradually increase the weights.

Stress controlled movements; no jerking or tugging.

Stress good body alignment and relate to everyday activities (keep back erect).

Stress widening the base of support and lowering the center of gravity.

Stress using all body forces and not just arms and back.

Skill Concepts Communicated to Children

Keep the back straight.

Bend the knees.

Spread legs apart forward and back.

Push or pull steadily and evenly.

Use one's whole body.

Movement Enhancement

Pushing and Pulling Enhancement Chart

	LEVEL		LEVEL		LEVEL
GAMES		GYMNASTICS			
Command Cards	I–III	Pull the Wand	I–III	Push the Donkey	
Parachute Play		Push the Wand Together		Pull the Donkey	
Follow the Leader		Push and Clap		Push-ups	
		Rocking Horse		Jack-in-the-Box	
Tug-of-War	II & III	Crocodile Crawl			
		Stand-up		Shoulder Wrestling	III
		Sawing Logs		Leg Wrestling	
Pull the Tail	III			Rooster Fight	
Circle of Friends		Elevator	II & III	Seal Slap	
		Elbow Wrestling		Push War	
		Stand-up		Foot Push	
		Going Down		Toe Push	
		Climbing Ropes		Crab Fight	
		Partner Pull-up		Pull-over	
		Push 'em Into Balance			

11

MANIPULATIVE SKILL THEMES

BALL ROLLING

Movement Description

Rolling consists of imparting force to an object that maintains contact with the surface. It is a fundamental manipulative skill that enables a child to learn how to control the speed and direction of the object. The body can be positioned in a sitting or standing posture. If standing, the ankles, knees, and hips will be flexed, head up, and the trunk inclined forward so the hands and the ball will be in close proximity to the ground during the swing.

Elementary Stage

In the elementary stage (Fig. 11-1) the child usually sits in straddle position and pushes or bats the ball with one or both hands. If both hands are used they seldom push evenly, thus causing problems with direction. If the skill is attempted from a standing position, the legs are straight or slightly flexed at the knees and the ball is pushed from between the feet with little or no attention paid to focus or follow-through.

Mature Stage

By the age of 6 years most children will demonstrate the mature stage (Fig. 11-2) as they roll a ball from a semicrouched position with the nondominant foot slightly in front of the other. The ball may be grasped with one or both hands held to the dominant side of the body. The arms are slightly flexed at the elbow as the child moves the ball toward the floor. The child focuses on the target. As the ball reaches the floor, both hands are placed at the back of the ball and move in a coordinated manner to propel the ball in the desired direction. Follow-through is in the direction the ball is going. Weight transfer is from back to front. At this stage the child is able to focus on the target area and be rather successful.

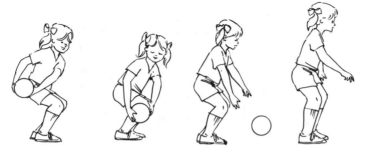

Figure 11-1 Elementary ball rolling.

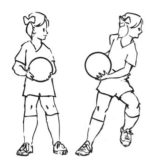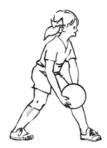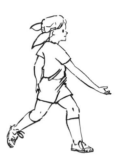

Figure 11-2 Mature ball rolling.

Movement Observation

Ball rolling is one of the first game skills a child masters. The first steps of understanding direction and force can be developed through activities and games that utilize ball rolling. Because a rolling ball only utilizes two dimensions of space (forward-backward and sideward) it is more easily controlled and caught than a thrown ball, which utilizes a third dimension of space (up and down).

Common Problems

1. Poor placement of hands (hands should be behind the ball; fingers pointing down);
2. Failure to transfer the weight backward and then forward (offer word pictures like shoveling dirt or mopping the floor);
3. Failure to release the ball at the proper time (slip the ball gently onto the floor);
4. Failure to step forward with the appropriate foot (foot opposite the ball side);
5. Lack of follow-through and/or focus on the target (reach for the target).

When assessing the ball-rolling pattern, the following check-sequence illustration (Fig. 11-3) may prove helpful to the teacher and child.

Movement Variability

Many elementary games require the skill of rolling a ball. The child needs to learn how to control the direction, force, and speed of the object being manipulated. Children should be encouraged to progress to the one-hand roll (from either side) as quickly as possible. Practice-variability should also include rolling the ball from a moving posture. A well-developed rolling schema can later be used in more com-

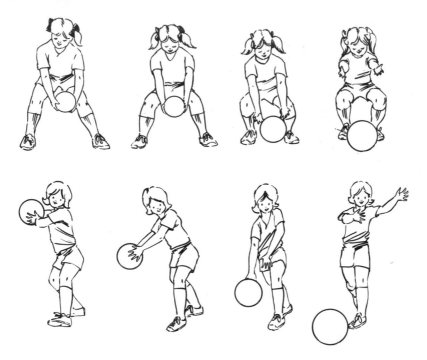

Figure 11–3   Check-sequence, ball rolling.

plex situations found in bowling, boccie, shuffleboard, curling, and team handball. The rolling-movement pattern also offers a foundation for the skill needed for horseshoes, jarts, and softball pitching.

Spatial

MOVEMENT-PATTERN VARIATIONS

Using two hands; one hand (left and right)
Straddle-sitting
Straddle-standing (feet parallel)
Stride-standing (alternate lead foot and rolling hand)
Crouched
Kneeling (both knees and one knee stride standing, feet parallel)
Arms positioned in front of body; at either side
While moving
Vary base of support (narrow to wide).

DIRECTIONS/PATHWAYS/LEVELS

Roll ball:

Straight ahead, diagonally left, right, backward (side and between legs), in a curved pathway;
While traveling (walking, running) forward, backward, and sideways;
While lying on floor, kneeling, standing, jumping (levels).

Time
Slow to fast   To a rhythmic beat

Force

Hard	Roll for distance
Soft	Roll for accuracy

Objects of various sizes and weights

ADDITIONAL MOVEMENT VARIATIONS

Roll a ball with a partner.
Roll to a moving target.
Combine other fundamental skills with rolling a ball.
Roll a ball down a balance beam, up a plank, around a large foam doughnut.
Have a bowling tournament.

SUGGESTED GENERAL PROGRESSION

1. Roll a ball from straddle position, ball held with both hands between the legs.
2. Roll ball from either side of the body while standing in stride position (two hands, then one).
3. Roll a ball diagonally from either side of the body.
4. While moving forward, roll a ball to a partner (target).

Teaching Hints

Use balls of different sizes and weights; however, do not use heavy objects such as a bowling ball during initial experiences.
Emphasize eyes on the target.
Work first on distance and moderate speed, then accuracy.
Provide quality variability of practice around suggested progressions and ability level.

Skill Concepts Communicated to The Children

Allow one foot to lead.
Coordinate shift of weight to back foot with backswing of arm.
Arm giving force is fully extended at completion of backswing.
Release the ball as it passes the forward foot.
Follow-through is in direction of desired pathway of the ball.
Eyes shift from target to ball.

Movement Enhancement

Ball-Rolling Enhancement Chart

	LEVEL			*LEVEL*
GAMES		Hit the Pins		II & III
		Roll Dodgeball		
Rat poison	I & II	Bowling Relay		
		Straddle Bowling		
Call a Guard	II			
Charlie Over the Water				

THROWING

Movement Description

Throwing is a complex manipulative skill in which one or both arms are used to thrust an object away from the body and into space. Depending on many factors (size of child, size of object, and so forth), the throw may be underhand, overhead, overarm, or sidearm. There is also a two-handed overhead throw that is used for projecting large balls. The mature throwing pattern is a complex skill requiring the coordination of many body parts. Of the three most common styles—overarm sidearm, and underhand—the unilateral overarm style is the form most commonly used and most thoroughly studied.

During the developmental stages, children demonstrate many different throwing patterns; however, Wickstrom (1983) reports an absence of any definite or precise order for the onset of the variations.

In normal-developing children 4 to 8 years of age, two distinct stages of throwing can be identified: elementary and mature.

Elementary Stage

First attempts at throwing are usually represented by the two-hand underhand (Fig. 11–4) and two-hand overarm (Fig. 11–5) throws. As the child's hands mature, a smaller ball will encourage the development of the basic one-hand overhand throw.

By 4 or 5 years of age most children demonstrate a throwing pattern in which

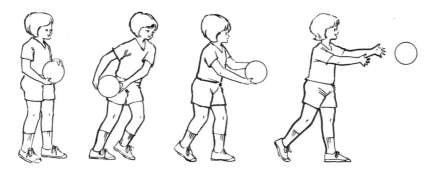

Figure 11–4   Two-hand underhand throw.

Figure 11–5   Two-hand overarm throw.

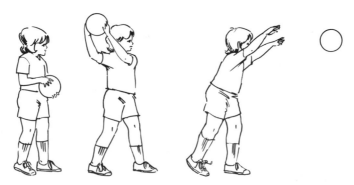

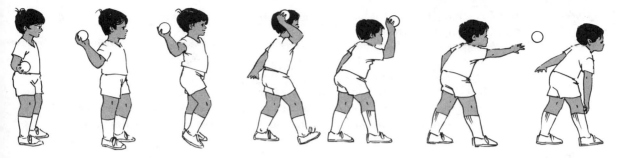

Figure 11-6   Elementary stage overarm throw.

the body more or less faces the target as the arm swings sideward, upward, and backward to a flexed elbow position with the hand held behind the head. There is some trunk rotation when the arm is swung backward as well as when the ball is thrust into space. The forward motion of the throwing arm is accompanied by a forward flexion of the trunk, resulting in a shift of body weight as a forward step is made with the leg on the throwing side of the body (Fig. 11–6). Follow-through is forward and downward.

Mature Stage

The mature stage of throwing (Fig. 11–7) is a coordinated sequence of moves in which the body is used to impart force and speed in an efficient and effective manner. Balance is assisted through the use of transfer of weight and the horizontal movement of the nonthrowing arm. The child assumes an open stance with the throwing shoulder pointed diagonally to the rear and slightly dropped. There is a marked increase in trunk rotation as the weight shifts to the rear foot, the arm swings backward, upper arm assumes a right angle to the body, and the elbow is flexed at a 90° angle. As the forward motion begins, the trunk rotates through the hips, spine, and shoulders, bringing the upper arm to a position straight out from the shoulder with the elbow leading the forearm (thumb pointing diagonally to the rear). At this point the forearm quickly extends followed by a snap of the wrist as the ball is released. The transfer of weight from the rear foot is completed by a step forward (and slightly lateral) of the opposite foot. The follow-through is forward and diagonally downward across the midline of the body. The following

Figure 11-7   Mature stage overarm throw.

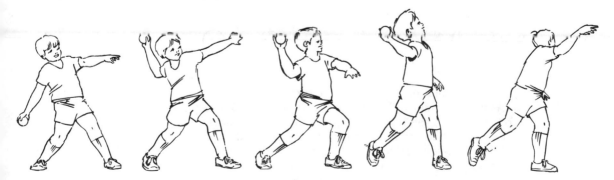

summary characterizes the general movements associated with the mature overhand throwing pattern:

Feet are slightly apart with forward foot opposite throwing arm.

Trunk rotates to throwing side and weight shifts onto rear foot.

There is a definite rotation through hips, legs, spine, and shoulders.

Weight shifts and there is a step with the opposite foot just before the ball is released.

Elbow extension occurs just before release as body continues follow-through.

Movement Observation

Research has provided considerable evidence describing improvement in throwing performance from late infancy through childhood. Although some children progress to the elementary stage of throwing without formal instruction and an abundance of practice, many do no attain mature pattern characteristics without some proper experiences (that is, practice and instruction). Although the skill of throwing requires the coordination of many body movements, throwing proficiency can be realized by the age of five or six by children engaged in play experiences (with meaningful feedback) that stimulate proper throwing behaviors.

Early analysis and correction of ineffective throwing behaviors will help children achieve this important game skill.

Common Problems

1. Beginning stance is "square" when facing the target (place contralateral foot more forward than foot on the throwing side of the body);
2. Failure to shift weight to rear leg (engage child in forward-backward, rocking-type movements—with and without ball play);
3. Failure to rotate the trunk (practice twisting and turning movements with head and feet in a stationary position; encourage a preparatory "reaching back" of the throwing arm to "open up" the stance);
4. Positioning the ball too close to head or behind head (90° elbow joint);
5. Positioning the upper arm close to the body (90° shoulder joint, elbow out);
6. "Palming" the ball (hold ball away from palm—grip with fingers);
7. Failure of elbow to lead the forward arm swing ("elbow out in front");
8. Releasing the ball too soon or too late (snap of the wrist and release of the ball occur simultaneously as forearm extends);
9. Failure to extend forearm quickly (fling the forearm, wrist, hand, ball);
10. Failure to follow-through ("reach for the target," back foot follows through, and weight is transferred to it; distance throws encourage this movement);
11. Inability to hit "target" (refrain from requiring children to throw for accuracy until they have acquired the mature throwing pattern);
12. When throwing underhand, failing to release the ball at proper time (reach directly for the target).

Trunk rotation is considered to be key in the development of overhand throwing proficiency. The gradual evolution from the trunk acting as a "block" with little or no rotation to the pelvic-initiated rotation will be encouraged by experiences that stimulate overhand throwing for long distances.

When assessing the throwing pattern, the following check-sequence illustration (Fig. 11–8) may prove helpful to both the instructor and child.

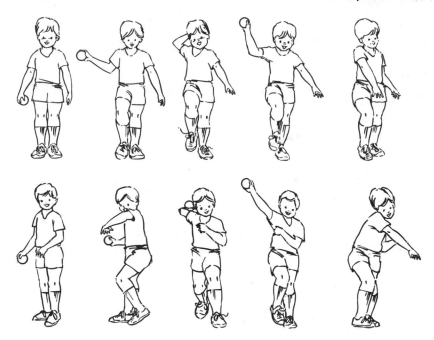

Figure 11-8 Check-sequence, throwing.

Movement Variability

Games at all levels offer opportunities for children to use either the underhand, sidearm, or overhand throw. The use of quality variability to provide a healthy throwing schema is very important if the child is to develop throwing patterns that allow success in dynamic game situations. The mature overhand throw movement is commonly used in lead-up games and in the following sports: softball, baseball, football, volleyball (serve), and the racquet games for smash and serve (tennis).

Spatial
MOVEMENT-PATTERN VARIATIONS

Two hands:
    Underhand (from front and either side)
    Overhand (overhead, chest pass, from either side)

One hand (right/left):
    underhand
    sidearm
    overhand
    variations

Vary base of support
    (narrow to wide)

DIRECTIONS/PATHWAYS/LEVELS

Throw up, down, forward, to side, at an angle
Throw while:
    squatting or sitting
    jumping or leaping
Throw while moving in various directions
    forward   sideways
    backward   diagonally

Time

Slow to fast   To a rhythmic beat

Force

Throw objects of various sizes and weights (whiffleball, fleeceball, softball, football, frisbee, playground ball).

Throw hard for distance.

Throw soft to medium.

Combine distance and accuracy.

ADDITIONAL MOVEMENT VARIATIONS

Throwing against a wall or other rebound material;

Throwing while maintaining a stiff posture (Tin Man);

Throwing while exhibiting an exaggerated relaxed posture (Raggedy Ann);

Throwing while performing locomotor skills (running, skipping, galloping);

Throwing to a partner;

Throwing balls at a stationary target;

Throwing balls at a moving target;

Throwing while moving to target (stationary/moving);

Throwing while being guarded.

SUGGESTED GENERAL PROGRESSIONS

1. Feet positioned and parallel, two-handed underhanded, overhanded, sidearm throws for short distances.
2. Feet in contralateral position (stride position—the foot opposite the throwing arm is in front).
3. Throw objects of various sizes, shapes, and weights.
4. Throw for distance.
5. Throw to a large target on the wall.
6. Throw to a stationary partner—short distance.
7. Throw to a stationary partner—long distance.
8. Throw to a moving partner, right and left.

Teaching Hints

Provide a quality variability of practice.

Encourage distance throws with balls easily gripped in one hand.

Provide "soft" balls (yarn, sponge) at the beginning and progress to more firm (whiffle, "soft" softball) balls.

Think of creative ways to help the children learn the necessary trunk rotation (rotating forward and out from under the ball).

Stress freedom of elbow from the body.

Stress speed of movement, hip rotation, and follow-through.

Emphasize the necessity for "leading the receiver" when throwing to a moving partner.

Work on distance and then accuracy.

Skill Concepts Communicated to Children

>Keep eyes on target.
>The leg opposite the throwing arm is out in front.
>Turn shoulder toward target.
>The shoulder of the nonthrowing arm should point toward the target.
>Elbow is held away from the body.
>Ball is held with fingers and thumb positioned near the ear.
>Body weight moves from back foot to forward foot as ball is thrown.
>The elbow leads the way, followed by wrist.
>Swing rear foot forward and follow through.

Movement Enhancement

Throwing Enhancement Chart

	LEVEL
GAMES	
Beanbag Ring Throw	I
I Don't Want It Ring the Tire	I & II
Ball Toss Gap Ball Individual Dodgeball One Step Poison Circle Sock-It-to-Me-Ball 25 Throws	II
Can Can Canoes and Rapids Club Guard Skeet Ball	II & III
Catch Up Hand Grenade Snowball	III

CATCHING

Movement Description

Catching is a fundamental manipulative skill that involves stopping the momentum of an object and gaining control of it by use of the hands. During the early stages of catching, moving objects are first trapped (stopped and held) with one or more body parts. The acquisition of eye-hand coordination enables the child to attempt the manipulative skill of catching in which an aerial object is grasped and controlled through the use of the hands and sometimes the arms. Basically, the mature stage of catching is characterized by placing the hands in a position for effective reception of the aerial object, which is grasped with the hands in such a manner that control is demonstrated. A functional understanding of time-space relationships and the coordination to make the necessary bodily adjustments must be achieved before the child will be able to demonstrate a proficiency in catching a moving object.

By the age of 4 years, most children can successfully catch an aerial ball from the frontal horizontal plane. This is, however, primarily a cradling movement of the arms (trapping a large ball against the chest) and generally does not involve just the hands. Depending upon experience, children generally acquire mature pattern characteristics between 5 and 6½ years of age.

Elementary Stage

By 5 years of age, most children have usually progressed to the elementary stage of catching (Fig. 11–9). Standing in a stationary position, the child tracks the incoming aerial ball, and the eyes close only as contact with the ball is felt or sometimes immediately preceding contact. The arms are held slightly bent in front of the body and the child attempts to make initial contact with the hands prior to ball-arm contact. The timing of the grasp with the flight of the ball and the immature coordination of the two hands working together often necessitate the continued use of the upper body to help secure the ball (Fig. 11–10). Ball size becomes increasingly important during this stage. During the transition stage from arms predominant to hands predominant, the use of smaller balls will encourage grasping of the hands rather than scooping attempts of the arms. It is not uncommon for a child who can catch a large ball with the hands to regress to the trapping movements against the body with the initial change to smaller balls.

Mature Stage

By the age of 6½ years, most children demonstrate the mature stage of catching proficiency (Fig. 11–11) with large balls. From a stationary position, the child tracks the incoming aerial ball to final contact with the hands. The elbows are slightly bent as the arms are held relaxed at the sides or in front of the body. The

Figure 11-9 Elementary stage, catching. **Figure 11-10** Trapping the ball against the chest.

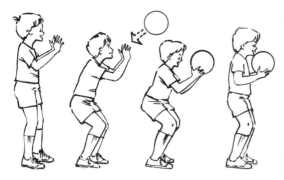

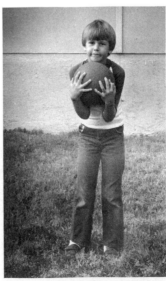

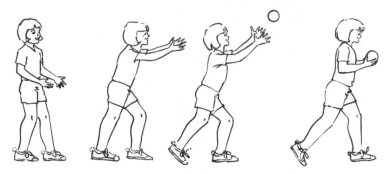

Figure 11-11 Mature stage, catching.

hands move forward to meet the approaching ball, which is caught solely with the cupped hands, as the force of the object is absorbed by hands and arms. At this stage, arm and body adjustments to variations in the flight of the ball are also attempted. The following characteristics summarize the movements associated with the mature catching pattern (ball traveling on the frontal horizontal plane):

Body is in alignment with incoming object.
Arms are held relaxed at sides and elbows flexed.
Hands and fingers are relaxed and slightly cupped and point toward the object.
Eyes follow the flight of the object.
Arms give upon contact to absorb the force, and fingers close around object.
Weight is transferred from front to back.

Both the elementary and mature stages of catching have all been characterized with the child in a stationary catching position. It should be noted that not until about 10 or 11 years of age are most children capable of perceptually judging flight projection from a nonpredetermined distance and angle. Such may be the case during many game and sport activities when the child attempts to catch a fly ball.

Movement Observation

Just as with throwing, many individuals fail to achieve the mature stage of catching because of lack of experience and/or lack of proper instruction. Along with varied practice conditions, children should be provided with feedback and reinforcement related to their performance. Several factors may affect catching performance: ball size, speed, and angle of approach. Although it is easier for children to catch a larger ball, their response tends to result in a more elementary form of catching, namely "trapping." The use of too small a ball may also produce undesirable responses. As a general rule, the ball should be large enough so that the child can cup it effectively, yet is not too small that a high degree of visual-motor control is required. Such factors should be kept in mind as the teacher observes catching performance. It is very easy to present tasks that are too difficult for the child to complete; thus appropriate tasks, keen observation, and feedback are vital to the attainment of optimal performance.

Common Problems
1. Failing to watch object until contact with hands ("watch the ball into your hands");
2. Failing to "give" with ball (as ball contacts hands, elbows should flex to "give" with impact);

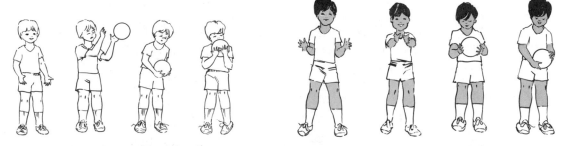

Figure 11–12 Check-sequence, catching.

3. Putting heels of hands together; thus object bounces out (hands should be held in opposition to each other, slightly apart to accommodate ball size, with thumbs held upward);
4. Keeping fingers straight and rigid; object bounces off and injury may occur (hands and fingers should be relaxed and slightly cupped);
5. Inability to vary the catching pattern for objects of different weights and sizes, and inability to adapt to objects approaching from various angles to the body (provide variability in practice);
6. Improper stance (feet should be slightly apart in forward stride position allowing weight to be transferred from front to back);
7. Reaching out to the side to catch; therefore not being in line with the incoming object (line body up with the object).

When assessing the throwing pattern, the following check-sequence illustration (Fig. 11–12) may prove helpful to the teacher.

Movement Variability

The importance of proficiency in catching to success in a variety of game and sport situations is obvious. Ample practice opportunities that are diverse and meaningful to the child are essential to the attainment of a mature schema and successful performance. The skill of catching can be utilized in numerous elementary game activities and in such refined sport areas as basketball, softball, baseball, soccer, team handball, and volleyball. Lacrosse requires an *absorbing* skill similar to that found in catching.

Spatial

MOVEMENT-PATTERN VARIATIONS

Catch with both hands; right hand; left hand.
Vary base of support (narrow to wide).
Overhand; underhand.
Catch object with hands at varied positions (examples):

Overhead (overhand)	Below waist (underhand)
Chest level (overhand)	At knees (underhand)
Body fully extended	To either side of the body

Body stationary
Body moving
Standing on one foot

DIRECTIONS/PATHWAYS/LEVELS

Moving: forward to catch an object
  backward to catch an object
  sideways to catch an object
  diagonally forward to catch an object
  diagonally backward to catch an object
  dodging (zigzag) prior to catching an object.
Low (sitting; full squat, back straight; lying-down positions)
High (jumping up)
Middle (partial squat)
Catching an object:
  incoming from front; side
  from various angles
  down from above.

Time

Reaction time/Rhythm
  Draw object to center of body quickly
  Draw object to center of body slowly
  Move slowly to catch an object
  Move quickly to catch an object
  Catch a slow- to fast-moving object
  Catch a bounced ball
  Juggling two or three objects.

Force

Vary weight and size of object caught   give with the object softly;
  (beachball, tennis ball,   forcefully
  Ping-Pong ball, playground ball,
  beanbag, volleyball, fleeceball,
  frisbee, football)

ADDITIONAL MOVEMENT VARIATIONS

Clap hands a number of times before catching objects.
Perform locomotor or nonlocomotor movement(s) before catching a released ball.
Throw and catch with a partner(s).
Catch a ball rebounding from the wall.
Catch and throw a ball to a rhythmic beat or music.
Catch a ball while rebounding from a mini-tramp.
Catch a deck tennis ring.
Catch a hula hoop rolling toward (away from, along side of) the participant.
Catch a bouncing ball; a rolling ball.
Catch with one eye closed.
Catch and toss lummi sticks with a partner (to rhythm).
Catch a small ball while playing jacks.
Catch with a scoop, glove, or carton.

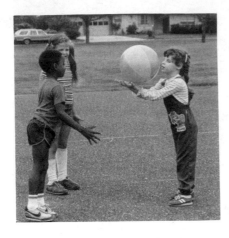

Sight-impaired children can play many games with verbal cues and appropriate equipment.

Teaching Hints

Use soft objects (beanbags, foam balls, yarn balls) with initial instructional periods.
Use objects that are highly colored.
Start with large objects and progress to smaller ones.
Let the students occasionally choose size of objects.
During initial learning experiences, provide the child with a background (from where the object is approaching) that does not provide complex figure-ground problems or distractions (auditory and visual).
Play games that emphasize catching and throwing.

Concepts Communicated to Children

Get in the path of the ball.
Stand with feet in forward stride position.
Curve fingers.
Keep one's eyes on the ball.
Reach for the ball.
Pull ball in toward body.
"Give" with the impact.

Movement Enhancement

Catching Enhancement Chart

GAMES	LEVEL		LEVEL		LEVEL
Ball Toss	II	Cross Over	II & III	Long Ball	III
25 Throws		Call Ball		Hot Ball	
Freeze Ball		Ring Toss		End-Zone Ball	
		Beach Ball		Overtake Ball	
		Bat Ball		Beanbags	
		Circle Ball		Hoop Activities	
		Beat Ball			
		Circle Stride Ball			
		Pass and Duck			
		Up the Field			
		One Step			

KICKING

Movement Description

Kicking is a manipulative skill pattern in which the foot is used to strike an object. The *placekick* (stationary ball) is the foundation for other kicking skills such as kicking a moving ball and punting. Good dynamic balance is critical to the development of successful kicking skills. *Dribbling* will also be discussed, because it represents a variable of the basic kicking pattern. The reader is reminded, however, that a consistently mature kicking pattern should be developed prior to attempting to dribble.

Elementary Stage

The elementary stage of kicking is characterized by the absence of a pronounced backswing as the kicking foot sort of jerks forward to push or punch at the ball. The arms are held sideways for balance and there is little follow-through as the arms are held sideways for balance (Fig. 11–13).

Mature Stage

In the mature stage (Fig. 11–14), the support foot is placed beside the object to be kicked and the kicking leg with knee bent swings freely from the hip through an arc toward the object to be kicked. The knee is quickly extended as the foot contacts the object and the body leans back for balance. The kicking leg continues its movement forward in the direction of the flight of the object. The eyes should be on the object at all times, and the arms should be relaxed and move in opposition with the legs.

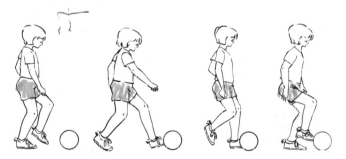

Figure 11-13 Elementary stage, kicking.

Figure 11-14 Mature stage, kicking.

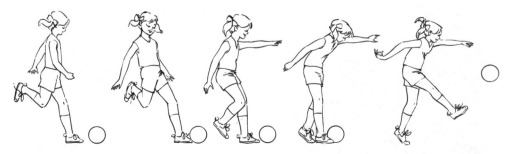

Movement Observation

Kicking is a unique game skill that requires dynamic balance from a small base of support. A general prerequisite ability to kicking is the ability to assume a balanced position on one leg (this occurs at approximately 2 years of age). As early as possible in the development of this skill, young children should be encouraged to kick for distance because this requirement encourages the child to move the kicking leg through a larger arc. The mature kicking pattern requires the kicker to use full range of hip and knee joints.

Children enjoy kicking, and when they are exposed to sufficient practice opportunities the skill can be acquired relatively early. However, the child often experiences difficulty when trying to kick in childhood games. When kicking a stationary ball, children are hampered by ineffective placement of the support foot. When punting, they experience difficulty controlling the drop of the ball, and when dribbling they experience difficulty controlling the path of the ball. The two main kicking skills—placekick and punt—require accurate foot placement of both support foot and kicking foot. In addition, the punt requires accurate timing of the kicking foot as it meets the descending ball. The dribble requires complex balance adjustments as well as a kinesthetic knowledge of the application of force placed on the ball. By the time children reach the age of 5 or 6 years, with appropriate experiences they should demonstrate the characteristics of a mature movement pattern. As the mature pattern becomes established and the ability to produce force increases (with age) the child begins to make more precise adjustments in accuracy with complex tasks such as punting and kicking a rolling, bouncing, and/or aerial ball.

Common Problems
PLACEKICK

1. Inadequate backswing (pushing action) from the hip of the kicking leg (encourage one or two steps prior to kicking);
2. Inaccurate placement of support foot (foot should be a "shadow" to the ball, that is, to the side and slightly behind);

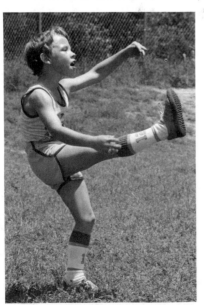

Full follow-through when punting.

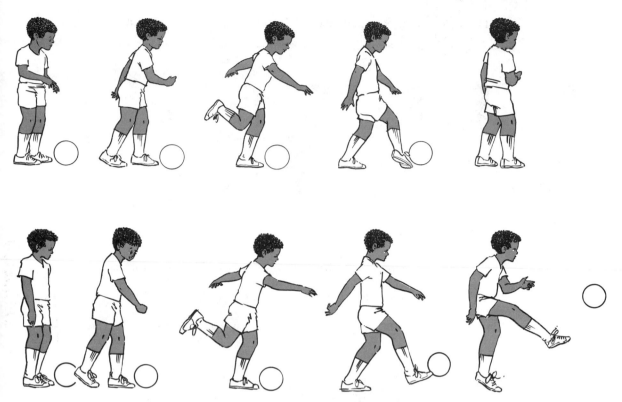

Figure 11–15   Check-sequence, place kick.

3. Lack of force (punching action) when striking the ball (leg should "whip" through the ball and arms should move in opposition);
4. Ball "pops up" (contact should be slightly below center; follow-through should be forward and toward the midline of the body);
5. Foot misses the ball completely (keep focus on the ball throughout the kick, and check position of body behind ball);
6. Ball rises dangerously soon after kicked (avoid placing toe "under the ball"; encourage "soccer type" side-of-the-foot kick).

When assessing the placekick pattern, the above check-sequence illustration (Fig. 11–15) may prove helpful to the teacher and child.

PUNT

1. Ball "pops" with little force (hold ball forward with outstretched arms and drop it straight down; contact is made on top of foot while leg is extended);
2. Insufficient force (take one or two preliminary steps, whip the kicking leg through the ball, look for the extended leg on follow-through);
3. Lack of balance while kicking and after kicking (hold ball in front of body, arms outstretched, move arms in opposition to legs during follow-through, lean trunk forward during follow-through, widen the base slightly);
4. Poor timing with the drop of the ball (arms are outstretched, ball is dropped—not pitched).

The following check-sequence illustration (Fig. 11–16) of the punt may prove helpful to teacher and child.

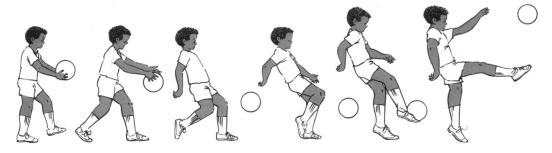

Figure 11-16   Check-sequence, punting.

DRIBBLE

1. Excessive force applied to the ball (take small steps and "tap the ball" using alternate feet);
2. Inability to control body balance (hold arms out for balance, take small steps, flex knees slightly);
3. Loss of control of ball (lightly "tap the ball," use side of foot nearest ball, avoid contact with toe of foot, "nudge" the ball in the direction of choice).

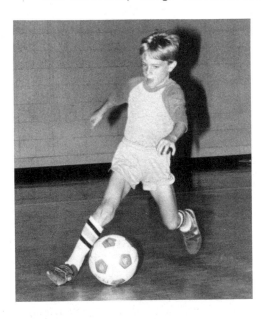

Dribbling.

Movement Variability

Children enjoy kicking objects and they should be encouraged to explore the various ways of kicking as soon as they have the balance required for running. A variety of objects of different sizes and weights should be supplied during practice variability, and kicking for distance should be encouraged initially as this promotes a full leg swing. Fundamental kicking skills are utilized in numerous low-organized and lead-up games as well as soccer and football. The kicking movement can also be found in dance and gymnastics.

Spatial
MOVEMENT-PATTERN VARIATIONS

(*Note*: Initial exploration should encourage the use of both feet for kicking.)

PLACEKICK:

Use inside, outside toe, heel, and instep of foot.
Kick from a prone position; supine position, crab position; squat position.
Kick standing; feet parallel (vary the distance apart).
Keep legs stiff.
Step into the kick (that is, run, walk).
Vary arm position (at sides, hands on hips, straight out in front).

PUNT

Stride stand; kicking leg back; arms straight forward; ball held with end of ball nearest the body; turned slightly to the kicking side.
Vary distance of feet apart.
Single step into the kick.
Multiple steps into the kick.

DRIBBLE

Use either side of foot and top of toe.

DIRECTIONS/PATHWAYS/LEVELS

forward
either side
diagonally right, left
under an object, through a hoop, over an object
zigzag pathway while dribbling
curved pathway.

Time

Execute kicking pattern slow to fast.
Kick to rhythm of music or drum.

Consecutive kicks (dribble).
Kick a ball repeatedly against a wall.

Force

Kick a light to heavy object lightly.
Kick a light to heavy object hard.

Kick for distance.
Kick for accuracy.
Kick for height.

ADDITIONAL MOVEMENT VARIATIONS

Kick a ball to barely avoid an obstacle.
Kick a ball to hit an obstacle.
Kick while running, leaping, galloping, sliding, or skipping.
Kick a ball back and forth with a partner.
Kick a ball to a person moving at various angles away and toward the ball.
Dribble a ball while maneuvering around objects and people.
Use imaginary movement stories that encourage kicking moves.
Use the kicking movement while dancing (see"Movement Enhancement").

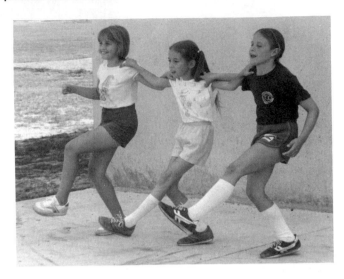

A kicking movement in dance.

Suggested General Progressions
(All tasks are for distance unless otherwise noted.)

1. Stationary child kicks a stationary ball forward.
2. Moving child kicks a stationary ball forward.
3. Stationary child kicks a ball that has been rolled straight to the child.
4. Moving child kicks a moving ball forward.
5. Stationary child punts a self-bounced ball.
6. While taking one step with nonkicking foot, child punts a dropped ball (emphasize distance, then accuracy, then distance/accuracy).
7. Child takes two steps (R, L) and punts (R) for distance, accuracy, distance/accuracy)
8. Stationary child kicks and punts ball to a partner.
9. Child dribbles in general space; no set pathways.
10. Child dribbles along a set straight pathway.
11. Child dribbles along a set curved pathway.
12. Child dribbles and passes laterally to a teammate repeatedly.
13. Child dribbles against an opponent.

Teaching Hints

Provide settings for distance kicking; mature kicking pattern should be established prior to focusing on accuracy.

Practice using both right and left foot.

Practice kicking in all directions.

Provide different sized, weighted, and shaped balls (round and elliptical; foam balls of all shapes are recommended).

Space children far enough apart so distance-kicking will be encouraged and safety hazards will be prevented.

When punting and placekicking, stress full follow-through.

When dribbling, stress short, soft, taps.

Frequently use the term "ball control" during dribbling practice.

Refrain from placing children in games until they have developed the control and balance necessary for safe and successful participation.

Encourage use of the kicking-movement pattern in combination with other fundamental skills (rhythmic locomotor/nonlocomotor work).

Relate kicking patterns used in dance to those used in maneuvering balls.

Provide additional balance work for those who need it.

Skill Concepts Communicated to Children

Keep eyes on the ball at all times.

Foot should contact ground ball just below midline of ball.

Drop (not toss) the ball to be punted.

Arms and legs work in opposition.

Kick "through" the ball for follow-through.

Inside-of-the-foot kick is best for controlling the height of the ball.

Center of gravity changes during a strong kicking movement, arms are important in maintaining balance.

Movement Enhancement

Kicking Enhancement Chart

	LEVEL
GAMES	
Circle Kick Ball	I–III
Hot Ball	
Kick the Pin	
Moon Soccer	
Boundary Ball	II & III
Place Kickball	
Crab Soccer	III
Battle Ball	
Circle Soccer	
Soccer Dodgeball	

The following dances can be used if the low kick (often combined with a hop) is used as a movement variation.

	LEVEL
DANCES	
Looby Loo	I & II
Hokey-Pokey	
Did you Ever See a Lassie?	
Hansel and Gretel	II & III
Seven Jumps	

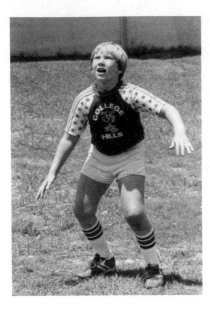

Figure 11-17   Good focus on the approach.

TRAPPING

Movement Description

Trapping is a receptive skill in which a ball is received and controlled by the body without the use of the hands. The trunk, legs, and feet are the body parts most frequently used to block the ball's flight and cause it to drop vertically to the ground and be controlled by the child. In the case of ground balls, the ball may be stopped or merely slowed down.

Elementary Stage

In the elementary stage the child meets the ball with an unyielding body. Only minimal attention is given to the direction of force of the object. The child's goal is simply to obstruct the ball's progress without using the arms or hands. Actual control is seldom accomplished during this stage.

Mature Stage

The mature stage of trapping is much like catching. The body is aligned with the oncoming ball and focus is maintained on the ball as the ball approaches the body (Fig. 11–17). Upon impact, the trunk, leg, or foot gives with the ball as the force is absorbed and the ball is controlled. As the ball falls to the ground the leg and/or foot is used to control the ball prior to it being propelled again. The arms are held relaxed and out from the body for balance.

Movement Observation

Trapping is a skill that is utilized in various games of low organization as well as the team sport of soccer. There are numerous ways to trap a ball. Initially, students should trap balls that come from directly in front of them. The sole-of-the-foot trap (Fig. 11–18a) and lower-leg trap (Fig. 11–18b) will offer the most control during this stage. Later progressions will include trapping a ball that is traveling along a diagonal path. The inside-of-the-foot trap will be more effective for balls traveling

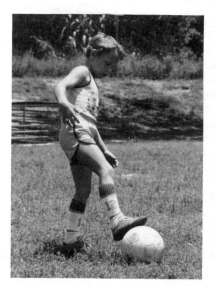
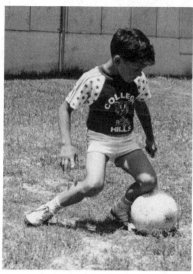

Figure 11-18   (a) Sole-of-the-foot trap; (b) lower-leg trap.

diagonally. As the child progresses to trapping moving balls while the body is also moving, considerable care must be taken to make sure the child maintains balance when making the necessary adjustments to receive the force of the ball effectively. When the ball is trapped with the sole of the foot, the child must understand the concept of retarding the force of the ball by allowing the foot to meet the ball softly, the object being to control the path of the ball and then to redirect the ball along a new path. An effective verbal cue such as "heel down, toe up" can serve as a skill-technique reminder. Whether using the sole of the foot or the inside of the foot, the child must be encouraged to absorb the force and then redirect the ball (that is, dribble or pass) as quickly as possible. When the ball is trapped with the leg or body, the concept of force absorption will help the child control the ball whose momentum is absorbed by the child's body and allowed to drop at the child's feet (Fig. 11–19).

Figure 11-19   Body absorption of force.

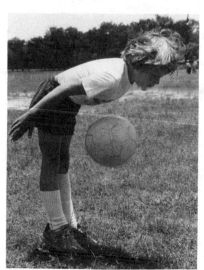

Common Problems

1. Failure to align the body with the path of the ball (keep eyes on the ball);
2. Inadequate visual tracking (eyes follow the ball until the ball contacts the body);
3. Failure to absorb the force of the ball, causing the ball to rebound off the foot (give as the ball contacts the body);
4. Transferring body weight to the ball, thus causing a fall (keep body weight on support foot and keep heel lower than the toe or sole-of-foot trap);
5. Failure to bend the knees when trapping with the legs (keep knees bent until ball is trapped between shins and ground).

Movement Variability

The similarities between catching and trapping should be emphasized as the child develops his or her trapping schema. With the growing interest in soccer in the United States, many elementary-grade children are very interested in their development of efficient eye-foot coordination skills. In soccer-type games the feet, legs, and body will be used to stop the momentum of the ball in a controlled manner.

Spatial
MOVEMENT-PATTERN VARIATIONS

Trap with chest, upper legs, lower legs, feet (right, and left)   Body stationary
Vary arm positions (up, horizontal, down)   Body moving
Vary the base of support (narrow to wide)

DIRECTIONS/PATHWAYS/LEVELS

While body is moving: forward, diagonally, sideways, and back to trap.
Body stationary and ball moving: toward, to left and right side, from behind, at angle toward.

> Levels: crouching the body to meet the ball
> high (springing into the air)
> middle (standing)
> low (partial squat, sitting, lying down).

Time

Trap while traveling in slow motion to a fast rate.
Trap a moving ball slowly to quickly.

Force

Trap a light to heavy object (fleeceball, nerfball, soccer ball).
"Give" lightly with the ball or forcefully trap it.

ADDITIONAL MOVEMENT VARIATIONS

Clap hands prior to the ball making contact with body.
Trap a ball and immediately send the ball sideways, diagonally, forward, backward.
Trap objects other than balls (beanbags, foam shapes).

Suggested General Progressions

1. While standing, trap a rolling ball coming from directly in front, using the sole-of-the-foot trap.
2. While standing, trap a rolling ball coming from directly in front using the lower-leg trap.
3. While standing, trap a rolling ball coming diagonally from the left or right, using the side-of-the-foot trap.
4. While standing, trap a bouncing ball coming from directly in front, from the left, from the right using the side-of-the-foot trap, thigh trap, or body trap.
5. While moving, repeat the traps described in items 1 through 4.

Teaching Hints

Provide a variety of different sized balls traveling at various speeds.

Use soft balls (yarn balls, nerf soccer balls, and partially deflated playground balls) in the early progressions.

Use soccer balls only after students are able consistently to trap lighter, softer balls.

Partially deflated balls are more easily controlled.

Use large beanbags at beginning of aerial ball-traps progression.

Keep children at lower progressions until contact with the ball is consistent (that is, consistently trap rolling ball, then bouncing ball, then aerial ball).

Emphasize the give of the body part(s) as contact is made with the ball.

Stress consistent eye contact with the ball.

Emphasize "heel down, toe up" for sole-of-the-foot trap.

Emphasize control of the ball after it is trapped.

Larger foot surface enables greater control.

Stress moving the ball immediately after the trap.

Skill Concepts Communicated to Children

Keep the eyes on the ball.

Line up the body with the path of the oncoming ball.

As the ball reaches the body part(s), "give" with the force of the ball; this may necessitate a slight jump backward.

Angle the body part(s) so ball will be deflected toward the ground.

Movement Enhancement

Trapping Enhancement Chart

	LEVEL
GAMES	
Circle Kick Ball Hot Ball	I–III
Boundary Ball	II & III
Crab Soccer Soccer Dodgeball Battle Ball Circle Soccer	III

BOUNCING/DRIBBLING

Movement Description

Bouncing and *dribbling*, manipulative skills requiring considerable eye-hand coordination, are means of propelling a ball in a downward direction. The development of bouncing originates as the child drops a ball, causing it to bounce, and attempts to strike the object repeatedly. As the child's ability progresses, control of the ball increases and the term *dribbling* is applied. It is at the dribbling stage that the child has learned to place the hand in relation to the center of the ball and meets the ball as is rebounds, maintaining contact with it as long as possible. Although few research studies have focused on this topic, the developmental sequence for ball bouncing/dribbling appears as follows:

1. Bouncing and catching;
2. Bouncing and "slapping" on the rebound;
3. Dribbling with the ball in control;
4. Dribbling with the child in control;
5. Advanced dribbling abilities such as utilized in basketball.

Along with the described developmental sequence, the child will generally exhibit the following proficiency characteristics (which may also be used as activity progressions):

1. Bounce with both hands and catch;
2. Bounce with dominant hand and catch;
3. Bounce with both hands repeatedly;
4. Bounce with dominant hand repeatedly;
5. Bounce with nondominant hand repeatedly;
6. Alternate hand while bouncing continuously;
7. Dribble (continuously and with control) with either hand and alternating;
8. Dribble and traveling.

While some 2-year-olds may exhibit a degree of proficiency in two-hand bouncing, it is not until approximately 5 or 6 years of age that the mature pattern is mastered.

Elementary Stage

At the elementary stage of development (Fig. 11–20) the child, while performing at a somewhat successful level, generally exhibits the following characteristics:

1. While striking the ball, the fingers are together and stiff.
2. The striking action is from the shoulder or wrist only, resulting in slapping.
3. The hand is repelled from the ball at time of contact.
4. Control of bouncing is not continuous.
5. Ball rebounds to a level other than at the waist.

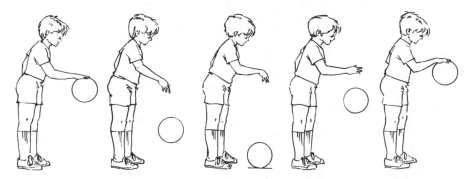

Figure 11-20 Elementary stage, dribbling.

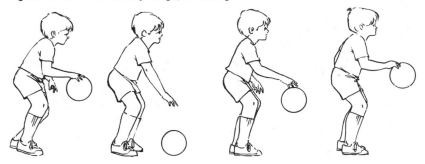

Figure 11-21 Mature stage, dribbling

Mature Stage

The following characteristics are found in the mature pattern stage (Fig. 11–21) of one-hand ball dribbling:

1. Feet placed in a narrow stride position and the body flexed at knees, hips, and waist, with a slight forward trunk lean.
2. The ball is contacted with fingers spread and propelled (pushed) to the floor by elbow extension and follow-through.
3. Height of bounce is maintained at waist level.
4. Focus is occasionally on the ball, but student is also able to focus away from the ball.

Two aspects of ball bouncing and dribbling—bouncing to another individual and foot dribbling—are discussed in separate sections ("throwing" and "kicking").

Movement Observation

As previously mentioned, while some 2-year-olds may exhibit some degree of ball-bouncing proficiency, it is generally not until approximately 5 or 6 years of age that the ability to repeatedly bounce a ball is acquired. At this stage eye focus is constantly on the ball and there is little locomotor movement. Both experience and visual-motor control in the form of eye-hand coordination are essential to the acquisition of ball-handling skills. A lack of coordination (that is, timing) between visual information and motor response may account for many of the problems associated with poor performance.

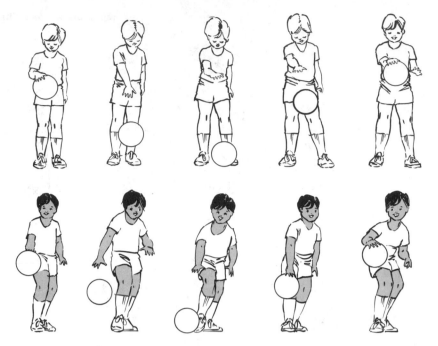

Figure 11-22 Check-sequence, dribbling.

Common Problems

1. Using the flat part of the hand to slap the ball (use fingers to push the ball and ride back with the rebounding ball);
2. Bouncing the ball too high or too low (consistent force should be applied to maintain ball at waist level);
3. Inability to maintain a stationary position while dribbling (if this is the desired task);
4. Poor concentration on the ball;
5. Insufficient follow-through, causing the ball not to return to waist level (the hand should meet the ball as it rebounds, maintaining contact as long as possible while the arm pushes with follow-through of arm, wrist, and fingers).

When assessing the bounce/dribble pattern, the following check-sequence illustration (Fig. 11–22) may prove helpful to both the teacher and child.

Movement Variability

While bouncing/dribbling are basically task-oriented game and sport skills, they do provide the child with opportunities for increasing the general schema, which is important to overall conceptualization and motor control of objects. Along with utilization in numerous elementary game activities, dribbling is also applied to the sport activities of basketball, speedball, and team handball.

Spatial
MOVEMENT-PATTERN VARIATIONS

Using two hands

Using one hand (dominant and nondominant)

Changing hands

While stationary

While moving

Vary base of support (wide to narrow)

DIRECTION/PATHWAYS/LEVELS

| While moving body: forward; backward sideward (left and right) diagonally changing directions | While moving body: over, under and around objects in circles zigzag curved line changing pathways | Low level (on knees, squatting, sitting) Medium level (standing) High level (on toes, while jumping) |

Moving the ball at various points from the body (in front, to side, under legs, around legs).

Time

While moving (traveling) slow to fast
Moving ball slow to fast

To music accompaniment or rhythmic beat

Force

Vary size and weight of ball (junior size basketball, volleyball, playground balls 7 to 10 in., rhythm balls).

Push soft to hard (ball at low to high level; below knees, waist).

ADDITIONAL MOVEMENT VARIATIONS

Outline letters, names, words.
Join with a partner(s); to the same beat; alternating balls.
Go through an obstacle course (chairs, hoops, cones, under and over ropes).
Perform while blindfolded.
Perform while following lines on the floor (straight, curved, zigzag, circles).
Play one-on-one with a partner.
Perform other movements between bounces (twist, spin, turn, squat, jump).
Use different locomotor skills while bouncing/dribbling (walk, jog, run, leap, skip, gallop, hop, slide).
Jump over and/or move under the ball as it rebounds.
Create a dribbling routine (music enhances this activity).
Dribble while moving up and down stairs.
On different surfaces (concrete, wood, carpet, tile, dirt).

Teaching Hints

Provide the child with a medium sized and weighted ball (8- to 9-inch playground ball) before force (weight and size) -variability activities are presented.
Keep in mind the stages of ball-bouncing progression and provide variability around these stages.
Do not use enhancement activities (games) that require a high level of ball control before such abilities are reasonably acquired.
After the child has achieved a degree of proficiency with the dominant hand, provide practice with the nondominant side.
Stress eye focus on the ball during initial learning periods and work toward kinesthetic (that is, a sense of "feel" for where the ball is) awareness with the advanced child.

Concepts Communicated to Children

Keep one's eyes on the ball.
Control the bounce with the fingers and wrist.
Push the ball slightly forward and downward.
Follow through.
Keep the level of the ball below the waist.

Movement Enhancement

Bouncing/Dribbling Enhancement Chart

GAMES	LEVEL
Ball Race Bounce Ball Call Ball	I & II
Two Square (and Four Square)	II & III
Bucket Ball Wall Ball	III

STRIKING

Movement Description

Striking is an action in which the hand(s) or an implement is used to give impetus to an object. As a skill, striking does not present well-defined sequences. The child may be confronted with numerous striking situations that require the use of the hand(s), head, or various implements to hit stationary or moving objects (usually balls). Striking patterns may be influenced greatly by the size, weight, and length of the implement, as will the nature of the object struck. Kicking, also considered a striking task, is treated separately because of its importance as a fundamental skill.

Striking develops in much the same sequential order as throwing in terms of general age-level performance. This is dependent, however, upon movement opportunities and availability of developmentally appropriate equipment (that is, weight and size). This skill appears to start from the overarm motion, as in throwing, with the child facing the object and primarily utilizing the arms and hands. This method of striking an object is replaced with the underarm and most commonly used sidearm pattern (across a horizontal plane); however, the initial selection of pattern is highly dependent on the position of the object in space. By three years of age, the child may be observed using the sidearm striking motion, with one arm being the primary initiator of the movement. The more common employment of both arms, such as in batting, is generally not exhibited even at a minimal proficiency level until the child is 4 to 5 years of age.

Children who are given special assistance with equipment of appropriate weight and size tend to progress faster from striking in a vertical plane (that is, facing the object squarely, extending the forearms, striking downward) to the more effective motion predominating in a horizontal plane.

Elementary One-Arm Striking Pattern

This pattern is generally performed with the use of the preferred hand or implement. The child exhibiting an immature pattern will (if attempting to strike an object directly in front) utilize an overarm motion (Fig. 11–23).

The legs are usually stationary, or a forward step is presented with a unilateral (that is, same arm-leg) pattern. The trunk is bent forward slightly, and little if any trunk rotation is present.

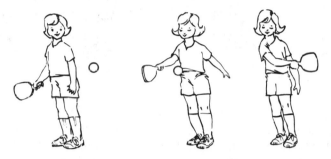

Figure 11–23 Elementary stage, one-arm striking.

Mature One-Arm Striking Pattern

Before contact is desired, weight is shifted to the back foot, while the trunk rotates approximately 45° to 90° to a cocked position. With the hand drawn back, force is delivered quickly as the weight shifts (forward), body rotates, and the arm moves horizontally to contact the object. Force is maximized as the child exhibits follow-through in the predetermined direction (Fig. 11–24).

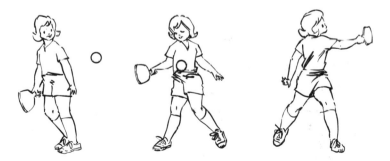

Figure 11–24 Mature stage, one-arm striking.

Two-Arms (Batting)

As with the immature one-arm pattern, initial attempts using both hands reveal a downward vertical swing (Fig. 11–25). The child faces the object squarely, bends forward at the trunk, and extends the forearms. Much of the force is delivered as the wrists are uncocked. As the skill develops, the child attempts to strike the object using a sidearm pattern. In the early attempts, the arms initiate most of the movement, for there is limited weight shift, hip and trunk rotation, and follow-through. The pelvis and trunk rotate as a unit, appearing to be a result of the forward arm motion rather than force initiated.

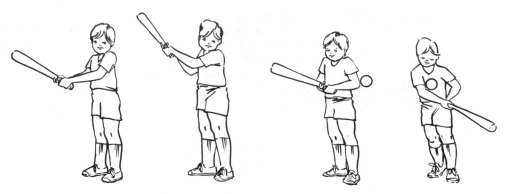

Figure 11-25 Elementary stage, batting.

Mature Batting Pattern

The child reveals characteristics of a mature pattern (Fig. 11–26) by initiating movement with a forward weight shift, rotation of the hips and trunk, followed by a smooth arm swing. The wrists are uncocked just before contact with the object.

In greater detail, the preparatory and executory phases of mature two-arm striking (horizontal) may be described (and used for assessment) as follows (Wickstrom, 1983):

1. Feet positioned approximately shoulder-width apart. Body position is perpendicular to the line of flight of the oncoming ball.

Figure 11-26 Mature stage, batting.

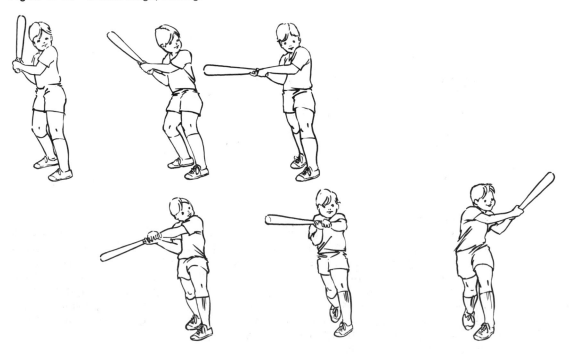

2. Trunk is rotated to the right (for right-handed batters); weight is shifted onto the right foot.
3. The lead elbow is held up and out from the body with the bat held off the shoulder. Striking arm moves back parallel to path of oncoming ball.
4. Eyes follow the flight of the ball until just before contact is made (visual tracking).
5. Body weight shifted forward (onto opposite foot) in the direction of intended hit.
6. Hips and trunk rotated in direction of intended hit with the hips leading.
7. Arms move "forward" into contact and follow-through action.

Wickstrom (1983) indicates that although each striking skill (one-arm, two-arm variations) has its own unique characteristics, all contain a basic sequence of three movements: step–turn–swing. Those movements are described as follows:

1. Body weight is shifted in the direction of the intended hit while shoulders and arms are coiled in the opposite direction.
2. Hips and spine are rotated in rapid succession in the same direction as the weight shift.
3. Arm(s) swings around and forward in close succession with the other rotatory movements.

Although not described in this section, other striking variations utilized by children such as striking in volleyball-type activities also contain elements of the basic sequence described.

Movement Observation

Although the young children may exhibit a proficient striking form, another developmental factor, *coincident timing*, especially of a moving object, may present difficulties in the performance outcome. Each striking task presents the child with a unique timing situation. Developmentally appropriate activities are essential for outcome success. It is highly unlikely that a child under the age of seven could successfully strike (with bat) a ball thrown fast by another child of the same age. This acknowledgment by youth-sport administrators may be observed in the form of a sport modification called T-Ball (that is, the ball rests on a stand). Children can, however, acquire with some degree of movement and outcome proficiency most striking skills (especially with slow or stationary objects) if given the advantage of developmentally appropriate equipment and practice.

Evaluation checklists may be developed from basic sequence items described, and descriptive components from one- and two-arm patterns; see Table 11–1 for an example.

Common Problems

1. Failure to contact object (if speed of the object is within the perceptual capability of the child, failure to focus visually on the object is a probable cause). Another is lack of practice with timing. Have the child practice watching the object and timing the act; first from a stationary position ("T"-stand or ball, on top of cone) and then suspended on a string;
2. Striking an object while standing with too narrow or too wide a base of support (approximately shoulder-width apart);
3. Rotating body too little; failure to rotate the body backward (twist the body away from the direction one plans to hit);

Table 11-1 Checklist For Striking

	Successful	Needs Extra Practice	Comments
STATIONARY/PITCHED BALL (ONE-ARM)			
Side-stride foot position			
Rotation through hips and torso			
Arms moves horizontally			
Ball contacted opposite forward foot			
Path of swing elongated with follow-through			

4. Keeping the elbow in too close to the body when arm action is involved (hold arms away from body, "wings up");
5. Striking a hard object with relaxed fingers and arm (if using hand only, think of the hand as a solid club head);
6. Failure to use sufficient backswing (the body should rotate approximately 90°, and the implement move through an arc of 180° before contact; bat should be held back during stance so less time is spent on backswing);
7. Failure to grip implement tightly (tighten–release–tighten grip for awareness);
8. Striking an object too far above (topping) or below, lifting its center of gravity (meet the ball squarely);
9. If striking a moving object, failure to get in line with it before contact (body weight should shift in the direction of the intended hit while shoulders and arms are coiled in the opposite direction; focus on ball and position the body appropriately prior to contact);
10. Failing to follow-through after the object has been contacted (move implement through the ball);
11. Lack of power (probable causes: facing incorrectly, poor weight shift, incomplete extension of forearms and wrists, weak grip, lack of follow-through, and improper contact with object).

Movement Variability

The diverse nature of striking requires the child to be familiar with several implements (varying in size and weight) in varying circumstances of object position and timing; therefore, variability in practice is essential for general striking competency. Such practice would allow the child opportunities to perform under a multitude of spatial, force, and timing conditions. Various forms of striking are fundamental to many primary movement activities, and they are used extensively in such advanced sports as volleyball, tennis, golf, racquetball, handball, baseball, and hockey.

Spatial
MOVEMENT-PATTERN VARIATIONS

Using one- and two-arm variations:
  overarm
  sidearm
  underarm
  oblique (golf-type swing)
  backhand
Ball:
  stationary
  swinging
  vertical bounce
  moving toward

vary foot placement:
  shoulder width
  narrow to wide

strike while in:
  personal space
  moving

DIRECTIONS/PATHWAYS/LEVELS

Vary level: (ground to reach height) and position of object in space
Vary level of body while striking:
  lying
  sitting
  kneeling
  squatting
Strike from above, below, side, and straight forward.
Lean forward, backward, and sideward while striking.
Strike object to fly in different directions.

Time
Striking: stationary object; swinging slow to fast
        an object moving toward slow to fast
        an object from various distances of origin

Force

Striking with: soft to hard impact
          light to heavy implements
          implements of varying sizes

ADDITIONAL MOVEMENT VARIATIONS

Strike: objects against wall
     objects over barriers (nets, ropes)
     objects to contact a target

Use of (examples):

either hand	beanbags
large paddles (plastic preferred)	balloons
Ping-Pong paddles	foam balls
racquetball rackets	whiffleballs
tennis rackets	tennis balls
badminton rackets	yarn balls
plastic bats	racquetball balls
plastic clubs (golf type)	Ping-Pong balls
plastic hockey-type sticks	shuttlecocks

Suggested General Progressions

Strike:

A stationary ball placed on floor with hand (alternate hands);

A ball being rolled back and forth between hands;

A ground ball with hand(s) to a partner;

A ball off batting tee (or cone) with hand(s);

A suspended ball with hand;

A balloon with hand(s) and lightweight implements;

A suspended ball with implements (moving from short handle to long handle);

A balloon with others (keeping it up);

An object held in hand;

A bounced ball first with the hand, then with lightweight racket;

A stationary ball off tee with lightweight bat;

A ball swinging suspended from a rope with hand, then with implement;

An object on floor with club (hockey stick or pillo polo club);

A thrown ball lightly after it bounces once;

A ball rebounding from a wall;

A moving object on floor with hockey-type stick;

A ball thrown underhand with implement (for instance, a scoop);

A ball thrown overhand with implement;

A ball that you toss into the air with implement;

A moving object hit with implement while moving.

Teaching Hints

Before learning striking skills, the child must demonstrate the ability to track an object approaching from various angles.

Prior to actual striking (with an implement), the child should be given opportunities to hold a short implement and make pathways in the air at various levels and in various directions from the body. Free-swinging movements should be emphasized.

Extensive work with short streamers will help the child acquire the relaxed swing necessary for effective striking.

Imagery such as "the arm acting like a swinging gate" is encouraged.

Objects to be hit should range from large to small, light to heavy.

Light objects such as balloons, nerf balls, and beach balls will help allay "fear of the ball."

Check frequently for proper grip.

Encourage "floating elbows" away from the body.
Stress follow-through in initial instruction.

Skill Concepts Communicated to Children

The top hand should touch the bottom hand when using both arms to strike.
Keep the eyes on the ball right up to contact.
Shift the body weight from back to forward when beginning the swing.
The bat should only have to be moved forward when the decision is made to strike.
Arms and wrists are extended on impact with the object.
Allow the arms to continue swinging after impact (follow-through).
Follow-through is in the direction one wants the object to go.
The swing should be level—like a swinging gate.
Feet remain in contact with the ground when contacting the ball.
The bottom hand is the last hand to let go as the bat is dropped by the side.

Movement Enhancement

Striking Enhancement Chart

	LEVEL
GAMES	
Beach Ball Nerfs Hot Rolls	I & II
Ball and Stick Relay Two Square (Four Square) Toppleball Call Ball	II & III
Bat Ball Fistball Tetherball	III

REFERENCE

WICKSTROM, R. L. (1983). *Fundamental motor patterns* (3rd ed.). Philadelphia: Lea & Febiger.

12

MOVEMENT-
AWARENESS THEMES

BODY AWARENESS

Movement Description

Body awareness is the impression the child has of one's own body parts and their capabilities for movement. Body awareness, sometimes called "body image" or "body schema," is essential to efficient movement and is the foundation of total movement awareness. Development of a child's body schema involves (1) identifying and locating one's body parts, (2) understanding their relationship to each other, (3) knowing how to use the body parts, and (4) understanding their capabilities.

An important part of the young child's vocabulary should be the names of body parts. The child's movement experiences should enhance body-part recognition and allow body-part relationships to develop the body schema progressively.

The young child first learns to identify body parts by name and then is capable of understanding their relationship to each other, how they are used, and the variety of movement capabilities for each.

Although most 5-year-olds can identify and locate the majority of their body parts, they should be evaluated on their ability to do so by means of a checklist before other body-awareness activities are attempted.

Movement Observation

A child's body-awareness capabilities can be evaluated by observing a game of "Simon Says" where the leader verbally asks the group to touch different body parts. Children should be able to locate the following body parts:

ears	mouth	nostrils	buttocks	fingers
eyebrows	chin	shoulders	arms	hands

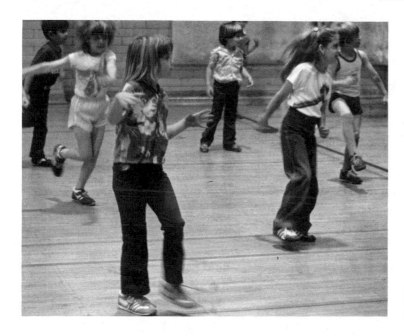

Body awareness involves a knowledge of how the various body parts can move.

eyelashes	cheeks	chest	elbows	wrists
hair	nose	back	thigh	waist
hips	stomach	forehead	knees	feet
toes	soles	heels	fingernails	scalp
ankles	trunk	spine	neck	earholes
lips	tongue	side	forearm	thumb
palm	knuckles	calves	legs	

Children can also be asked to use various parts of the body to do something, as in the following examples:

Stamp your feet	Twist your neck
Clap your hands	Nod your head
Wiggle your nose	Snap your fingers
Open your mouth	Shrug your shoulders
Bend your knees	Close your eyes
Bend your elbows	Wiggle your toes

The teacher can very effectively use a checklist to help identify children who have problems with the above activities.

Common Problems

1. Errors or slowness in response to touching and using the correct body parts (physically move the correct body part as a cue for the child);
2. Hesitancy in movements (give positive feedback immediately when beginning correct responses);
3. Inability to extend or contract different body parts fully (physically manipulate the body part for the child until the child gets the feel of the full range of motion);
4. Inability to coordinate the movement of two body parts at the same time.

Movement Variability

Development of a solid body schema is essential to all motor-skill development. Body-awareness activities will serve to enhance the following:

1. A vocabulary and awareness of names and location of essential movement parts of the body;
2. The relationship of one body part to another;
3. The ability to move and be aware of the role and capabilities of body parts (understanding what and how we move);
4. The ability to contract and relax specific muscle groups.

These are all essential components of meaningful movement and, as such, comprise the fundamental basis of all game, dance, and gymnastic activities.

Combining Body Awareness With a Motor Program
Spatial

MOVEMENT-PATTERN VARIATIONS

Move as many different body parts as possible while:
sitting,
standing,
lying on back, stomach,
lying on side,
kneeling,
balancing on one, two, three, four, or five body parts.
Move one part at a time all around as many different places as it will reach, then move several different parts the same way.
Move different body parts while moving across the floor using different locomotors (walking, running, skipping, hopping; try some novel patterns too).

DIRECTIONS/PATHWAYS/LEVELS

Move individual body parts:
forward,
backward,
sideways,
at a high or low level,
tracing different pathways in the air; try straight, curved, zigzag.
Move two different body parts at the same time:
both in the same direction,
in opposite directions,
at the same level,
at different levels,
with the same pathway,
tracing different pathways.
Move different body parts at one time in the same direction; in different directions.

Time

Move individual body parts:
fast,
slow,

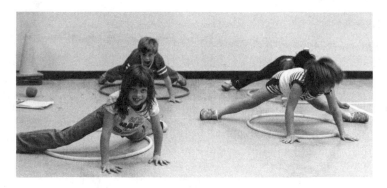

Children place body parts in relationship to hoops.

accelerating their speed,
decelerating their speed,
in time to musical accompaniment,
to a drum beat.
Move two different body parts at:
the same speed,
different speeds.
Contract and extend different limbs quickly, then very slowly.

Force

Move individual body parts:
smoothly,
roughly or jerkily,
hard,
soft,
while airborne,
with a stable base.
Move two or more body parts with the same force or different force.
Extend a body part farther then before.
Hold a body position longer and longer each time.

ADDITIONAL MOVEMENT VARIATIONS

1. Use flash cards to:
   a. Show figures with missing body parts; children move missing part.
   b. Show individual body parts; children identify and move shown body part or try to hide the diagrammed part. Children can try to touch shown body parts with a partner's same body part.
   c. Show body in relation to walls or objects; children imitate the position shown on the card: O is a hoop, X is the child.
   d. Show the direction different body parts face in relation to objects and walls: O is a hoop, → represents the direction the body part should point.
2. Using verbal commands, have children show body part relations to different walls. Use wall identifications like:
   a. pictures
   b. outstanding physical features
   c. outside objects
   d. geographic locations; north, south, east, and west.

Examples:
a. Sit with elbows pointing toward the number wall.
b. Lie down with head toward the animal wall.

3. Move body parts in relation to other body parts; for example, move with elbows behind feet; move with feet higher than head.

4. Move an object in relation to body parts. Move beanbag around knee.

5. Move body in relation to an object. Move under the rope feet first. Balance with hands inside and feet outside the hoop.

6. Move body in relation to an object and a wall. Balance with one foot inside the hoop pointing toward the north wall and one hand inside the hoop pointing toward the east wall.

7. Play "one behind." Instructor touches body parts and children stay one behind by beginning to touch the same body part after the instructor has touched the second body part. Use verbal cues also.

8. Laterality (left-right recognition) may be enhanced by asking the children to move right- and left-side parts ("Lift your right leg," "Close your left eye"). Example: With children lying on their backs, ask them to move various parts, such as:
Lift your legs
Lift your arms
Touch your elbow to your chest
Lift your right arm
Touch your ankles together
Touch your knees
How many parts can you lift off the floor at one time?

9. Paste one part of a body such as the eyes or nose (cut out from magazines) on paper and have the child draw the rest of the person. Draw incomplete faces or stick people on paper to be mimeographed and distributed for completion.

10. State and ask the children to complete the following:

I comb my	(hair)	I snap my	(fingers)
I shrug with my	(shoulders)	I smell with my	(nose)
I squat with my	(hips, knees)	I throw with my	(hand, arm)
I kneel on my	(knees)	Food goes to my	(stomach)
I write with my	(fingers)	I hear with my	(ears)
I taste with my	(mouth, tongue)	I wave with my	(hand)
I clasp with my	(hands)	I walk with my	(feet)
I bend at the	(waist, elbow, knee)	I lick with my	(tongue)
I brush my	(hair, teeth)	I catch with my	(hands)
I sleep on my	(back, side)	I jump with my	(feet)
I kick with my	(feet)	I see with my	(eyes)
I chew with my	(teeth)	I wear earrings on my	(ears)
I wear a belt around my	(waist)		

11. Identify the following joints by name and ask the children to move them in as many positions as possible; then ask the following:
How many ways can you move your neck? What movements can you make with your toes? Will your fingers move side to side? Up and down? Can you move your hips around in a circle shape? Which body part can be moved the least, your shoulders or waist? Show me how your knees move when you run, walk, skip, jump.

12. Cut pictures of people from magazines and then cut into smaller pieces and have the children reassemble. Paper dolls may be cut and reassembled also.

13. Have the children outline each other on large sheets of paper. Instruct them to color a designated part of the outlined body in a specific color.

14. Have the children make people using vegetables (carrots, corn, peppers), marshmallows, gum drops. Attach paper parts for the body with glue, or use toothpicks if preferred.

15. *Space*
Make shadow designs using an opaque projector or other light source. The child stands with back to the light and casts a shadow on the screen or wall. Ask questions, or direct activities such as:
    a. "Move only your fingers, now your toes, your head, your elbows. Keep watching your shadow as you move them in many ways."
    b. "How many different ways can you make your arms bend? What part of your arm bends? [elbow] Can you make your arms bend at the elbow and then stretch them out again? Watch your shadow as you move." Same sequence, but with legs (bend at the knee), head (bend at the neck), feet (bend at the ankle), hands (bend at the wrist), body (bend at the hips).
    c. "Can you make a design with your shadow? What else can you make your shadow do? Can it jump up? Can it hop? Can it walk? Can it run in place? Can it leap? Can it skip?"
    d. "See what else your shadow can do."

16. *Human Sticks*
Six children work together to make the shape (with their bodies) of a human stick figure lying on the floor. At first, parts may be assigned: "John, you be the head." "Sara, you be the right arm."
Once the body is made, the parts may move. "Sara, you are the right arm. Can you make it stretch? How else can you make the arm move?" Do the same with other children. You may ask the children to respond to commands such as: "Bend the right leg. Raise the right arm. Bend the left arm."

17. *Body-Part Jumping*
Draw a large stick figure of a person (use tape or chalk) on the floor for each child. The children are asked to hop or jump from one body part to another.
    a. "Can you stand on the head and jump to the neck?"
    b. "Can you jump from the neck to the right hand?"
    c. "Jump from the right hand and see if you can land on the waist."
    d. "Can you jump from the waist to the left hand?"
    e. "Now try jumping from the left hand to the left foot."
    f. "See if you can jump from the left foot to the right foot."
    g. "Stand on the right foot. Can you walk up the right leg, jump to the head, and then walk backwards to the left foot?"
    h. "Stand on the right hand. Can you hop on one foot to the left hand?" Many other variations are possible and should be used.
    i. "Stand in front of your stick figure. I will call out the name of a body part, and you run and stand on it as fast as you can. When I blow the whistle come back and stand in front of your stick figure ready for the next call. Head!" Pause long enough to be sure that every child has responded correctly, then blow the whistle. "Leg!" And so forth.

18. *Build a Floor Body*
Using beanbags, boxes, cans, hoops, balls, wands, ropes, build a body on the floor.
    a. "Can you build a human body using the boxes, hoops, cans, beanbags, and other materials you see here?"
    b. When the children have finished, ask them to study for several minutes the body they created. Afterward, take the different parts, stack them in a pile, and see how quickly they can put the body back together again. For added interest let the children give their body a name (Fred, Sam, Hazel, Lucy). "Let us take 'Sam' apart and stack him in a pile. When the whistle blows, see how fast you can put 'Sam' back together again."

19. *Space Walk*

Use a gym floor, sidewalk, or other open area on which patterns may be painted or taped. Directions may be painted beside each floor pattern, such as: hop right, hop left, and so forth. Children start at the beginning and follow the painted space walk. The space walk may include anything the teacher deems necessary. If directions are placed on movable cones instead of being painted on the sidewalk they may be changed periodically. Children unable to read may be talked-through the space walk by the teacher.

20. Discovering body awareness is a partnership. Divide the children into partners. Explain that together they have 4 hands, 4 feet, 2 heads, 4 elbows, and so forth. Moving across and attached in any manner, the children must solve a series of movement problems. Examples:

a. "Can you [both] move across the mat with only three feet touching the mat?"
b. "With six parts of your body touching?"
c. "Can you move to the other side without touching the mat with your feet?"
d. "Show me a movement with one elbow touching the other's ankle."
e. "Move across knee to knee and try to be different from the others."

21. *Relationships with Mirror Activities*

Have a child stand in front of a full-length mirror. The other children give directions to locate body parts. The child can only look at his or her reflection in the mirror when touching the designated part with one hand. Upon making a mistake, the child giving the last instruction takes the mirror position.

a. Repeat the above activity, but have the child use both hands to touch the body.
b. Repeat the above activities but indicate the right or left parts of the body in the mirror reflection.

Teaching Hints

Use physical manipulation and touching of different body parts to help children identify their parts.

Have children draw pictures of the movement of different body parts.

Use flash cards to cue children on body parts and positions.

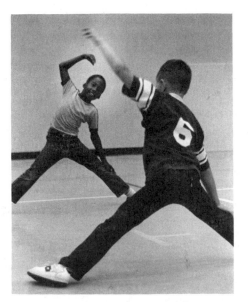

Mirror games enhance body awareness.

The use of rhymes and songs help children remember their body parts. Use a jointed doll to demonstrate where the body bends.

Skill Concepts Communicated to Children

All body parts have specific names.
One body part can lead a movement.
Muscles can contract and relax.
A contraction makes muscles shorter.

Movement Enhancement

Body Awareness Enhancement Chart

	LEVEL		*LEVEL*		*LEVEL*
GAMES		*GYMNASTICS*		*DANCE/RHYTHMS/RHYMES*	
Command Cards	I–III	Blow Up the Balloon	I & II	Tall and Small	I & II
Beanbags		Jack in the Box		Reach to the Skies	
Follow the Leader		Pogo Stick		Two Little	
				My Hands	
Hoop Hop	I & II	Stand Up	II & III	This Is the Circle	
Charlie Over the Water		Turk Stand		That Is My Head	
		Knee Walks		Make a Fist	
Hot Ball	II & III	Balance Stands		Rest Rhyme	
Chinese Hurdle		Tripod		Hokey-Pokey	
Skin the Snake		Wring the Washrag		Looby Loo	
Frozen Beanbag		Tummy Balance		Did You Ever See	
Deep Freeze		Rocking Horse		a Lassie?	
In the Creek		Egg Sit			
		Balance Board Activities		Heads, Shoulders,	II & III
		Human Bridge		Knees, and Toes	
		Side Balance		Where Is Thumbkin?	
		People Pyramids		Seven Jumps	
		Thread the Needle			

SPATIAL AWARENESS

Movement Description

The ability to orient oneself to the position of other people and objects in space and the knowledge of how much space the body occupies is fundamental to all movement. *Spatial awareness,* an extension of body awareness, relies on and may be considered a primary element of the visual modality. Children possessing this awareness are more likely to become adept at maneuvering themselves in a constantly changing environment without collisions. An extension of spatial awareness, namely *directional awareness,* which enables the child to perceive the dimension of objects in space and their position in relation to themselves, is considered to be an important readiness skill for both reading and writing as well as fundamental movement. Directional awareness and its components—*laterality* and *directionality*—are discussed in a separate section of this chapter because the development of this awareness is vitally important to both academic and movement success.

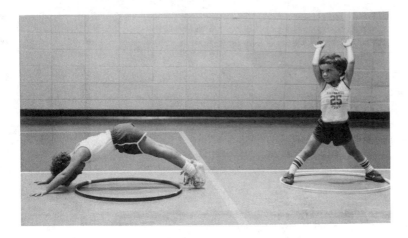

Movement Observation

The child's spatial awareness is developed to a degree upon entrance into kindergarten; however, a heightened awareness is essential to success in the school environment. Children should exhibit a knowledge of how much space their bodies occupy, an internal awareness of left and right, the ability to move their bodies into general space without collisions, and the ability to locate objects in space in relation to themselves and other objects. The key to spatial awareness is developing a keen visual perception of the position of objects in space in relation to oneself and other objects.

The development of spatial awareness occurs in two phases; thus evaluation of this awareness should also be divided into two parts. The child is first able to locate objects in relation to his or her own body position in space (*egocentric localization*). This ability can be observed by positioning the child in relation to an object in space. A school desk, a chair, or a bench is a good object to use as these provide a full range of relationship possibilities. The child should demonstrate the following body-position relationships:

over	near to
under	far from
beside	around
in front of	across and between (two desks or objects)
behind	

The second phase, *objective localization*, is the ability to locate two or more objects in relation to each other and independent of oneself. The child demonstrates the development of this awareness by positioning two different objects in space and observing the following relationships of the objects to each other:

behind	under
next to	between
close to	in front of
far from	inside of
over	outside of

Two balls of different sizes may be used or any two different objects of choice. The use of a hoop or box as one object provides for the inside-outside projection to be demonstrated. Again, when observing these two phases of development the teacher would do well to maintain a checklist (see Chapter 8, "Evaluation") of each relationship to keep track of when the child achieves the desired response.

Generally, children exhibiting poor spatial orientation have difficulty judging position in space, estimating distance, knowing the dimensions (coordinates) of space, and perceiving relationships between objects.

Common Problems

1. Errors or slowness in positioning oneself or an object (physically position the child or object so that the child may better visualize the relationship required);
2. Difficulty in judging distance from a target (person or object) from self;
3. Clumsiness in movement or collisions with others and objects in space (check visual acuity and reinforce movement without collisions);
4. Lack of understanding of the relationship possibilities (demonstrate the various terms).

Movement Variability

A good understanding of spatial relationships is fundamental to all meaningful movement and is important in the acquisition of academic skills. Spatial awareness activities will reinforce the following:

1. The ability to move in general space without collisions.
2. An understanding of how much space one's body occupies.
3. The ability to locate objects in space in relationship to oneself and other objects.

Without the development of this awareness, children's movements will appear clumsy and awkward as they attempt to move through space.

Combining Spatial Awareness With a Motor Program
Spatial

Explain the difference between *personal* and *general space*. A hoop can be used to demonstrate this when stationary; the area inside the rim and one or two steps outside is one's personal space; if the hoop is rolled over the floor, then it is in general space.

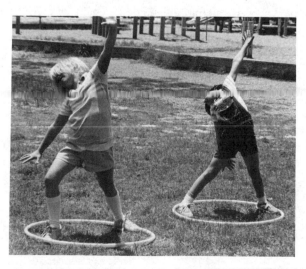

Developing an understanding of symmetry.

In general space:

Stand with front toward, back, side, and other side of teacher.

Lie on back, stomach, side, and other side.

Make the body:

tall—small

wide—narrow

curved—stretched

twisted—straight

Move into general space using various locomotor patterns; move:

forwards   diagonally

backwards   following a curved, straight, or zigzagged path

sideways

Move to something near; far.

Move to something larger or smaller.

Walk the outline of various geometric shapes: circle, square, triangle, and so forth.

Roll across a mat and observe how much space the body occupies.

Try this with body narrow, then wide, and observe the difference.

Place foot in one spot and stretch the body as far as it will go—forward, backward, sideward, and upward.

Time

Move slowly and quickly through space, staying as far and close from everyone as possible.

Vary the speed (by accelerating then decelerating) through space without collisions; make quick changes in direction on signal, then try changing in slow motion.

Force

Cross the room taking first large steps, then small. Estimate the least number of steps necessary to cross the room.

Step very lightly or forcefully.

ADDITIONAL MOVEMENT VARIATIONS

1. In the classroom or gym, walk carefully among desks, chairs, or cones without touching the objects. Use different locomotors. Move fast, then slow, and change directions, levels, and pathways periodically.
2. Set out various-sized objects to step *over* (boxes, chairs, balls, hoops, cones, milk cartons, others).
3. Set out objects at various heights to go *under*.
4. Design obstacle courses using tunnels, chairs, cones, ladders, boxes, and other objects that challenge the child to adjust to a variety of objects in space. Allow children to design their own obstacle courses.
5. Set out balls or blocks of various sizes at various points in the play space. Direct children to:

   walk to the farthest small ball,

   walk to the closest large ball,

   run to the nearest medium-sized ball, and so forth.

   Vary the locomotor pattern used.
6. Line up the entire class in a straight line, shoulder to shoulder, then have children spread out to arm's length apart. Do this also in a square or circle figure.

7. With a ladder flat on the floor:
   Move forward between the rungs; backward.
   Creep on hands and knees between the rungs.
   Jump, hop, or run between the rungs. Go over two at a time.
   Bounce a ball between the rungs.
   Toss a beanbag back and forth between stepping between the rungs.
   Walk on the rungs or sides of the ladder. Go forward, backwards, and sideways
   Place the ladder on its side. Creep in and out of the space going forward and backward.

8. Using a hoop flat on the floor:
   Move in and out of it going forward, backward, and sideways. Find as many different ways of doing this as possible.
   Have a partner hold the hoop on edge or flat off the ground and explore different ways of going in and out of the middle.
   Roll the hoop and go over it or through it before it stops rolling.

9. With a partner:
   Stand: side by side,
          facing each other,
          back to back.
   Move about the room, maintaining this relationship with the partner.
   Move away from the partner; now toward the partner.
   Move far from and close to the partner.
   Walk around the partner.
   Have the partner lie on the floor and then step over and into the spaces formed by the body parts.
   Have the partner make a shape and go under it. Explore different ways of doing this.

10. Jump rope in place, then move across the floor (see Chapter 9 for ideas on jump-rope techniques).

11. Gymnastic (and jumping) activities (see "Vestibular Awareness" section in this chapter for more ideas).

12. Place a rope on the floor in different directions and then go over it in various ways.

Teaching Hints

Use a variety of objects of different shapes and sizes when schema is being developed.

Use flash cards to show the various relationship variations.

Obstacle courses should provide variety in spacing of objects as well as size and shape of objects to maneuver in and out of.

Have children trace their body shape and then observe or measure how much space they occupy.

Skill Concepts Communicated to Children

The body can be maneuvered through space by altering its size, shape, direction of travel, and level.

The body has certain relationships with other people and objects according to its location in space.

An understanding of the following terms:

near	around	below
far	center	between
close	in front	in
over	behind	out
under	above	

Movement Enhancement

Spatial Awareness Enhancement Chart

GAMES	LEVEL		LEVEL		LEVEL
		Jump the Shot		Chimes of Dunkirk	
		Over the Brook		The Muffin Man	
Follow the Leader	I–III	Frog in the Pond		Turn the Glasses Over	
Hopscotch Games		In the Creek			
		Islands		Children's Polka	II & III
Brownies and Fairies	I & II	Rattlesnake		(Kinder polka)	
Hoop Hop		Man From Mars		Round and Round	
Rescue Relay		Cut the Pie		the Village	
Cat and Rat				Seven Jumps	
Charlie Over the Water		DANCE/RHYTHMS/RHYMES			
Gardener and Scamp				Crested Hen	III
Seven Dwarfs		Bluebird	I & II	Greensleeves	
Squirrels and Trees		Loobie Loo		Lummi Sticks	
Jet Pilot		Did You Ever See		Grand March	
		a Lassie?		Skip to My Lou	
Eyeglasses	II & III	Farmer in the Dell			
		Hokey-Pokey			

DIRECTIONAL AWARENESS

Movement Description

Closely associated with body and spatial perception is the awareness of the body with regard to location and direction. *Directional awareness* consists of two awareness components: laterality and directionality.

Laterality is defined as an internal awareness that the body has a left and right side. In the hierarchy of awareness development, body awareness is thought to emerge first, followed by the emergence of laterality. Laterality is also thought to be a basic prerequisite for the subsequent emergence of directionality.

Directionality is the external projection of laterality. This component of the awareness gives dimension to space. A child possessing good directionality is capable of conceptualizing left-right, up-down, front-back, and various combinations.

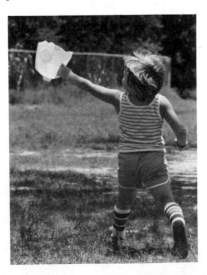

Catching over the shoulder is an advanced directional-awareness task.

Movement Observation

Children with a good sense of laterality do not need to rely on cues such as a ribbon or watch around their wrist or a ring on their finger to provide information about left and right. Without a fully established awareness, children may, along with movement difficulties, encounter problems in discriminating between various letters of the alphabet (for example, b, d, p, q).

Although it is not unusual for the 4- and 5-year-old to experience confusion in direction, teachers should be concerned for the older child who consistently exhibits such difficulties.

The following signs are easily recognizable by the teacher and may indicate a deficiency in a child's directional awareness:

1. General difficulty with responding to instructions emphasizing direction (conceptualizing and producing a motor program);
2. Inability to shift weight to maintain balance when jumping, hopping, or leaping;
3. Difficulty in using feet alternately;
4. Difficulty in maintaining rhythm while performing locomotor skills.

Movement Variability

It is through movement experiences that the child has the opportunity to conceptualize and respond to directional information. Both laterality and directionality give dimension to space and facilitate the child's determination of where he or she is in relation to other phenomena in the environment. A variety of movement experiences is essential to enable the child to develop a strong schema that reflects a diverse conceptual foundation.

Combining Directional Awareness With a Motor Program
Spatial

A variety of locomotor, nonlocomotor, and manipulative-skill movement activities should be performed that emphasize the following aspects of directional awareness:

left-right	over-under-around
up-down	clockwise-counterclockwise
front-back	curved
forward-backward	zigzag
sideward-diagonally	

Time and Force

Movement experiences incorporating diversity in the spatial dimensions just mentioned may also be enhanced through movements that vary from slow to fast (that is, object and person), through musical accompaniment, and through varying levels of force production (weak to strong).

Examples of General Movement Experiences

Using a finger, point as directed; examples: to the right, left; in front, in back, behind, to the side, to the top and bottom (of objects), over your shoulder, between your legs.

With the eyes closed, point to (examples): objects in the gym, the door, the stage, the clock.

Move below, over, under, and between objects in the gym (chairs, beams).

Move body parts in a specific direction (examples): Put your arms in back of you; put your hands in front of you; put your arms in back of your legs; put both of your hands on the same side; point both of your hands to one side; put your arms between your legs; put your fingers under your feet; put your elbow below your hips; put your feet over your head.

Using a designated locomotor skill, move to (balls are placed at specific points in the area): the nearest large ball, the nearest small ball, the farthest small ball, the farthest large ball.

Relationships (people): Step over (*Johnny*); stand near (*Sally*); stand between (*Joe*) and (*Pat*); touch another child's right hand; touch another child's left ear; touch another child's right shoulder; touch another child's left knee; touch another child's right foot.

Using hoops, beanbags, or carpet squares, stop in the direction instructed.

Move through an obstacle course that has written and/or visual directional instructions.

As the teacher presents a flash card indicating directional term or arrow, respond with a series of movements in that direction.

Using hoops, move around, inside, over, through, and in and out.

Place a number of parts inside the hoop (two or three).

Move on scooter boards through an obstacle course (consisting of cans, cartons, chairs, other objects).

Follow lines or maps drawn on the gym floor.

Using a ladder lying flat, follow directional cues such as, walk *between* or *on* the rungs; walk *forward, backward*; step *over*; walk *beside*; lead with the foot, and so forth.

Walk in different directions with coffee-can stilts.

European rhythmic activities:

Run in circular formation. On signal, change places with the student opposite.

When the tamborine sounds, run away from the circle and scatter in all directions; on the second signal, return to the circle.

On signal, run in clockwise, circular formation while circling the right hand above the head (repeat activity counterclockwise with left hand circling).

Elementary directionality task.

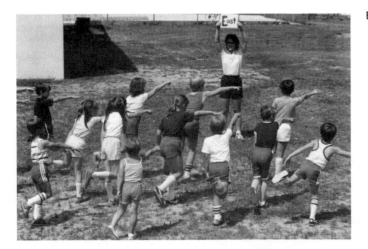

On signal, run backward in circular formation; on signal, run toward the center in four steps, turn around in place four steps, run away from the circle in four steps, and continue to run in clockwise, circular formation. Repeat sequence each time new signal is given.

Angels in the Snow (lying on backs):

Slide both arms along the floor and touch hands together overhead.

Slide both legs apart as far as possible.

Slide arms and legs along the floor at the same time.

Move the left arm overhead.

Move the right leg to the side.

Move the left arm overhead and the right leg to the side at the same time.

Relationships (partner):

Move around your partner to the right; to the left.

Move over your partner.

Move under your partner.

Move under some of your partner's body parts.

Touch the top of your partner; the bottom.

Stand behind your partner; beside; in front of.

Touch the body parts of your partner that the teacher names (left wrist, right hip).

Beanbag activities:

Hold the beanbag in the right hand; the left hand.

Place the bag on the left shoulder; the right shoulder.

Place it on the lowest part of the body; the highest part.

Try to place the beanbag on the floor in front; in the back.

Move around the beanbag at a low level.

Move over the beanbag at a high level.

Activities with balls:

Bounce with the right hand; the left; with both hands.

Bounce the ball twice with the right hand; twice with both hands, and twice with the left hand and continue.

Change directions while bouncing the ball.

While bouncing the ball, change hands.

Chalkboard activities:

Draw vertical and horizontal lines as directed; up, down, right, left

Twist board activities:

Twist, moving arms in the direction given; for example, both to one side; one forward, one back; one up, the other back making clockwise and counterclockwise movements.

Teaching Hints

Ask children to repeat directional terms practiced (Level I).

Use a variety of equipment to reinforce directional concepts (scooters, cones, hoops, tape, cans, cartons, chairs, balls).

Emphasize directional terms with locomotor movements (especially during skill development, games, and dance activities).

Skill Concepts Communicated to Children

The body can move through space in several directions.
An understanding of the following terms:

up/down	clockwise/counterclockwise
forward/backward	diagonal
right/left (sideways)	straight/curved/zigzag

Movement Enhancement

Directional Awareness Enhancement Chart

GAMES	LEVEL		LEVEL	DANCE/RHYTHMS/RHYMES	LEVEL
		Mousetrap			
		Cat and Rat			
Command Cards	I–III	Beater Goes Round		Jack in the Box	I & II
Follow the Leader		Ship Wreck		Turn the Glasses Over	
		Indian Running		Chimes of Dunkirk	
Back to Back	I & II	Go Tag		The Muffin Man	
Partner Tag		Islands		Loobie Loo	
Scarecrows and Cranes		Here to There		Hokey-Pokey	
Squirrels in the Trees		Guard the Toys		Jack in the Box	
Catch the Witch		Hop Tag		Right Hand, Left Hand	
Cat and Rat		In and Out			
Hot Ball				Orchestra Leader	II & III
Birds and Cats		Mousetrap	III	Round and Round	
Cars		Exchange Dodgeball		the Village	
		Roll Dodgeball			
Race Around the Bases	II & III	Balance Dodgeball		Greensleeves	III
				Skip to My Lou	

VESTIBULAR AWARENESS

Movement Description

The ability of the child to maintain body position while counteracting the force of gravity is *balance.* Proficiency in balance requires the child to maintain control of the body both in *stillness,* as in maintaining held positions, (standing on one foot or performing a head stand), and in *motion,* as in locomotor, nonlocomotor, and manipulative skills. Both static balance and dynamic balance are essential to all meaningful movement.

Static balance is generally accomplished before *dynamic balance.* A young child learns to stand unassisted before attempting to take his or her first steps. Consequently, children need to experiment with a variety of held positions (Fig. 12–1) before they can be expected to try different body positions in motion (Fig. 12–2). For example, a child who cannot balance on two hands and one foot could not be expected to experience success with the lame-dog walk.

A child's stability is greatly influenced by muscular control, fitness of the inner ear, ability to concentrate, and by past experience with balancing activities. It is necessary for the child to sense a change in the relationships of the body parts and then to compensate rapidly and precisely for those changes in order to maintain balance.

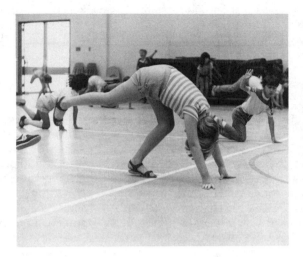

Figure 12-1   Static balance.

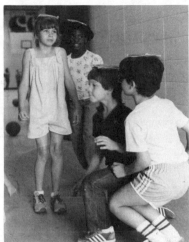

Figure 12-2   Dynamic balance.

Movements that indicate an ability to compensate for changes in body-weight distributions include:

1. Raising of both arms to catch balance;
2. Bending of knees or lowering of whole body to maintain balance;
3. Using stepping patterns where the weight is transferred from one foot to another without hesitancy along a straight line or balance board.

Movement Observation

Keen observation of both static and dynamic balance will ensure maximum motor development of these two perceptual motor abilities. Research indicates that evaluation of dynamic balance can best be accomplished by observing children moving on a balance beam or a line on the floor that is approximately 6 cm wide × 2.5 m long (10 cm high if off the ground). Static balance can be evaluated by timing and observing children standing on a balance stick 1″ × 1″ × 12″ with the foot placed lengthwise on the long axis.

Common Problems
STATIC BALANCE

1. Failure to use arms to catch balance (extend arms out to the side to aid in balancing);
2. Consistent use of only one arm or one side to regulate body weight (stress the use of both sides by practicing bending to one side then the other).

DYNAMIC BALANCE

1. Failure to use arms and consistent use of only one arm or one side (see above for static balance);
2. Need to walk or run very fast to maintain balance (slow down walk and focus eyes at the end of the beam);

3. Being unable to use a steplike pattern and constantly leading with the same foot when moving forward (stress stepping pattern on a line on the floor first);
4. Looking down at the feet (eyes should focus up or at the end of a balance beam);
5. Hesitancy and looking backward to maintain balance (stress good straight posture and body weight over the center of gravity while moving slowly at first).

Movement Variability

The fundamental stability skills of infants are for the most part maturationally determined. Control of the head, neck, and trunk, as well as sitting and standing, is usually accomplished when the child develops sufficient strength. However, development of the basic stability necessary to accomplish locomotor, nonlocomotor, and manipulative skills requires a variety of experiences and opportunities to explore both static and dynamic balancing activities on and off equipment.

Training should take place through several kinds of balance tasks including those in which some kind of visual stress is imposed (for instance, an eyes-closed balance task), in tasks where the child is asked to move and maintain equilibrium (beam walking), as well as in activities in which the child's center of mass remains relatively fixed (static balances of various sorts).

Balancing may be made increasingly difficult for a child by imposing stresses of several kinds.

1. The area on which the child is balancing may be made smaller (decrease the width of the balance beam).
2. Some kinds of visual stress may be imposed, ranging from the easiest (watch a stable point), through increasingly difficult (specific instructions about what should be done with the eyes) to requiring the child watch a moving point that moves from left to right across the line or beam which the child is attempting to walk.
3. The platform on which the child is asked to balance may be made increasingly unstable. An example would be to ask the child to balance on a small board with some kind of runner or knob underneath it.
4. In static balances, the child's base of support may be decreased or the center or mass may be raised, that is, "Stand on one foot . . . lift your arms [or knee] higher."

Spatial
MOVEMENT-PATTERN VARIATIONS

Balance on:
  one body part; foot, knee, seat, shoulders, stomach;
  two body parts; feet, hand and foot, knees, knee and hand, seat and foot;
  three body parts; 2 feet-1 hand, 2 hands-1 foot, 1 knee-2 elbows, and so forth;
  four body parts;
  five body parts; and try
  six body parts.
Change base of support from wide to narrow.
Move on the above combinations of body parts.
Change the body shape while balanced on different parts; use curled, stretched, and twisted shapes.

DIRECTIONS/PATHWAYS/LEVELS

While balanced on different body parts, move another:
  forward

backward
left to right (sideways)
in a circular, zigzag, or straight pathway in the air.
Balance on different parts at high, medium, or low level.
While moving on different body parts and combinations, go:
forward
backward
sideways
in a zigzag, straight, or curved path.

Time

Change balance shapes or move with different body parts on the floor:
quickly
slowly
accelerating
decelerating
evenly
jerkily
on a drum beat
hold one position long, one short, and one medium.

Force

Take a body shape that is strong- or weak-looking.
Feel the force of the muscles when holding positions for longer and longer periods of time.
Move into different balances very slowly then quickly.

ADDITIONAL MOVEMENT VARIATIONS

Stability can be greatly enhanced by balancing and moving on various equipment. This section will include a progression of problems for each piece of stability equipment.

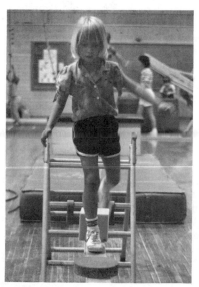

BALANCE BEAM

(About 4 inches wide; a tape line on the floor may be used.)

1. Walk forward, sideways, and backward.
2. Balance on different body parts and move from one balance to another without falling off.
3. Try turning around at different levels.
4. Use different locomotors—run, jump, hop, leap, and skip along beam.
5. Carry different objects as you move: beanbags, hoops, wands, balls.
6. Balance beanbags on different body parts.
7. Pick up objects placed on beam as you move along it.
8. Step over different objects on the beam: hoops, beanbags, blocks. Vary the height and distance between objects.
9. Go under obstacles placed over the beam.
10. Manipulate objects as you move along the beam; toss and catch a ball, bounce it on the floor, move it around your body and so forth.
11. Play follow the leader.
12. Find different ways to get on and off the beam.

TIRES

(Old truck and car tires work well. Place them flat on the ground.)

1. How many ways can you move around the tire?
2. Go over the tire; use the center as you go over; first put one foot in.
3. Now try both feet.
4. Bounce on the tire.
5. Bounce off and on in different directions.
6. Place tires in a sequence flat on the ground and move across without touching the ground, without touching the tires, or by stepping only in the middle of each tire. Use different locomotor patterns.

BALANCE BOARD-ROCKER BOARD

1. Balance on your feet; use a wide base, then a narrow base.
2. Balance on different body parts and different combinations, maintaining your balance as you change positions.
3. Balance with a partner; try to change levels and still stay on.
4. Manipulate different objects; toss and catch a beanbag to yourself, then to someone else; bounce a ball around you, a hula hoop.
5. Pick up objects on your board while balancing.

TRAMPOLINE

Creative use of the trampoline* can result in the development of endurance, coordination, balance, and self-confidence. Rebound stunts like the knee drop, seat drop, and front drop should be reserved for the older child. Trampoline activities should be organized for small groups so that there is maximum opportunity for turns, and a few safety rules need to be

*Note: Close supervision by the teacher is important when using the trampoline.

established. To ensure safe use of the trampoline, children should (1) jump alone and (2) crawl onto and off of the trampoline bed.

The following problem variations are designed to enhance the development of the child's overall balance.

1. Crawl around the bed.
2. Walk on the bed forwards, sideways, and backwards.
3. Roll on the bed; log-roll then try forward rolls, backward rolls, egg rolls.
4. Bounce with two feet in the middle of the bed, feet close then apart.
5. Teacher holds a 4-foot pole or stick across and close to the bed. The child first steps over the stick then jumps over it. The stick can be raised or lowered as the child desires.
6. Jump making quarter turns, half turns.
7. Hop on alternating feet.
8. Find different ways to hold the arms while jumping; try moving them.
9. Find different ways to hold and move the head and jump.
10. Touch different body parts while jumping.
11. Try doing some jumping jacks.
12. Grasp different objects while jumping: beanbags, hoops, balls. Try to toss and catch these while jumping.
13. Try jumping rope or other rope maneuvers while jumping.
14. Count the number of times one can jump out loud.
15. Try jumping to different jump-rope songs and chants.
16. Jump and face different positions on a compass or a clock.
17. Play Simon Says and have children face different directions on command.
18. Jump with light weights on hands or ankles.

LADDER

(Horizontal on the floor or at a slight incline.)

1. Cross on hands and feet or knees front first, then back first.
2. Cross using just the feet forward, backwards, and sideways.
3. Step, jump, or leap between the rungs only.
4. Use only the side rails to cross; vary directions.
5. Carry different objects while traveling across.
6. Manipulate different objects when crossing.
7. Try to pass a partner without losing balance.

HOOPS, WANDS, OR ROPES

(These can be laid on the floor.)

1. Walk along your equipment forward, backward, and sideways.
2. Change the shape of the rope and travel on it.
3. Use different body parts as you travel on your obstacle.
4. Make interesting bridges over your obstacle by using different body parts.
5. Combine with a partner to bridge both your obstacles.

BEANBAGS

1. How long can you balance on a beanbag? Try eyes closed, on one foot.
2. Make bridges over a beanbag.
3. Balance your beanbag on different body parts as you find different balance positions.
4. Balance your beanbag on different parts as you move through space with different locomotor patterns. Create your own locomotors.

PARTNERS

(Use a mat underneath.)

1. How many ways can you balance on a partner when the partner's base is:
   a. hands and knees*(Fig. 12-3)
   b. back or (Fig. 12-4)
   c. upright—knees bent and feet spread wide (Fig. 12-5)?

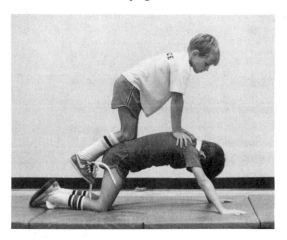

Figure 12-3 Hands and knees base.

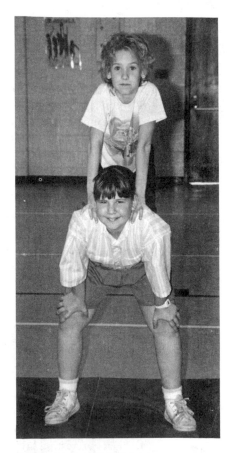

Figure 12-5 Upright base.

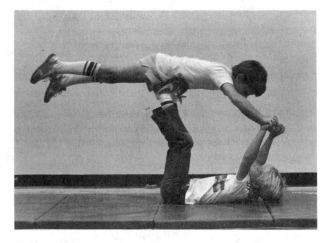

Figure 12-4 Back-lying base.

*Note: Weight should be placed only over the hips or shoulders, never on the small of the back.

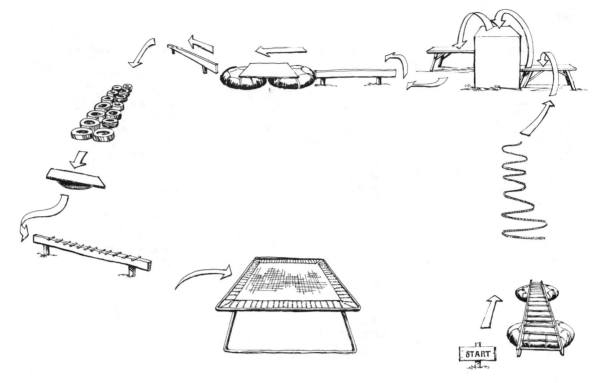

Figure 12-6

OBSTACLE COURSE

1. How many ways can you move over the equipment without losing your balance? (See Fig. 12-6.)

Teaching Hints

Have children experiment with differnt arm positions as they attempt to balance.

Practice balance activities on a line on the floor before going on a balance beam.

Hold up numbers for the child to identify as he or she moves forward and/or backward to encourage proper focus.

Start activities at a lower level and progress to high levels as skill improves.

You may offer a hand to assist in balance each time, thus encouraging the child to grasp less tightly.

Stress squeezing muscles to maintain held positions for longer periods of time.

Skill Concepts Communicated to Children

Look at something out in front of you as you balance.

Extending the arms out to the sides will help maintain balance.

When walking on a beam, alternate the feet as you go.

If you lower your body or widen your base you will balance better.

Balancing the body in different positions is like balancing a scale: one must be equal on both sides of the center.

Movement Enhancement

Balance Enhancement Chart

	LEVEL			LEVEL			LEVEL
GAMES			Hand Wrestling			Spanker	
			Stand-Up			Stiff Knee Pick-up	
Command Cards	I – III		Rocker			Mule Kick	
Follow the Leader			Rooster Fight			Bent Knee Hop	
Whistle Stop			Wheel Barrow			Jump Foot	
			Row Boat			Frog Dance	
Hoop Hop	I & II		People Pyramids			Frog Stand	
Kneeling Tag			Mule Kick			Head Stand	
			Rabbit Jump			Hand Stand	
Balance Dodgeball	II & III		Seal Crawl			Forearm Balance	
Over the Brook			Forward Roll			Thigh Balance	
Deep Freeze			Ankle Walk			Angel Balance	
Frozen Bag Relay			Step Over the Wand			Sitting Balance	
Islands			Bear Walk			Three-Man Mount	
Spoon and Ball Relay			Balance Stand			Backward Roll	
Hopscotch Games			Inch Worm			Backward Extension Roll	
Freeze Ball			Dog Run			Eskimo Roll	
In the Creek			Duck Walk			Cartwheel	
Kangaroo Relay			Egg Roll				
			Egg Sit			*RHYTHMS AND DANCE*	
GYMNASTICS			Heel Slap				
			Kangaroo Jump			Hokey-Pokey	I & II
Lame-Dog Walk	I–III		Thread the Needle			Loobie Loo	
Frog Jump			Turk Stand			Mulberry Bush	
Animal Walk Obstacle Course			Tripod				
Leap Frog			Double Knee Balance			Round & Round the Village	II & III
Human Ball			Stoop and Stretch			Jump Jim Joe	
Log Roll			Crane Dive			Limbo	
			Cork Screw			Seven Jumps	
Measuring Worm	I & II		Coffee Grinder				
Wring the Washrag			Twister			Horah	III
			Blind Touch			Zip Code 001	
Crab Walk	II & III		Tummy Balance			Cats Meow	
Frog Squat			Tightrope Walking				
Bouncing Ball							
Churn the Butter			Push-ups	III			
Double Walk			Single Squat				
			Sit-Up				

EYE-HAND–EYE-FOOT COORDINATION

Movement Description

As a group, rhythmic awareness, eye-hand coordination, and eye-foot coordination represent the teaching themes related to the development of temporal awareness. As the child's spatial world is developing, so is the time structure that is responsible for the coordinated interaction of various muscular and sensory components.

Visual-motor coordination, the ability to coordinate effectively the hand and/ or feet with that which is perceived visually, begins very early in a child's life. Through appropriate movement opportunities this ability develops into the gross- and fine-motor control of eye-hand and eye-foot movements that are the end products of synchrony, rhythm, and sequence. The development of eye-hand and eye-foot efficiency demonstrates the presence of an established time structure within the body of the child. This perceptual process of seeing a stimulus and effectively responding with the hands and/or feet encompasses more than the fundamental manipulative skills of throwing, catching, volleying, striking, bouncing, and kicking that are covered in separate skill chapters. This ability is the basis upon which the fundamental skills mentioned are effectively performed; therefore its inclusion into the curriculum for children is vital.

Eye-hand coordination as described in this chapter is the perceptual motor awareness that enables the child effectively to touch, grasp, release, flick, and tap objects with the hands. Effective *eye-foot coordination* enables the child to step in specific patterns and maneuver objects with the feet and toes.

Movement Observation

The child's eye-hand and eye-foot coordination, like other controlled movements, develops from the midline of the body to the periphery. Therefore gross movements involving mostly the shoulder become more refined as the elbow, wrist, and hand develop strength and coordination. By 7 years of age the child (with a varied activity background) can be observed manipulating with moderate levels of success objects such as jacks, marbles, and puzzles.

Children performing at the elementary stage (Fig. 12–7) of eye-hand coordination may be observed making very deliberate movements with their hands toward objects they wish to touch or grasp. When they release an object there is a tendency to release too early or too late. Attempts at tapping or flicking objects result in more of a punching movement due to their lack of synchrony of the body parts involved. At the less than mature stages of eye-foot control, children attempting to step in specific patterns (for example, stepping on the rungs of a ladder resting flat on the floor) will exhibit great concentration and deliberate movement with their feet. As a child's eye-hand and eye-foot coordination matures, the movements will become more reflexive.

Figure 12-7   Children's movement at the elementary
stage requires considerable concentration.

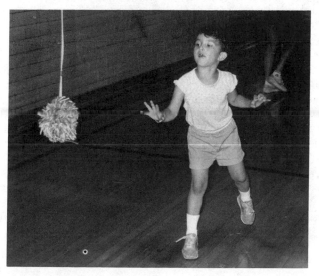

Children with poor eye-hand and eye-foot coordination are going to exhibit performance problems with those activities in which they must visually track and manipulate either an object or themselves in response. While the gross-motor manipulative skills (striking, kicking, throwing, catching, bouncing) and fine-motor movements (sorting, rhythm sticks, tracing, tapping) are most frequently associated with these abilities, other common movement skills such as jumping, walking, running, and climbing depend upon an adequate visual-motor efficiency. A lack of coordination between visual information and motor response may account for many of the problems associated with poor performance. The difficulties encountered by the child frequently stem from a general integration, which may be the basis for immature performance across a number of fundamental skills, such as those previously mentioned.

Common Problems

Examples of general visual-motor (that is, eye-hand and eye-foot coordination) integration problems are:

1. Difficulty in keeping eyes on the ball as it crosses midline of the body;
2. Moves head instead of eyes;
3. Inability to touch or hit ball as it moves;
4. Difficulty in receiving objects;
5. Reaching out for ball and moving head back; closing eyes as ball approaches;
6. Hesitancy in deciding which foot to use to step; always trying to see where to step;
7. While walking across ladders or objects on floor, the child has problems adjusting length of step to varying distances.

Movement Variability

Visual-motor efficiency, being the essential component in the majority of gross- and fine-motor-skill proficiency, demands a diversified movement experience foundation. Because of its importance to performance, programming should begin early in the child's education before gross-motor manipulative skill movement-pattern concentration. Eye-hand and eye-foot coordination experiences should include (but certainly not be limited to) the commonly accepted gross-visual-motor skills of throwing, catching, kicking, and striking. Climbing horizontal and vertical ladders, walking on rungs of a ladder placed flat on the ground, tagging peers in games, tapping musical instruments, stepping in and out of hoops, and playing hopscotch—all enable the child to experience variability of practice that will result in an enhanced general eye-hand and eye-foot coordination. With a strong schema the child can concentrate on movement-pattern proficiency and be more likely to acquire the skills needed for advanced activities such as juggling, combatives, select folk dances (for example, tinikling), and frisbee. With a background of varied experiences, the child is also equipped to respond effectively to the constantly changing sport-skills environment.

The authors would like to emphasize that the experiences suggested for schema enhancement stress the visual-motor component of performance. This entails the use of a focal point; for example, throwing at a target, hopping from square to square, and stepping (walking) between the rungs of a ladder.

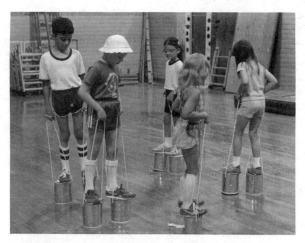

Combining Eye-Hand Coordination With a Motor Program

Spatial

Movement-pattern variability with movement variations in different directions and at low to high levels from the ground should include:

GROSS–MOTOR MANIPULATIVE SKILLS

Rolling balls to a designated target (bottles, bowling pins);
Throwing/tossing objects to a designated target (picture, bucket, hoop);
Catching (with hands, scoops) objects of various sizes (balls, beanbags, rings);
Striking objects of various sizes (balloons, drums, balls) with the hand(s) and implements (rackets, paddles, bats, sticks);
Ball bouncing using various ball sizes;
Grasping (climbing ladders, poles, ropes);
Clapping.

JUGGLING

The following progressions are suggested in the teaching of juggling:

1. Practice tossing and catching one object—using the dominant hand, then the nondominant hand—until consistency of toss height is achieved. Children should quietly chant "toss, catch" during this stage.
2. Using an object in each hand, practice tossing and catching. Children quietly chant "toss, catch"—(dominant hand); "toss, catch"—(nondominant hand). Repeat this unilateral exercise until toss height and rhythm have been established.
3. Using two objects, toss and catch bilaterally. Children quietly chant "toss" (dominant), "toss" (nondominant), "catch" (nondominant), "catch" (dominant). The second object is tossed as the first object starts to fall.
4. Using two objects, toss and catch using only one hand. One object is held in the fingers and the second one is secured by the thumb in the back of the hand. As object held by fingers is released, the second object rolls toward fingers to be tossed as first object starts to fall. Students quietly chant "toss, toss," "catch, catch." Repeat with nondominant hand.

5. Three-object juggling begins with two objects being held in the dominant hand (as in item 4 above) and one object held in the nondominant hand. Begin by tossing object A from the dominant hand, followed by object B from the nondominant hand. Practice in cycles of three tosses, three catches, then begin again. When three tosses can be successfully caught, move to four, then five, and so on. Concentration becomes very important, and it is best to have a set number in each cycle until the movements become more reflexive.

TEACHING HINTS

1. Small, firm beanbags or commercial "juggling cubes" should be used (weighted paper balls wrapped with tape are also effective).
2. Height of toss should be no higher than where child can comfortably reach overhead.
3. Catching should be between waist and shoulders (closer to waist).
4. Facing about $2\frac{1}{2}$ ft. to 3 ft. from a wall will help to stabilize the toss (Fig. 12–8).
5. Insist that students master the two-object bilateral juggle with consistency in toss height as well as rhythm before progression to three-object juggling.
6. Appropriate music ($\frac{2}{4}$ or $\frac{4}{4}$ time) can help to establish the rhythm of juggling.
7. Set the number of tosses and catches low at first so students can experience success without losing control of the objects. This will help to eliminate repeated struggling with inconsistent tosses.
8. Refrain from rushing the students into a new phase before they have mastered the present phase.
9. Establish 25 "toss-catches" without dropping an object as the goal for each phase prior to moving onto the next progression.
10. Focus should be on the apex of the tosses (Fig. 12–9).
11. Early success is very important if students are to be intrinsically motivated to continue practicing.
12. Teachers should juggle frequently to give the students a role model.

Figure 12-8   Facing a wall to help stabilize the toss.

Figure 12-9   Focus is on the apex of the toss.

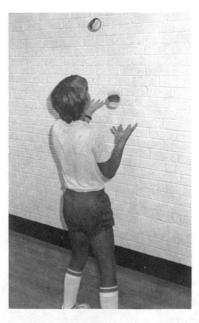

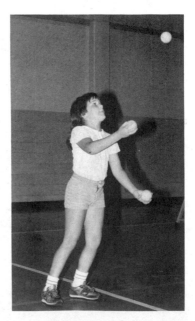

Time and Force

The experiences described thus far may be enhanced through movements that also vary from slow to fast (that is, object and person) with musical accompaniment, and through varying levels of force production (soft to hard).

EXAMPLES OF GENERAL MOVEMENT EXPERIENCES

Roll a ball underhand using two hands (then one) to knock down tennis ball cans.

Throw a beanbag underhand to a bucket or within a hoop.

Throw a fleeceball at a target on the wall.

Catch a large playground ball on the right side, left side, overhead and below the knees.

Catch a beanbag with both hands; the right hand, left hand.

After blowing soap bubbles, catch and pop them.

Bounce a playground ball with two hands, then one hand.

Bounce a ball between the rings of a ladder.

Shoot a small playground ball through a lowered basketball goal.

Hit a balloon with the hand to try to keep it in the air.

Hit a balloon back and forth with a partner.

Roll a hula hoop and keep it going by hitting it with the hand.

Using a plastic bat or racket, hit a whiffleball suspended from a string.

Hit a foam ball with the hand back and forth on the floor with a partner.

Beat designated points (X's) on a drum with a stick to a rhythm.

Climb play apparatus that includes various types of ladders.

Climb cargo nets and playground fire poles.

Clap hands with a partner using rhymes (pat-a-cake).

FINE-MOTOR MANIPULATING SKILLS

Stacking objects

Dropping small objects on targets   Pegboard

Marbles

Jacks   String activities

Finger symbols

Combining Eye-Foot Coordination With a Motor Program
Spatial

Movement-pattern variability with movement variations in different directions and at low to high levels from the ground should include:

GROSS-MOTOR MANIPULATIVE SKILLS

Kicking objects of various sizes

Hacky Sack activities (kicking)

Trapping (with feet) objects of different sizes

LOCOMOTOR SKILLS

Walking and running across, through, and on pieces of equipment (ladders, ropes, hoops, cones, obstacle course);

Leaping, jumping, and hopping over, onto, and between various points (equipment, lines, squares, marks on surface).

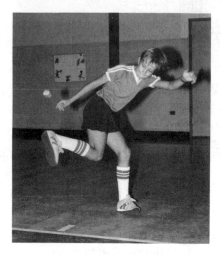

Time and Force

The experiences mentioned may be enhanced through movements that also vary from slow to fast, with musical accompaniment, and through varying levels of force production.

EXAMPLES OF GENERAL MOVEMENT EXPERIENCES

Kick a large playground ball around the room.
Dribble a soccer ball between a course of cones.
Punt a lightweight ball into the air.
Hit a suspended ball with the foot.
Push a beanbag around the room with one foot while sitting,
Keep a balloon in the air by using the feet.
Trap a large playground ball with both feet while standing and sitting.
Walk on lines drawn on the floor.
Walk on a balance beam.
Walk between and on the rungs of a ladder.
Run in and out of a course of hoops without touching one.
Leap over a low hurdle.
Leap from hoop to hoop.
Play hopscotch
On a letter grid, jump on the letters representing your name.
Air-write with feet.
Pick up marbles with feet.

Teaching Hints

Select fundamental skills that best accommodate the developmental level of the child: rolling a ball underhand using two hands, before one-hand throwing, and simple jumping before hopping, and so forth.
Provide large focal points (targets, balls, other objects).
Encourage use of both right and left hands and feet.

Stress concentration on the focal point (keeping eyes open.).

Use eye-hand activities when confined in classroom, (that is, bad weather).

Skill Concepts Communicated to Children

Keep the eyes on the object (focal point).

Movement Enhancement

Eye-Foot Coordination Enhancement Chart

	LEVEL		LEVEL		LEVEL
GAMES		Long and Short Combo Soccer Steal		DANCE	
Boundary Ball	I & II	Formation Jumping		Marching	I–III
Hoop Hop		Crab Soccer	III		
Hot Ball				Bluebird	I & II
Train Station		GYMNASTICS		Oats, Peas, Beans, and Barley Grow	
Traffic Cop					
		Rope Stunts	I–III		
Kick the Beast Relay	II	Lazy Rope		Bleking	III
Potato Race		Snake Rope		Zip Code 001	
		Circle Rope			
Hopscotch	II & III	Straight Rope			
Jump the Shot		V-Rope			
		Rope Rings			

Movement Enhancement

Eye-Hand Coordination Enhancement Chart

	LEVEL		LEVEL		LEVEL
GAMES		Ball and Stick Relay		Three Little Monkeys	
				This Little Clown	
Circle Stride Ball	I & II	Hand Soccer	III	Over the Hills	
Hot Potato		Jacks		Row, Row, Row	
Beanbag in a Can Relay		"Lamb Over the Wall"		Dig a Little Hole	
Throw and Go		"Eggs in the Basket"		Ten Fingers	
Clothespin Drop		"Around the World"		Little Fish	
		"Cherries in a Bucket"		Bunny	
Cat and Rat	II	"Lazy Susan"		If I Were a Bird	
		"Pigs in a Pen"		Two Little	
B-B Ball	II & III	"Fast Charlie"		Left and Right	
Agents and Spies		My Doll			
Magic Wand		Par Three		Names in Rhythm	II & III
Blue and Gold		Scoot to the Hoop		Rhythm Echo	
Brownies and Fairies		Sweep-up Relay		Dance of Greeting	
Kneeling Tag				Morse Code	
Seven Dwarfs		DANCE/RHYTHMS/RHYMES			
Finger Toss				Lummi Sticks	III
Over and Over		Peas Porridge Hot	I & II		
Top Hat Tag		Itsy Bitsy Spider			
Pebble Flip		Here Is the Beehive			
		I'm a Little Teapot			

RHYTHMIC AWARENESS

Movement Description

All meaningful movement takes place in a time structure, which, when organized, is rhythmical. *Rhythmic awareness*, therefore, refers to the child's ability to move (utilizing fundamental movement skills) or to make sounds that are repetitive, patterned, and result in balance and harmony of movement or sound.

Children develop rhythmic awareness through experiences that stress (1) moving to or singing with already established rhythms (for example, recorded music, drum beat, singing, chanting, or clapping) and (2) creating movements or sounds in their own time structure. The beauty of rhythmic activity is that it is inherently pleasurable for the child. One has only to observe children at play to notice their frequent use of chants (nonsensical and meaningful) and repetitive movements, which give them great enjoyment. Rhythmic activities using songs and chants (for instance, alphabet song, "Ten Little Indians") enhance the learning of many fundamental academic skills and contribute greatly to the development of fundamental motor abilities. Musical accompaniment may be a valuable teaching technique for the teacher instructing children to coordinate their movements in such activities as skipping, galloping, or bouncing a ball.

To develop rhythmic awareness in children is to develop an internal time structure that is consistent and meaningful to the child. The basic elements of rhythm are pulse beats, accents, measures, patterns, and qualities that are internalized and reinforced through selected movement activities.

Pulse beats are the division of time into equal intervals. The intervals between pulse beats may vary depending on the speed of the piece (music or other accompaniment), but the amount of time that each interval between pulse beats occupies must be exactly the same. A child who can time the climax of a movement with the exact moment of the beat is said to be moving in response to pulse beats. This is no simple feat even for many adults.

The first step in helping children understand this difficult element is to offer many opportunities to move to a musical accompaniment without requiring an accurate response. Not only is the frequent use of music with movement motivating but it provides the necessary experience of moving within a time structure, which will later enable the child to adapt to an established rhythm. The kindergarten and even the first-grade child should not have his or her attention drawn to an inaccurate response to pulse beats, but rather should be encouraged to develop movements that are regular and repetitive in the child's own time framework. Children at this age develop the awareness of pulse beats by repeating similar movements over and over with an accompaniment much like chanting a nursery rhyme repetitively. Simply using locomotor movements for expressive purposes will accomplish this goal. Once children can repeat movements like clapping, tapping, or walking in place at regular intervals, then they are ready to attempt to order their movements around established beats.

All movements can be timed to coincide with established pulse beats. In locomotor skills, the moment of contact of the foot or other body parts with the floor is timed to coincide with the beat. In rhythmic running, for example, the foot should touch the floor at the same time as the pulse beat occurs. With non-locomotor skills and other creative movements, the beginning of the movement should coincide with the beat. Manipulative movements should be timed so that contact of the object either to the floor or to the body coincides with the beat.

For example, bouncing a ball to a pulse beat would require that the ball contact the floor or the child's hand at the moment of the beat.

Accents are the extra impetus placed on certain beats that divide pulse beats into a series of equal groups, called *measures*. There is an innate tendency to accent alternate beats to create a strong-weak sequence, which simulates the body's heart beat or respiration. In all movement there is a point at the beginning, middle, or end at which added force is applied or released. For example, an accent naturally occurs at the beginning of pushing or pulling movements and most locomotors. However, the accent of a stretching movement is at the end of the complete stretch rather than at the beginning. In more continuous movements there is an accent in the middle of the movement. Swinging and swaying are examples of this, with the accent at the bottom or middle of the swing as opposed to either end of the movement. In most common dance steps, as well as locomotor movements, the primary accent occurs at the beginning of the movement. Children respond to accents first by learning to clap on the accented pulse beats and then by making some other forceful movement or step instead of clapping. Large, forceful movements and, of course, stamping and clapping are the simplest response to accents. Changes in direction, level, and size of movement can also delineate an accented pulse beat.

Measures are equal groupings of pulse beats that are marked by accents. The major accent generally occurs on the first beat of each measure and a lesser accent may occur on the third beat of a four-beat measure. The number of beats in each measure defines the *meter*. A measure that has two beats is a *duple meter,* and one that has three beats is a *triple meter*. The meter established by music or other accompaniment will dictate the types of movements possible. The most common meters used in children's dance and locomotor skills are the *quadruple meter* (four beats; used for walk, run, jump, hop, leap, and other even-movement patterns) and 6/8 meter (six beats in two groups of three; used for skips, slides, gallops, and other uneven-movement patterns).

Counting out the amount of time and duration of music and movements is an important skill in developing an awareness of the element of measures. For example, in quadruple meter the beats are counted 1-2-3-4, 2-2-3-4, 3-2-3-4

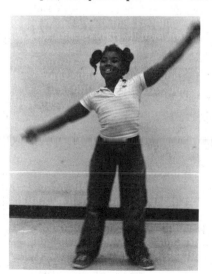

Children can make a strong movement on an accented beat to show their understanding of this element.

and so on for the number of measures required. In this way the child and teacher can keep track precisely of the amount of time a particular movement sequence occupies. This is especially important when children are trying to coordinate group-movement sequences, repeat movement patterns exactly, or the teacher is designing a sequence for a program. The key concept here is that children learn to count out measures and keep accurate track of the duration of a particular sequence. Naturally, this skill is somewhat advanced and should not be required of the kindergarten or even the first-grade child. By second grade the children may begin counting measures and ordering movement sequences to those measures. It is suggested that the quadruple and 6/8 meters be worked with first, as these are the simplest and most common in children's dance.

Patterns are achieved when movements or sounds are put together so that they are not equal to each other in time. One part of the movement will take longer than another. When skipping, the step part takes two pulse beats and the hop portion takes one, totaling three beats and two movements. Any time a movement is uneven, a rhythmic pattern occurs, as with the gallop, slide, two-step, and polka. Another possibility is to have a pulse-beat interval that is divided equally (for instance, two or three equal parts) followed by an undivided interval that spans the same amount of time. The resulting pattern follows a two-to-one ratio with the first movements being half as long as the second. Two runs followed by a walk, or two walks followed by a slow walk are examples of an even-movement pattern. Very simply, unless one movement is continued in exactly the same way for a long time, a movement pattern usually results. The movement pattern, then, is a combination of movements that occupy varying amounts of time.

Qualities are attributes that distinguish rhythmic movements from each other. Two children can perform the same movements in the same time structure and yet the performances can appear totally different. One has only to vary the size and/or speed of movement to change the quality of the performance. A child who is swinging his or her arms in a wide arc will appear very different from another who is swinging the arms in a small arc, and yet both may be performing the same skill in the same time period. This difference in "quality" of rhythmic movement is the result of variations in the intensity (that is, size and force) and tempo (speed) of the movements. These variations that distinguish one child's movements from another represent the beginning of creative expression.

The terms used to describe the elements of rhythm are presented for the teacher's clarification only and will not necessarily be used with the children. Words easily understood by the children should be substituted for the terms presented here.

For example, the concept of accents can be conveyed by using words like loud and soft beats or strong and weak movements. Tempo can be communicated as fast or slow movements. The idea of meter can be described as skipping (uneven) beat or walking (even) beat. In this way children can develop an understanding of the elements of rhythm through movement experiences that are commensurate with their ability to understand terminology, thereby developing a functional movement vocabulary. It is not necessary for them to memorize definitions for the technical terms or even to know those terms; what is most important is that their schema is reinforced in such a way that they can respond accurately to and create movement sequences to a variety of rhythmic accompaniments. If this is accomplished then the later learning of specific folk and square dance steps, as well as other more complicated skills that demand rhythm and timing, will be much easier for them.

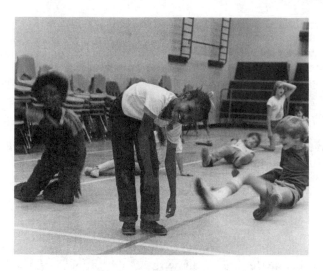

Childen use movement to express emotion.

Creativity

Fostering creativity in the child is a very important task that is often overlooked by teachers who are anxious to "teach." Creativity is not something that can be taught as such, but rather must be stimulated and then given room to grow. It is sometimes very difficult for a conscientious teacher to step back and allow the children to move as they feel, and yet this very freedom is crucial for the development of creative expression. The following are some practical suggestions to help the teacher foster blossoming creativity in children.

Begin with *imitative activities*. Children are very adept at pretending to be familiar animals, people, fairy caricatures, objects, and events. It is important to choose a stimulus for imitation that is familiar to all and suggests movement possibilities. The following list of categories offers some ideas:

Living creatures
(animals and people; real and imaginary)
Natural events
(weather, climate, and nature activities)
Objects
(transportation, machines, toys)
Familiar events
(movies, sports, circus)
Poom, fairytale, simile, and double simile
(move as a pelican, move as a pelican just after lunch).

Remember that the children themselves may be your greatest source of ideas. They have been playing "let's pretend . . . " since they were two, and certainly haven't forgotten how.

Allow children to move first without accompaniment and then add a rhythmic structure (drum beat, piano, record, other sources).

Progress to *interpretative activities*. These stimuli should encourage children to express moods, feelings, and actions. There should be a lot of variations in movement as each child expresses his or her own ideas about surprise, for example.

Have children interpret art through movement. Variations in texture, shape, size, and color provide stimulus for creative-movement activities.

Use props like ribbons, scarves, wands, and hoops that enable children to shed their self-consciousness about movement by focusing their attention on the prop.

Encourage movement patterns that demonstrate a wide variety of space, time, force, and relationship variations.

Movement Observation

The ability to "keep time" and move rhythmically demands three basic skills. Children must be able to *attend* to the accompaniment, *identify* the pulse beats, and then *order* movements around them.

Five- and 6-year-old children may find it hard to synchronize their movements with an accompaniment, especially when the pulse beats deviate from their own natural rhythm. Consequently, these children should be exposed to an accompaniment often in a way that is relaxed so that their movements can occur with the accompaniment and without tension. It is particularly important to avoid continual drilling on this matter and to allow the child to develop his or her own "timekeeping ability" through free-movement activities.

The 7- and 8-year-old (second and third grader) can be expected to order their movements more accurately to pulse beats. The child will find a walk in place easier to control than a walk forward, skips and gallops easier than a run, and small jumps easier than hops to an accompaniment. At this point it may be necessary to motivate the child to try to identify and order movements around pulse beats, because the child may be more interested in moving only for movement's sake. Children's development will be greatly enhanced by the use of gamelike activities that challenge them to be accurate. Working with lummi sticks and tinikling poles are particularly useful in motivating children toward accuracy.

Once the child has mastered an accurate response with simple movements of arms and legs to a series of beats, the teacher can then expect to see accents and rhythmic patterns, movements with equipment, partners, and in different directions, levels, and so forth (Murray, 1975).

Movement Variability

Discovering the inherent rhythm in movement and being able to move rhythmically greatly enhance the child's motor-skill development. The discovery of the child's internal rhythm should result in more fluid and coordinated movement patterns. A child who has not developed a basic level of rhythmic awareness may exhibit movement patterns that appear awkward and clumsy, characterized by a stumbling, uneven walking pattern as opposed to a smooth and even transfer of weight.

In the skill chapters, rhythm is a part of the time variable used to provide the child with a repetitive signal for movement. Depending on the child's age and experience, success in ordering movements to the accompaniment will vary. Regardless of the success exhibited, the teacher should continue frequently to use an accompaniment with fundamental movement skills.

When developing rhythmic awareness through movement, activities should be provided that follow a progression.

1. First allow the child to explore movement patterns (both creative and established, locomotor, nonlocomotor, and manipulative) in the child's own time structure. That

is, the child determines his or her own pulse beats and accents, and moves accordingly.

2. The child should be encouraged to establish sequences of movements and repeat them.
3. The child may then work with a partner and use small equipment.
4. Group activity should be organized by the teacher until the child is able to demonstrate proficiency.
5. Once the child is comfortable creating movement patterns without accompaniment, then rudimentary clapping, slapping, and stomping should be encouraged to an established rhythm (music, poem), followed by locomotor and nonlocomotor movements.
6. Keeping time can then be expanded to using small manipulative equipment, instruments, and then working with a partner.
7. Finally, a sequence of movements to established rhythms can be expected.

Auditory Rhythmic Activities

Rhythmic awareness is also developed through the use of singing rhythms, finger plays, and rhymes. These activities "offer opportunities for combining movement and socialization to rhythmic patterns" (Gallahue, 1982). Use of these rhythmic activities demands movement responses that serve to reinforce the child's internal awareness of pulse beats, accents, patterns, and tempo in an enjoyable manner. A further benefit of auditory rhythmic activities is that they heighten children's ability to attend to an accompaniment as they listen for the action directions and sing along.

Singing rhythms are those songs that appeal to youngsters and suggest action possibilities by telling a story. Children will sing along as they create movements to go along with the songs in this category. As they sing the song over and over, they internalize the rhythm of the song through enjoyable repetition.

Finger plays incorporate singing or chanting short and simple rhymes with specific hand and finger actions. These rhymes are easy to learn and help to develop the accompanying finger dexterity in children.

Rhymes and *poems* present further stimulus for developing rhythmic auditory awareness. Most kindergarten youngsters are familiar with a variety of nursery

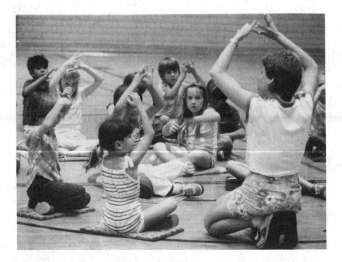

Finger plays are fun.

rhymes and learn new ones easily as they perform actions to them. These differ from finger plays in that they may involve whole-body movements as the children "act out" the words to the rhyme or poem.

The enhancement section of this chapter contains a list of appropriate singing rhythms, finger plays, and rhymes.

Combining Rhythmic Awareness with a Motor Program

The following activities stress moving in response to a pulse beat and, by necessity, require an accurate motor response. There is, however, another aspect of dance that stresses interpreting and expressing feelings and ideas through movement without attending to an external time structure. This is called *creative dance*. Creative dance experiences are usually the first exposure a child has to the world of dance. As the child explores the fundamental-skill and movement-awareness themes, he or she should be encouraged to key-in on the quality of the movements that communicate different feelings and emotions.

For example, a strong, forceful stretch as opposed to a slow, smooth stretch will communicate a totally different feeling. Children need to experience the full range of their creative-movement capabilities by being encouraged to try new and different actions that they have not yet explored. Communication experiences should be followed by sequencing and phrasing or patterning activities where the child must combine various movements to make a statement. Finally, the child will be able to create a total dance by putting together several sequences that express an idea, feeling, activity, or movement awareness.

It is difficult and probably unwise to isolate rhythmic experiences from creative experiences because of the many possibilities for movement which exist. Therefore, this section on rhythmic practice should be utilized in such a way as to encourage individual creative expression following the above progression. The use of a variety of stimuli will greatly enhance the child's creative capabilities. We suggest:

A variety of music and sounds;
Instruments created by children;
Reading poems and stories to interpret;
Viewing art work to interpret;
Creating movements around props.

Spatial

Perform at the moment of beat:

Clap hands or floor.
Slap different body parts.
Tap feet.
Make small hand gestures.
Make large arm gestures.
Bend and extend different body parts: knees, elbows, fingers, wrists, neck, waist, hips; shrug shoulders.
Push and pull, swing and sway, twist and turn on the beat.
Walk in place.
Perform the various locomotors moving forward.
Change directions every fourth beat or accented beat.

Change movement patterns (skip, gallop, slide) on accents.
Move only on accented beats, pause on other beats, freeze (shape) on accented beats.
Combine locomotor and nonlocomotor movements into a pattern and perform over again.
Experiment with all movement possibilities and body parts in this dimension.

Time

Move slowly so that one movement occupies more than one beat (half as fast).
Let one movement last an entire measure.
Move quickly so that more than one movement occupies one beat (twice as fast).
Combine different speed movements into a pattern (that is, two steps and a slow walk = 4 beats); try different combinations.
Make movements that accelerate from half as fast to on beat to twice as fast.
Make movements that decelerate from twice as fast to half as fast.
Make movements that are sustained (last two or more beats).
Make sudden movements that last only part of a beat.
Move body in sustained (slow) maneuver; let a body part(s) (head, arms) move on accents.

Force

Vary the quality of movements by contrasting actions that are:

strong, then weak
hard, then soft
heavy, then light
firm, then fine or loose.

ADDITIONAL MOVEMENT VARIATIONS

Try the following partner relationship possibilities for rhythmic-movement sequences:

advancing-retreating	together-apart
meeting-parting	above-below
mirroring-matching	behind-in front of
following-copying	over-under
questioning-answering	on-alongside

In a large group move in succession or unison.
Create rhythmic movement sequences that utilize the following:

hoops	scarves
wands	flags
streamers	rings
balls	other props of the children's creation

Create rhythmic sequences in relationship to large apparatus

use:
   ladders
   mats

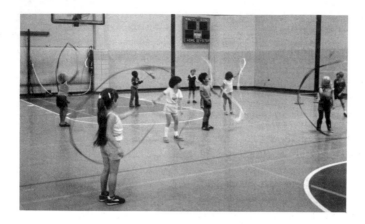

    beams
    bars
    other
go:
    over-under
    through, inside, outside
make shapes:
    around
    under
    over
    between

Create tapping sequences in 4/4, 3/4, 2/4, and 6/8 time using lummi sticks. Work alone, in pairs, then in a group.
Remember to vary the direction, level, and speed of the sequence.
    Use rhythm instruments in a movement sequence:

    bells
    triangles
    sand blocks
    tambourines

Teaching Hints

1. Use simple, uncluttered sounds to establish rhythms; consider using:
   a. your voice (singing or chanting)
   b. a rhythm drum
   c. a tambourine
   d. a xylophone
   e. lummi sticks
   f. finger cymbals
   g. records with an unchanging beat (Country and western, marches, and simple rock-and-roll music works well.)
   h. homemade instruments

2. Avoid too much loud drumming; use other percussion instruments for variation.
3. Always require a movement response when exploring rhythms.
4. Hand waving, tapping on and off the body, shaking the head are all good responses to begin with.
5. The ability to create a movement pattern demands time and encouragement. Allow sufficient time for the children to explore, stand back, and don't interfere except to support the work in progress.
6. Allow children time to perform their creations.
7. You need not be a dancer to teach creative rhythms, so don't be afraid to try.
8. Use props and imagery like scarves, hoops, picture, sounds, and feelings to stimulate creative movement.
9. Avoid telling the children how something moves, but rather allow them to decide on their own movements.
10. When children seem inhibited, try outlandish similes ("How would you move if you were a piece of bacon on a really hot sidewalk, a stork walking in peanut butter, a grasshopper on top of a moving bowl of jello?").

Skill Concepts Communicated to Children

All movements occur in a time structure.

When movements are ordered and repetitive, then they are rhythmical.

Pulse beats and accents can be identified in movements and sounds.

Movement Enhancement

Rhythmic Awareness Activity Chart

	LEVEL		LEVEL		LEVEL
RHYTHMIC GAMES		SINGING RHYTHMS		Ten Little Indians	II
				How Do You Do, My Partner	
Marching	I–III	A Hunting We Will Go	I – III		
The Crazy Clock		You Can		Clap Your Hands	II & III
Levels		Little Miss Muffet	I		
Orchestra Leader		Look! See!		Bingo	III
Lummi Sticks		Yankee Doodle	I & II	FINGER PLAYS	
Rhythm Echo	II	Keep It Moving			
Threes and Sevens		Hinges		Here Is the Beehive	I & II
		Butterfly		The Little Clown	
Names in Rhythm	II – III	Up, Down, Turn Around		I'm a Little Teapot	
		Teddy Bear		Over the Hills	
Reverse Ranks	III	Toot the Flute		Row, Row, Row	
Line or Circle Clap		Jack in the Box		Dig a Little Hole	
RHYTHMIC GYMNASTICS		The Little Green Frogs		Ten Fingers	
		Top of the Morning		Little Fish	
Balls	III	Spinning Tops		Bunny	
Hoops		Mulberry Bush		If I Were a Bird	
Wands		Ten Little Jingle Bells		Two Little	
Ribbons		Loobie Loo		Left and Right	
		Farmer in the Dell		Itsy Bitsy Spider	
		Did You Ever See a Lassie?		Three Little Monkeys	

Nursery Rhymes (I & II)

The following familiar nursery rhymes are listed in order of difficulty. Start with the first line and devise a movement sequence that is true to the rhythmic pattern. Use locomotor, nonlocomotor, and various body movements that may suggest the words, but not necessarily. Add succeeding lines one at a time. Choose rhymes familiar to the children because the rhythmic sequences for those will be well established.

Twinkle, Twinkle Little Star
Hot Cross Buns
Sing a Song of Sixpence
Baa, Baa, Black Sheep
Pussy Cat
Ding Dong Bell
Pease Porridge Hot
Fe Fi Fo Fum
One, Two, Buckle My Shoe
Diddle Diddle Dumpling
One, Two, Three O'Leary
Tom, Tom, the Piper's Son
Hickory Dickory Dock
Humpty Dumpty Sat on a Wall
Little Miss Muffet
Ride a Cock Horse

Rhymes and Sayings (I–IV)

The following sayings and rhymes provide stimulus for short movement compositions. Children should be encouraged to create their own movement patterns to the lines.

"April showers bring May flowers."
"Birds of a feather flock together."
"A bird in the hand is worth two in the bush."
"All is not gold that glitters."
"The early bird catches the worm."
"An apple a day keeps the doctor away."
"Rain, rain go away, Little Johnny wants to play."
"A stitch in time saves nine."
"Early to bed, early to rise, makes a person healthy, wealthy, and wise."

Chants (I–III)

Chants provide a rhythmic pattern that is continuous and enables children to create movement sequences or just move various body parts rhythmically to their accompaniment. Chants may be created by the children out of nonsense syllables or familiar words.

Who Put the Cookies in the Cookie Jar?
Ice Cream
I Went to the Store
Valentines
Tim Tam Toes Tap

Rhythmic Awareness Activity Chart (continued)

	LEVEL		LEVEL		LEVEL
DANCES		Danish Dance of Greeting		Oh, Susanna	III
London Bridge	I & II	Seven Jumps		Bleking	
Chimes of Dunkirk		Hansel and Gretel		Badger Gavette	
Hokey-Pokey		This Old Man		Glowworm	
Jack the Giant Killer		The Popcorn Man		Skip to My Lou	
Oats, Peas, Beans, and Barley		Paw Paw Patch		Klapptanz	
I See You		Kinderpolka		Danish Schottische	
Birds in the Nest		Ach Ja		Crested Hen	
Round and Round the Village		Hobby Horse		Horah	
		Fool's Jig		Grand March	
Sally Go Round the Moon	II & III	Shoo Fly		Gustaf's Skoal	
		Limbo		Little Brown Jug	
Jolly Is the Miller		Bow Belinda			
Jump Jim Joe		The Wheat			
		Maypole Dance			

VISUAL AWARENESS

Movement Description

A child's ability to perceive and react to visual stimuli is crucial to his or her future academic achievement. Unfortunately, many children entering school are deficient in at least one of the three types of perception necessary to good visual awareness.

Good visual awareness involves effective functioning of depth, form, and figure-ground perceptions.

Depth Perception

This is the ability to judge distances in three-dimensional space. Development of depth perception increases the child's ability to utilize external cues in determining depth, distance, and size.

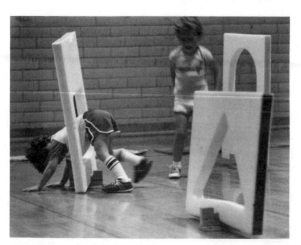

A sound visual awareness is necessary to maneuver through obstacles of varying sizes and shapes.

Form Perception

This is the ability to recognize forms, shapes, and symbols. Related to form perception is perceptual constancy: the ability to recognize categories of shapes regardless of size, color, texture, or angle of observation. The young child may have difficulty perceiving that the huge airplane on the field is the same size and shape as the one several thousand feet above in the sky. Research indicates that children 4 to 7 years of age may rely on different perceptual information to identify objects. Four-year-olds generally rely on form or shape, rather than color, whereas 5-year-olds tend to use color for identification. By the time children are in the second grade (7 years), color and form are utilized more equally to identify objects. Progression in development proceeds from ill-defined globulous masses to the differentiation of elements within objects.

Children with inadequate form perception may have difficulties in such activities as differentiating letters, numbers, sorting objects, and engaging in movement activities that involve moving objects or boundary lines.

Figure-Ground Perception

This refers to the ability to perceive and distinguish a figure separate from its ground: being able to select specific stimuli from a mass. The child who attempts to catch a thrown ball must be able to screen out obstructive stimuli (sky, clouds, children, buildings, trees) while sighting and concentrating on the ball.

These three perceptive abilities account for approximately 80 percent of the information received as stimuli. Therefore, a sound visual awareness is fundamental to success in most fundamental movement skills.

A child with poor visual awareness may appear clumsy and may have problems with academic subjects. Movement is an excellent medium for enhancing the development of visual awareness. A good visual schema will form the basis for all future learning.

Movement Observation

The following signs are easily recognizable by the teacher and may indicate a deficiency in visual awareness:

1. clumsiness in daily activities
2. difficulty in coloring large symbols
3. difficulty in matching symbols and shapes
4. inability to recognize and interpret symbols correctly
5. difficulty in form and depth perception
6. inability to reproduce letters, numbers, and symbols correctly

If remedial work is indicated, the teacher may select from a number of specially designed programs to aid in the correction of deficiencies.

Movement Variability

A sound visual awareness is essential to the learning of all motor skills. Consequently, visual awareness training should begin when the child is preschool age to ensure maximum development. In public education the kindergarten child should

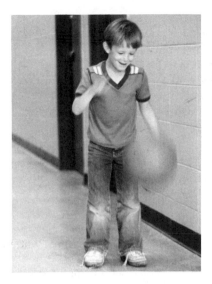

Figure-ground perception.

receive visual training at the beginning of the school year and should be evaluated periodically throughout the year to determine possible weaknesses. Visual training should continue through the primary grades to ensure a readiness for learning.

Parents should be encouraged to participate at home with the child in some of these activities.

Combining Visual Awareness With a Motor Program
Spatial

Move through space staying as far from everyone as possible.

Move as close to everyone without touching as possible; vary the size of the space.

Vary the direction of travel.

Place one body part close to someone and another part far away.

Try different body parts and combinations of parts.

Trace the path of different shapes on the floor:

circles	ovals
squares	straight, curved, and zigzag lines
rectangles	alphabet letters
triangles	numbers

Move at different levels while traveling through space.

Move one body part at three different levels: high, medium, and low.

Make the body into the above shapes both flat on the floor and while standing up.

Trace the above shapes in the air with different body parts; try fingers, hands, feet, head, elbows, knees.

Go toward a wall that has animal pictures on it, pick out one animal, and try to imitate it with your movement.

Find someone in the class wearing the same color tennis shoes as you and go to them.

Time

Move through space as quickly or as slowly as possible *without collisions.*

Match movements to a drum beat while traveling through space.

Move the body into different shapes first quickly then as slowly as possible; try this first while standing then while lying down.

Change shapes and levels on a drum beat.

Force

Move about the room with very smooth/jerky motions without collisions.

Move about, sometimes exploding into the air then staying very close to the ground, without touching anyone.

Move quietly and loudly.

ADDITIONAL MOVEMENT VARIATIONS

1. Have children sort different objects into like piles; use buttons, toothpicks broken into different lengths, geometric shapes, colored objects, etc.
2. Have the child catch a balloon thrown by the teacher then progress to large balls and beanbags, then small balls and other objects.
3. Try to juggle first two beanbags, then two balls, then three objects.
4. See if the child can bounce a ball with different body parts: elbow, knee, head, wrist, etc.
5. Keep a balloon aloft by batting it with different body parts.
6. Leap across different objects placed on the ground without touching them. Leap over a hula hoop, a jump rope or two placed parallel, a wand, a traffic cone, etc.
7. Move in and out, and over and under different obstacles that are off the ground without touching them.
8. Push a small object while creeping across the floor.
9. Expose a picture to the child, then hide it, and have the child recall as many things as he or she remembers.
10. Have the child duplicate a pattern you have just drawn after you hide it from view.
11. Find as many different ways as you can to sort a group of objects like buttons; groceries, beads, clothes, kitchen items, and so forth.

Teaching Hints

Plan many and varied spatial dimensional cues and reference points for judging distance (depth perception).

Stress recognizing similarities and differences among shapes.

Have students reproduce a variety of shapes with their bodies.

When teaching figure-ground perception, first limit the number of stimuli in the background and use white or light solid colors.

Gradually add stimuli to the environment.

Skill Concepts Communicated to Children

The body can recognize a variety of shapes that one can see.

One can move through space without collisions.

One can locate specific objects in space.

Movement Enhancement

Visual Awareness Enhancement Chart

GAMES	LEVEL	GYMNASTICS	LEVEL	DANCE	LEVEL
What's Missing? Peripheral Vision Finding Different Objects	I–III	Animal Walk Obstacle Course	I–III	A Hunting We Will Go	I–II
Nuts and Bolts Letter Race	I & II	Partner Stunts	II & III	Did You Ever See a Lassie?	I & II
Clothespin Drop Ping-Pong Bounce	II & III			Round and Round the Village Jolly Is the Miller Shoo Fly Paw Paw Patch	II & III
I Pass These Scissors to You	III				

TACTILE AWARENESS

Movement Description

Tactile awareness involves the ability to discriminate among objects through touch and the ability to remember the feel of various objects in order to categorize them. Tactile perception is a very basic component of all manipulative skills and plays an important role in all exploratory learning. Through feeling and manipulating objects, the child experiences a variety of sensations that not only have a survival value but also contribute to a better understanding of the environment. The sense of touch enables children to distinguish objects with different feels and further enables them to manipulate a variety of objects more effectively.

Fundamental tactile awareness begins in infancy when a baby first grasps objects at about 3 months of age. The child very quickly learns to differentiate among soft and hard objects, hot and cold, and rough and smooth objects. The total sum of these preschool experiences will determine the child's tactile awareness when he or she enters kindergarten. A child who has been offered a variety of different textured and shaped objects to manipulate through the preschool years will be better equipped to relate to novel objects in grade school than one who has been deprived of these experiences.

By the time children enter school they should be able to describe and identify familiar objects without the aid of a visual cue.

Movement Observation

Children with tactile awareness problems can be easily identified through simple observation in tactual discrimination activities. The teacher should look for the following behaviors:

1. Inability to discriminate tactually (without visual cues) between different-sized coins, or fabrics with different textures. Other objects may be used here;

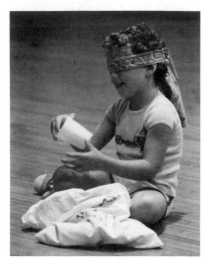

Identification of objects without visual cues
develops a keen tactile awareness.

2. Complains of clothes irritating the skin; may avoid wearing a coat;
3. Craves to be touched or held;
4. Avoids touch and reacts negatively to physical contact;
5. When the child's eyes are closed, child is unable to identify fingers as they are touched.

Movement Variability

Developing tactile awareness is necessary to learning both fundamental manipulative and primary educational skills. Tactual awareness can be practiced very effectively through a variety of movement activities.

Combining Tactile Awareness With a Motor Program
Spatial

Move on different surfaces while barefooted:
    hard floors
    lawns
    beaches, sandy and rocky
    balance beams
    mats.
Use different locomotors and move at different levels and directions.
Blindfold children and have them:
    follow tape marks (while barefooted) that form different paths: straight, curved, and zigzag; identify the pathway;
    feel a cardboard shape, then walk that shape and name it;
    feel different textures, then move like that texture, and label the texture.
Perform isometric exercises using different amounts of pressure.
Trace different shapes on the child's back and have the child move in those shapes.

Time

Move at varying speeds on different surfaces.
Accelerate and decelerate on different surfaces.
Move on a drum beat on different surfaces.
On signal, make sudden changes in direction on different surfaces.

Force

Move like different heavy objects/light objects.

Move up high in the air or close to the ground on different surfaces.

Make jerky or smooth movements on various surfaces.

ADDITIONAL MOVEMENT VARIATIONS

1. Touch the various parts of the body of a child with various objects. Ask the child to name or move the parts touched and to identify the characteristics of the objects used for touching.

2. Have children perform isotonic and isometric exercises with various objects: balls, hoops, wands, and beanbags can be used.

3. Have children climb ropes, cargo nets, ladders, and other playground equipment that have different textures.

4. Have children move through, over, or under a variety of obstacles, including tires, trampoline beds, mats, playground equipment, boxes, benches, beams, etc.

5. Have blindfolded children feel the position of another child while he or she is in movement, then ask them to name the skill or reproduce it.

6. Have blindfolded children identify, discriminate between, and categorize different objects.

7. Have children work in pairs and push each other across the room slowly, with one child providing just enough resistance for the pushing child to move the other child slowly. Try this:
   a. with palms touching.
   b. standing back to back.
   c. standing shoulder to shoulder.
   d. using any other pair of body parts.

8. Have the children stand about 10 inches from the wall, facing it. They lean toward it and pretend to push it back with their hands.

9. Have the children press against the floor or other rigid surface with the whole body in both face-up and face-down positions, first with eyes closed, then with eyes opened.

10. Have children kneel with hands on floor below shoulders and slightly turned inward, thighs at right angles to the floor, back straight. Ask the children to press "holes" in the floor with the hands. Hold while the teacher counts to three, then relax.

11. Have children stand with back about four to six inches from a wall. Tell them to lean backward and press against the wall with the back as hard as possible. Still pressing, tell them to slide down to a position as if sitting on a chair, with knees bent and back flat against the wall. Slide up to the original position.

12. Use different body parts to manipulate different objects. Use hands, feet, elbows, wrists, knees, heels, etc.

Teaching Hints

Utilize familiar objects for tactual discrimination tasks.

Encourage children to label objects by the feel of them.

Use objects with homogeneous shapes, textures, size, or weight for sorting.

Skill Concepts Communicated to Children

Objects can be hard, soft, rough, smooth, sticky, slimy, and so forth.

The feel of an object can be determined by body parts other than the hands.

The shape of an object can be determined just by feeling it.

Movement Enhancement

Tactile Awareness Enhancement Chart

	LEVEL		LEVEL		LEVEL
GAMES		GYMNASTICS		Egg-Sit	
				Forward Roll	
The Feely Bag	I–III	Bear Walk	I & II	Backward Roll	
		Inch Worm		Trampoline	
Partner Tag	I & II	Egg Roll			
		Log Roll		Shoulder Wrestling	III
Back To Back	II & III			Leg Wrestling	
Put in Order		Eskimo Roll	II & III	Push War	
Memory Ball		Bridge		Foot Push	
Sandpaper Numbers		Rocking Chair		Toe Push	
and Letters		Corkscrew		Rhythmic Ball Gymnastics	
		Thread the Needle			

AUDITORY AWARENESS

Movement Description

Auditory awareness refers to the ability to discriminate, associate, and interpret auditory stimuli in order that such information may become meaningful to the individual. More specifically, the following is involved:

1. The ability to locate and identify sounds;
2. The ability to retain and respond to auditory commands;
3. The ability to respond to a rhythmic accompaniment;
4. The ability to distinguish between sounds that are both similar and dissimilar;
5. The ability to comprehend verbal communication.

Four components of auditory awareness appear to be relevant to enhancement by movement activities. These are discussed below.

Auditory Figure-Ground

This component is the ability to distinguish and concentrate on relevant auditory stimuli while ignoring irrelevant stimuli within an environment containing general auditory information. Children with inadequate functioning of the *auditory figure-ground* component have difficulty concentrating on verbal instructions and responding to directions.

Auditory Discrimination

This refers to the ability to distinguish between different frequencies and amplitudes of sounds. Included in the *auditory discrimination* component is *auditory constancy,* namely the ability to recognize auditory information as the same under varying circumstances. Children with poor discrimination abilities usually exhibit problems in rhythmic activities, games, and dances, all of which are dependent on such skills.

Sound Localization

Sound localization involves the ability to determine the source or direction of sound. Being able to locate individuals, animals, or objects (for example, ears, horns) with limited or no immediate visual information is something that must be experienced in order for the child to be effective and safe in his or her environment.

Temporal Auditory Perception

This component refers to the recognition and discrimination of variations of auditory stimuli presented in time. Especially relevant during the presentation of rhythmic and dance activities, inadequacy in *temporal auditory perception* may hinder the child's movement as she or he attempts to interpret tempo, rate, emphasis, and order of auditory stimuli.

The existing variations of abilities in auditory perception may be attributable to differences in ability or differences in early parental training (awareness depends upon learning). Therefore, unless training occurs many children will have difficulty in hearing and following the teacher's instructions in school. Further problems in listening and reading comprehension may occur because the child cannot distinguish between, and attend to, auditory cues.

Movement Observation

A child who is deficient in auditory awareness will appear to be inattentive and at times disobedient. Some behaviors that suggest poor listening skills include:

1. An inability to identify common sounds without visual cues;
2. An inability to follow simple directions that are clearly stated;
3. Poor performance in dance activities;
4. An inability to understand verbal commands.

Although all children benefit greatly from auditory training, the child who is deficient needs to be placed in a remedial program to ensure future ability to learn in the classroom.

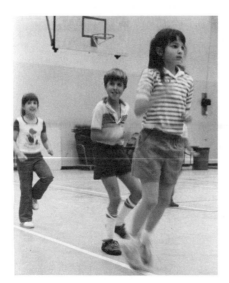

Auditory awareness is a key component of rhythmic awareness.

Movement Variability

Movement provides an excellent medium for practicing listening skills. When learning to follow directions it is more motivating for the child to actually show understanding through movement than to demonstrate understanding verbally.

Teachers must stress that noise be kept to a minimum so that their voices can be heard by all children when giving directions. Following directions should be made a challenge for the children.

Combining Auditory Awareness With a Motor Program
Spatial

On command, have the children:

touch or move different body parts;
form different shapes with their bodies;
move across the floor with different locomotors;
move at different levels: high, medium, and low;
trace curved, straight, and zigzag pathways as they move through space;
change directions as they move;
touch the floor with different body parts.

Time

On command, the children should be able to:

stop and start movement;
accelerate and decelerate movement;
go at different speeds;
move different body parts in time to a rhythmic accompaniment (try a drum beat, tambourine, lummi sticks, or recorded music that has a simple beat);
imitate different clapping patterns and sequences.

Force

On command, the children should be able to:

move with jerky movements;
move with smooth movements;
move with heavy or light movements;
move close to the ground or high in the air;
make hard and soft gestures with the arm or other body parts.

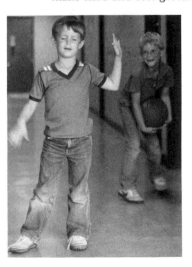

Identifying common sounds and directions without visual cues.

ADDITIONAL MOVEMENT VARIATIONS

1. Have children identify with their eyes closed the following common sounds:
   a. sharpening a pencil
   b. closing a window
   c. turning on the water fountain
   d. turning on a light
   e. knocking on a door.

2. Have children identify with their eyes closed an object when it is dropped or how many times a ball bounces when dropped.

3. Have children point with eyes closed in a direction where they believe a designated sound (ringing bell, ticking clock, etc.) is coming from.

4. Have children identify with eyes closed various rhythm instruments.

5. Have children move in conjunction with changes in volume of music. Loud music would suggest large movement, and soft music would suggest small movement, for example.

6. Repeat different rhythmic patterns and sequences using lummi sticks, ribbons, or poi pois.

7. Have blindfolded children try to identify the voices of other children in the class.

8. Have children follow simple directions, for example:
   a. march loudly for five steps
   b. bounce the ball eight times
   c. clap hands twice.
   Make this into a game and challenge the children to be accurate in their responses.

9. Jump rope to music.

10. Give commands as children perform on apparatus.
    (The following activities are to be performed blindfolded or in a dark room:)

11. Ask children to move toward or away from a voice or other auditory signal.

12. Provide children with paper cups or other objects. Have them throw the objects a particular distance and then find them as quickly as possible.

13. While in a restricted space, have children move about without touching each other. They may make their own sounds while moving. Make the activity more difficult by further restricting the space.

14. Ask children to roll balls to each other on the grass.

15. Ask children to throw objects at a sound. For example, children may shoot baskets by aiming toward an audible beeper.

16. Arrange an obstacle course in which the order of direction is dependent upon sound. For example, sounds emitted from tape recorders, electronic beepers, or record players may be used. In addition, children may be stationed at various obstacles to lead youngsters in the correct order by calling, clapping, or creating sounds with objects.

17. Associate a movement such as hopping, jumping, rolling, or skipping with a particular sound. For example, a clap may mean a hop; a bell may mean a jump; a horn may mean a skip; a strike of a triangle may mean a squat. Make sounds in a particular order and ask children to respond with appropriate movement in the same order.

Teaching Hints

Keep noise to a minimum so that all children may hear the directions.
Use a variety of vocal notations; sometimes loud, sometimes soft.
Use different sounds to signal different types of movement.
Challenge the children through games that demand good listening skills.
Use music during activity.

Skill Concepts Communicated to Children

Sounds may come from a variety of places.

One can replicate auditory commands in movement.

One can tune into one sound among other sounds and respond to just one cue.

Movement Enhancement

Auditory Awareness Enhancement Chart

	LEVEL		LEVEL		LEVEL
GAMES		Little Red Fox		Chimes of Dunkirk	
		O'Leary		Farmer in the Dell	
Prui	I–III	Attention Relays		Hokey-Pokey	
Go Touch It		Knock-Knock		Looby Loo	
Kitty, Kitty		Colors		Did You Ever See	
				a Lassie?	
Giants, Dwarfs,	I & II	Math Merriment	III		
and People				Ten Little Indians	II
Just Now		*DANCE AND RHYTHMS*			
Cat and Rat				Klapptanz	III
		I'm a Little Teapot	I & II	Bingo	
Indian Chief	II & III	Row, Row, Row			
		If I Were a Bird			

REFERENCES

GALLAHUE, D. (1982). *Developmental movement experiences for Children.* New York, N.Y.: John Wiley & Sons.

MURRAY, R. L. (1975). *Dance in elementary education* (3rd ed.). New York: Harper & Row.

SUGGESTED READINGS

ANDREWS, G. (1976). *Creative rhythmic movement for children.* Englewood Cliffs, NJ: Prentice-Hall.

BARLIN, A. (1979). *Teaching your wings to fly.* Santa Monica, CA: Goodyear.

BRUCE, V. R. (1970). *Movement in silence and sounds.* London: G. Bell & Sons.

DIMONDSTEIN, G. (1971). *Children dance in the classroom.* New York: Macmillan.

GALLAHUE, D. L. (1982). *Developmental movement experiences for children.* New York, N.Y.: John Wiley & Sons.

HARRIS, J., PITTMAN, A., WALLER, M., (1978). *Dance a while.* Minneapolis: Burgess.

JOYCE, M. (1980). *First steps in teaching creative dance to children.* Palo Alto, CA: Mayfield.

JOYCE, M. (1984). *Dance technique for children.* Palo Alto, CA: Mayfield.

KIRCHNER, G. (1985). *Physical education for elementary school children* (6th ed.). Dubuque, IA: Wm. C. Brown.

LOGSDON, B. J., BARRETT, K. R., BROER, M. R., McGEE, R., AMMONS, M., HALVERSON, L. E., & ROBERTON, M. A. (1984). *Physical education for children.* (2nd ed). Philadelphia: Lea & Febiger.

MURRAY, R. L. (1975). *Dance in elementary education.* (3rd ed.). New York: Harper & Row.

SCHURR, E. L. (1980). *Movement experiences for children.* (3rd ed.). Englewood Cliffs, NJ: Prentice-Hall.

13

PHYSICAL FITNESS ACTIVITIES

INTRODUCTION

Physical fitness is an integral cornerstone of this text. Elementary physical education programs in which fitness is considered a high priority are more apt to produce students who possess and value healthy, agile bodies capable of functioning at high activity levels. As discussed in Chapter 4, fitness cannot be left to chance. The optimum physical education program will not permit fitness to be viewed only as a by-product of daily lessons, but will have planned instruction and adequate practice time so that stated goals for fitness development can be achieved.

The intent of this chapter is to provide a selection of exercises and activities that may enhance the development of health-related fitness components (muscular strength/endurance, optimal body composition, flexibility, and cardiorespiratory endurance) of children. The authors believe that the skill-related components of fitness (agility, speed, power, coordination, reaction time, and balance) will be enhanced as children participate in the variability of practice activities planned for each skill theme; therefore such activities are excluded from this discussion. Health-related components of fitness, on the other hand, are task specific and must be dealt with in a direct manner if a difference is to be realized. Optimum physical fitness will be achieved only if muscle groups and organic functions are stimulated on a regular basis. Programming for fitness development should involve the specific utilization of muscle groups that are frequently isolated so that the effort requirement is focused on a specific muscle (for example, the bicep), a group of muscles (abdominals, upper body, etc.), or organs (circulatory system—heart, lungs, blood vessels). Fitness development for children should concentrate on the entire body; thus teachers must plan accurately to ensure that all of the major muscle groups (legs, trunk, arms and shoulder girdle, cardiorespiratory systems) are exercised regularly.

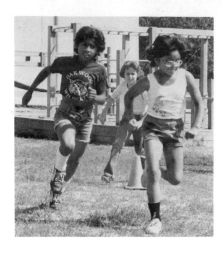

A vigorous program facilitates the development of physical fitness.

Planning for fitness begins when the yearly plan is being developed. Thus we strongly suggest that several days be allowed after the tenth class day for assessment of the children's level of fitness at the beginning of each school year. In late April or early May another block of time is set aside for a reassessment of health-related fitness capabilities.

The second opportunity to make specific plans for fitness development is during the construction of each theme packet in which a minimum of five fitness activities that are appropriate for use during that theme are listed.

Finally, implementation of these plans is realized during each daily lesson in the following ways:

1. Approximately one-third of the total lesson time (that is, 12 to 15 minutes of a 45-minute period) is devoted to the fitness phase with specific component objectives.
2. Utilize equipment, methods, and organizational strategies so students can be constantly active during the entire fitness phase.
3. Pace each daily lesson (that is, plan the vigorous and not-so-vigorous events of the lesson) in such a way that the students are stimulated to a realistic level of involvement so as to cause an acceptable overload and thereby keep the heart rate within an acceptable range (126 to 172 beats/minute depending on age and fitness level; Table 13–1). The children should experience a labored demand on their bodies (rosy cheeks, perspiration, fast heart beat, rapid breathing). The teacher should enhance the students' awareness of these physiological changes by reinforcement: "Wow, Tommy, I can tell by your breathing that you are working hard. Keep up the good work!"

TABLE 13-1 Recommended Working Heart Rates

		INTENSITY LEVELS		
Age	Max Hr (220-Age)*	Level I 70%	Level II 75%	Level III 80%
5	215	150	161	172
6	214	150	161	171
7	213	149	160	170
8	212	148	159	170
9	211	148	158	169
10	210	147	158	168
11	209	146	157	167
12	208	146	156	166

*By subtracting the child's age (in years) from 220, the estimated predicted maximum heart rate is determined. The intensity level (%) should be maintained for a period of 15–30 minutes.

TABLE 13-2

MONDAY	TUESDAY	WEDNESDAY	THURSDAY	FRIDAY
Cardiorespiratory	Upper body strength/endur. Flexibility	Cardiorespiratory	Flexibility Abdominal strength/endur.	Cardiorespiratory
Cardiorespiratory	Flexibility Upper body strength/endur.	Cardiorespiratory	Abdominal strength/endur. Flexibility	Cardiorespiratory

Physical fitness activities are presented during the fitness phase of each daily lesson on a rotational basis so that all of the health-related components are covered in a systematic manner (Table 13-2). The authors would like to note, however, that although the 10 to 20 minutes (approximately one-third of the total lesson time) allocated for the fitness period present a strong stimulus for the development of fitness, it should not be perceived as a thorough treatment. This period of the lesson promotes ideas for activities, a physiological stimulus, and the development of a positive attitude toward fitness. A thorough fitness program (as mentioned in Chapter 4) utilizes other periods of the day (for example, recess, noon, before and after school) to supplement fitness development. Of course, the more active the children are kept the more the body is taxed; hence, the greater the opportunity for the body to become more fit.

Pacing

Many adults worry about working children too hard, and therefore allow them to "stop" and rest. Children need not *stop* to rest! It is important that daily fitness activities are sequenced in such a way to allow *pacing* of effort (that is, alternating moderate- to high-intensity efforts with low-intensity efforts). Children should be taught the reasons for pacing as they participate in activities that alternate between intense and less demanding activities. To accommodate an understanding of workload, children should learn to monitor their heart rate. Young children (preschool to first-grade level) can be taught to determine heart rate most effectively at the carotid artery in the neck area, whereas older students can usually monitor the heart rate at the brachial artery at the wrist. This cognitive understanding can then be transferred to individual play situations in which pacing may be implemented by the child. Children can be taught pacing techniques (lower lift of knees, modified movement of arms, smaller stride, walking) that will allow them to adjust their own expenditure of effort so that their body may recover without a complete cessation of movement, and they may persist in the activity for the length of time required.

Overload

The *overload principle* is in effect when a muscle(s) is required to exert more than normally. In order for health-related fitness to improve, each student must experience some degree of overload when participating in fitness activities. The authors believe that children will most often reach their individual overload threshold if they enthusiastically participate in a variety of fitness-oriented activities and if the duration of their participation is sufficient to tax genuinely the various muscle groups and systems of the body. The teacher can encourage children to reach beyond past performances by challenging them: "Can you jump five more times [frequency] than you did yesterday, David?" "Sue, see if you can continue skipping for 30 more seconds [duration]." "Jim, can you jump rope and keep up [intensity] with this fast music?" Each of these challenges has the capability of overloading the muscles and systems of the body, and the more often that muscles and body systems are required to exert more than normally, the stronger they become. Once again the teacher is reminded of the difficulty of achieving overload in a short 10- to 20-minute fitness period. Only through intelligent planning is this apt to occur.

Motivation

Children perceive their world as a playground. Thus, *motivation* toward activity is generally not a problem for teachers—appropriate focus of that wonderful energy becomes the teacher's primary task. The enthusiastic, creative, active teacher will use the imaginative world of children to channel youngsters' natural energy into appropriate activities that will enhance their fitness level.

The teacher's personal response to activity and fitness in general (as demonstrated by the teacher's personal level of fitness as well as frequent participation in the activities) is a very potent motivator for students. Feedback and recognition are also effective motivators and should be used liberally.

General Activity Suggestions

1. Activities should be chosen and presented to allow for maximum participation of all students.
2. Elimination-type games and activities should be changed so that no child is removed from the activity and required to wait. For example, rather than sit out after being tagged, the child can go to the sideline, complete 25 successful jumps with a jump rope, and then reenter the game.
3. Plan carefully to exercise all major muscle groups and systems (that is, legs, trunk, arms and shoulder girdle, and cardiorespiratory system).
4. Assign partners of comparable size.
5. Present activities according to progression based both on level of required exertion and acquired motor-skill level.
6. Accurate performance of all exercises is not only desirable but also essential for maximum benefit.
7. Begin with a small number of repetitions and add to that number every third day.
8. When 20 repetitions of an exercise can be completed efficiently, the next most difficult exercise should be assigned (for example, when 20 modified pull-ups on a low horizontal bar with heels resting on ground and body at 60° angle can be completed, the child should begin working on regular pull-ups).
9. Early success and praise will encourage a continued interest in the fitness activities.
10. Tag games and tumbling activities offer excellent dynamic challenge possibilities for all of the fitness components.
11. Opportunities for student leadership should be considered for children above the second grade (for example, children leading the exercises).
12. When possible, the fitness components that are not stressed during the fitness phase should be stimulated in another part of the lesson.
13. Children should be motivated to give 100 percent effort as they participate.
14. Cognitive information regarding names of muscle groups, proper techniques, and exercise concepts should be provided to the students at their level of understanding. For example, when lining up to return to their classroom, the children could be asked, "What muscle helps me to do push-ups or push open a door?" (triceps); "What part of my anatomy will I land on if I fall backwards?" (gluteus maximus).
15. Many of the fitness activities for children in Levels I–II may be presented in a rather informal manner (through story plays, challenges, and similes), whereas students at

Level III and above are usually capable of participating in a more organized fitness program (structured exercise routines, aerobic dancing, mass calisthenics).

Calisthenics

The authors believe that, although presentation of individual exercises can benefit the young child, highly structured calisthenic routines are not appropriate for children at Levels I and II for the following reasons:

1. Highly structured exercises are generally not compatible with the child's physical, emotional, and cognitive development.
2. Too much time is lost when children are required to perform en masse to a structured routine (for example, "All touch your right toe with your left hand on one, stand tall on two, touch the left toe with your right hand on three and stand tall on four").
3. Young children respond more exuberantly to imaginative challenges (for example, "If you were an inchworm, how would you move?" "While lying on your stomach, can you make your feet move toward your hands without moving your hands?" "What happens to your body if you keep your knees straight?"). The next time the inchworm movement was desired, the challenge could simply be, "Move like an inchworm."
4. Synchronized performances eliminate the opportunity for students to perform at their own pace.

The activities in this chapter are grouped according to their fitness and muscular group focus. The teacher should choose appropriate activities according to the motor-skill and fitness levels of the students. Variations can also be implemented to increase or decrease the effort requirements of the activities. Each child should be encouraged always to put forth his or her best effort; therefore, it is important that what children are asked to do is commensurate with their developmental level.

The method of presentation for Levels I and II will be more informal than the presentation for Level III and above. All teaching strategies should be in keeping with the needs and abilities of the students. For example, the use of guided discovery and problem-solving teaching styles in the informal presentation of fitness activities for children at Levels I and II may include locomotor and nonlocomotor challenges and story plays. The command teaching style is also appropriate for locomotor and nonlocomotor challenges.

The remainder of the chapter contains specific exercises and activities as outlined:

Starting Position for Exercises

FLEXIBILITY ACTIVITIES

Legs
Trunk
Arm and Shoulder Girdle
Neck

MUSCULAR STRENGTH/ENDURANCE ACTIVITIES

Legs
Trunk
Arm and Shoulder Girdle

CARDIORESPIRATORY ENDURANCE ACTIVITIES
ACTIVITIES REFERENCE CHART (Table 13–6)

STARTING POSITIONS FOR EXERCISES

Various starting positions are used for the activities presented in this chapter. The following illustrations are offered for clarification.

1. Supine

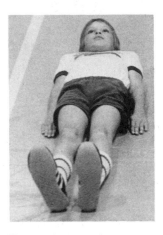

Figure 13-1

2. Prone

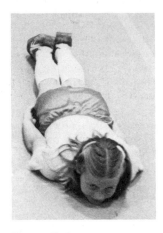

Figure 13-2

3. Hook Lying

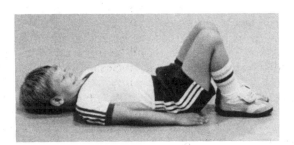

Figure 13-3

4. Long Sit

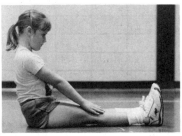

Figure 13-4

5. Straddle Sit

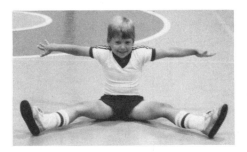

Figure 13-5

6. Hook Sit

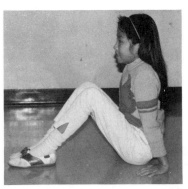

Figure 13-6

7. Cross-Leg Sit

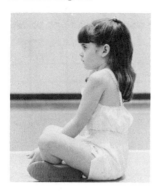

Figure 13-7

8. Sitting on Heels

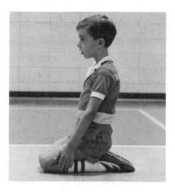

Figure 13-8

9. Standing

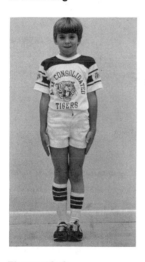

Figure 13-9

10. Straddle Stand

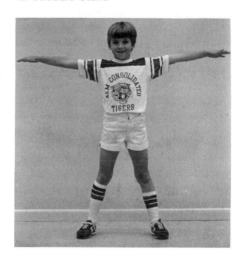

Figure 13-10

11. Front Leaning Rest

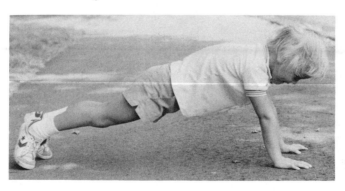

Figure 13-11

12. Side Leaning Rest

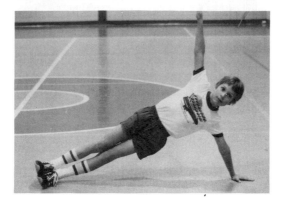

Figure 13-12

13. Hands and Knees

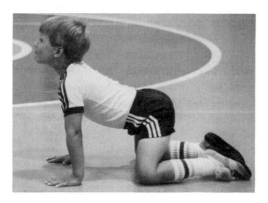

Figure 13-13

14. Crab

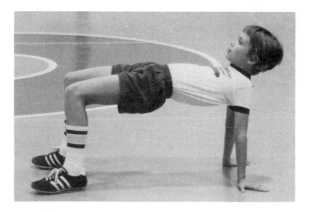

Figure 13-14

Commands that ask the children to change from one starting position to another can be a flexibility, strength, reaction-time, endurance, and cognitive activity in itself. The stronger and more agile the child, the faster the challenges can be stated, thereby causing a stronger effort requirement from the child. An example of this activity follows.

> Class, as I call out the various starting positions we have learned, I want you to assume that position as quickly as you can. Ready?
> Long sit—supine—prone—straddle sit—prone—hook lying—front leaning rest—prone—supine—hook sit—supine—standing—straddle stand—hands and knees—crab—hands and knees.

Various sequences can make this activity appropriate for any ability level.

FLEXIBILITY ACTIVITIES

The importance of overall body flexibility has been clearly established (Chapter 4) as an essential component in one's health-related fitness. The experiences presented here are suggested as appropriate to improve both static and dynamic levels of flexibility as well as joint strength. Another fitness consideration—posture—is also directly influenced by the child's degree of flexibility.

Teaching Hints:

1. Movements should be deliberate, with focus upon a full range of motion. Bouncing movements are to be discouraged. Stretch to a point of pain and then back off a little and hold.
2. To maximize the benefits from stretching activities, hold the stretch position for a minimum of 30 seconds (Level III and above).
3. At the beginning, each exercise should be repeated for six repetitions, with the overload increments occurring gradually.
4. Encourage children not only to be aware of the extent of their flexibility ("How far can you reach down your leg?"—today to the ankles, days later to the toes, then palms flat on the floor) but also to strive for daily improvement.
5. Incorporate games that require extended flexibility moves (for example, "Over and Under Tag").
6. Use flexibility as a pacing technique inserted between strength and endurance activities.

Through the medium of "movement stories," children can be stimulated to execute many moves that will serve to test out and improve the range of motion of their joints. As the teacher verbalizes a fairy tale or short story, the students act out the roles of various people or animals in the story. Through the use of variability of time, force, space, and relationships, the children can be required to perform stretching, agile moves that will both stretch and strengthen the various joints of the body. The joints most often used in such imaginative activities are the spinal vertebrae, hips, knees, ankles, shoulders, elbows, wrist, and fingers (especially if climbing apparatus is available).

Wands also offer excellent challenges for flexibility as the body attempts to move over and under individually held wands. (See Fig. 13–15.)

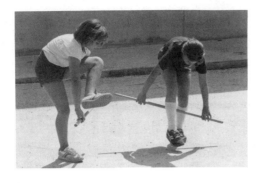

Figure 13-15

LEGS

1. Hamstring Stretch:
   Starting Position: back lying
   Procedure: Extend one straight leg up toward the ceiling; later grasp toes and try to keep knees straight.

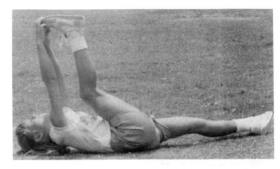

Figure 13-16

2. Groin Stretch:
   Starting Position: straddle stand
   Procedure: Move the feet further apart inch by inch then bend over and place palms on the floor and hold the position for as long as possible, being careful not to lock the knees.

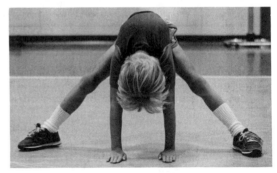

Figure 13-17

3. Groin, Hamstring, Low Back Stretch:
   Starting Position: wide straddle stand
   Procedure: Bend forward front, center, right, left, and behind feet.

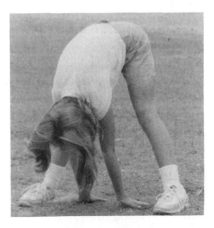

Figure 13-18

4. Quadricep Stretch:
   Starting Position: prone position
   Procedure: Alternate pulling each lower leg toward the buttocks; both legs can also be pulled simultaneously.

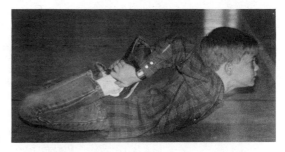

Figure 13-19

5. Foot to Head:
   Starting Position: crossed-leg sit
   Procedure: Alternate pulling each foot to head.

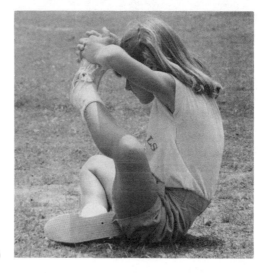

Figure 13-20

6. Calf and Arch Stretch:
   Starting Position: standing—arms held out in front
   Procedure: Slowly squat while keeping heels flat on the floor; place hands on floor in front of feet and continue to stretch calf and feet muscles; rock slowly back and forth, allowing heels to rise only if necessary; emphasize keeping heels in contact with the floor as much as possible.

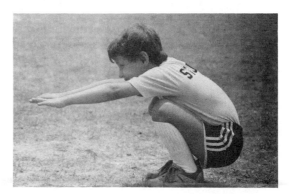

Figure 13-21

7. Leg, Foot, Back Stretch:
   Starting Position: hands and knees, tops of feet resting on floor
   Procedure: Alternate sitting back on heels while extending the arms forward; emphasize keeping entire surface of lower legs and tops of feet in contact with the floor.

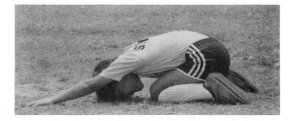

Figure 13-22

8. Hamstring Stretch:
   Starting Position: standing
   Procedure: Bend forward and grasp toes (knees may bend); slowly straighten legs; hold at maximum stretch; emphasize not locking the knees.

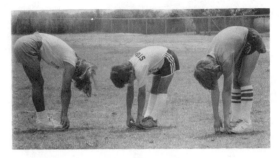

Figure 13-23

9. Calf Stretch:
   Starting Position: front lean against wall, standing 1½ to 2 feet from the wall
   Procedure: Lean forward to bring chest as close to wall as possible (head may be turned to one side) while keeping back and knees straight and heels flat on floor. Increase standing distance from wall as flexibility permits.

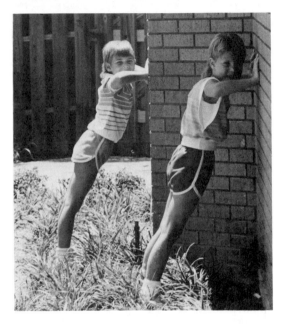

Figure 13-24

10. Heel Walk:
    Starting Position: standing
    Procedure: Walk on heels with legs straight and toes pointing toward the ceiling; first attempt should be two sets of 10 yards each.

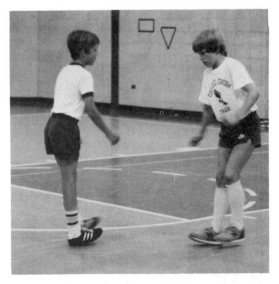

Figure 13-25

TRUNK

1. Low Back Stretch:
   Starting Position: straddle sitting
   Procedure: Alternate pulling torso toward
   each leg; torso can also be pulled straight forward through legs. Close legs and pull torso
   forward over knees; hold each position a minimum of 10 seconds.

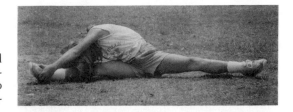
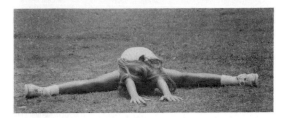

Figure 13-26a,b

2. Low Back Stretch: (pelvic tilt)
   Starting Position: hook lying, arms at sides
   Procedure: Inhale while arching back; exhale
   while pressing back to the floor ("Use abdominal muscles to push your backbone into the
   floor"); continue pressing until all air is exhaled; repeat the procedure four to six times.

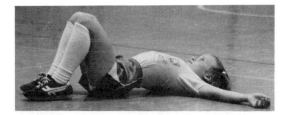
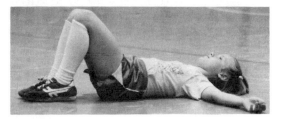

Figure 13-27a,b

3. Mad Cat:
   Starting Position: hands and knees, head up,
   focus straight ahead, back relaxed
   Procedure: Arch back up by pulling in the abdomen, tightening the buttocks, lowering the
   head, and exhaling; hold until exhalation is
   completed, then relax, letting the back and
   abdomen sag while inhaling, head returns to
   starting position, repeat cycle rhythmically for
   six repetitions.

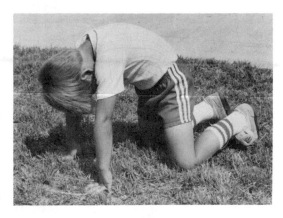

Figure 13-28

4. Psoas Stretch:
   Starting Position: long lying
   Procedure: Alternate hugging each knee to
   the chest while keeping outstretched leg flat
   to the floor; emphasize keeping low back in
   contact with floor.

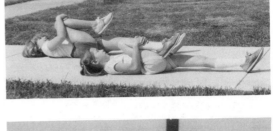

Figure 13-29

5. Trees:
   Starting Position: moderate straddle stand,
   arms by sides or held straight overhead
   Procedure: Slowly allow the upper body to
   bend right, left, forward, and backward; when
   arms are held above the head more weight resistance will be experienced.

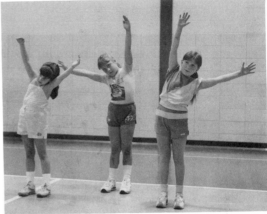

Figure 13-30

6. Washing Machine Twist:
   Starting Position: straddle standing
   Procedure: Slowly twist the body rhythmically from right to left; arms may be held in
   various positions, and head should turn in direction of twist.

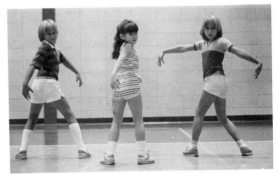

Figure 13-31

7. Trunk Twister:
   Starting Position: wide straddle, trunk bent
   forward (parallel to the floor), knees straight
   (but not locked), hands behind head, elbows
   back
   Procedure: Twist trunk to right (left elbow
   points to the floor), then left (right elbow
   points to the floor); repeat four twists, then
   stand upright; repeat four times.

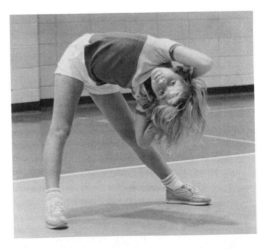

Figure 13-32

ARM AND SHOULDER GIRDLE

1. Shoulder Stretch No. 1:
   Starting Position: standing, arms at sides
   Procedure: Alternate pulling shoulder blades
   together while rotating arms outward and
   back (thumbs point to rear) and pulling shoulders forward while rotating shoulders and
   arms forward and inward.

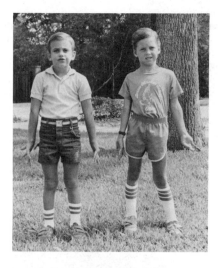

Figure 13-33

2. Shoulder Stretch No. 2:
   Starting Position: straddle standing
   Procedure: Hold the hands behind the back,
   bend the trunk forward until parallel to the
   floor, and then left arms behind back as high
   as possible. Do not lock the knees.

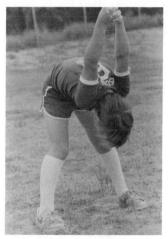

Figure 13-34

3. Arm Circles:
   Starting Position: moderate straddle standing,
   arms out to side
   Procedure: Circle arms (large circles—forward
   and backward) utilizing full range of motion;
   abdomen and buttocks held firm to minimize
   lumbar curve.

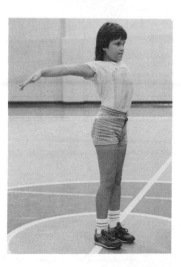

Figure 13-35

4. Lateral Arm Pulls:
Starting Position: moderate straddle standing
Procedure: Move one arm shoulder high across midline of body; free arm reaches under and grasps extended arm right above elbow; pull arm to maximum position; repeat with other arm.

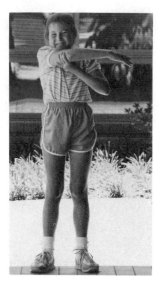

Figure 13-36

5. Vertical Arm Pulls:
Starting Position: moderate straddle standing
Procedure: One arm reaches up the back to meet other arm reaching over the shoulder; grasp hands and hold in maximum stretch, alternate arms.

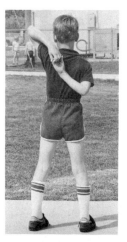

Figure 13-37

NECK

1. Yes, No, Maybe:
Starting Position: moderate straddle standing, hands at sides
Procedure: Stand tall in good posture; alternate rotating the head as far as possible to the right and then to the left (4 times), forward and backward (4 times); no circular rotations (that is, front, right, back, left in rapid sequence).

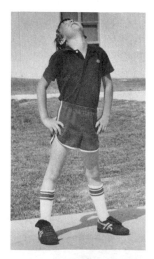

Figure 13-38

2. Neck Pulls:
   Starting Position: moderate straddle stand or cross-leg sit
   Procedure: Stand or sit tall in good posture; place left hand on top right side of head and gently pull head to the left; repeat with the right hand pulling head to the right; place both hands on back of head and gently pull chin to chest; move head up and backward so face is toward the ceiling. Keep back straight during entire exercise.

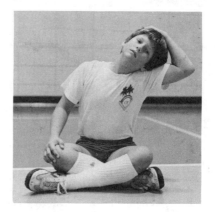

Figure 13-39

MUSCULAR STRENGTH/ENDURANCE ACTIVITIES

Muscular strength is demonstrated by the amount of force (intensity) that can be exerted by a muscle or group or muscles working against resistance. For the child, the resistance is often simply the movement of body parts against gravity. *Muscular endurance* is demonstrated by the length of time (duration) that a muscle(s) can persist in exertion. With slight modification (intensity and duration), most of the same exercises can be used to develop both muscular strength and endurance. The teacher is reminded that although strength can be present without endurance, the reverse is not true. To train for endurance, the resistance (intensity) is reduced so the duration of participation can be lengthened sufficiently to cause an overload (overtime) on the muscle(s) and/or organic system.

Teaching Hints:

1. Stress proper form and explain to students why good form is essential (that is, improper form causes wasted effort and can also contribute to injury).
2. Simply lifting their own body weight offers enough resistance for strength building for students at Levels I and II. Level III (and above) students can engage in partner activities that permit an increased resistance.
3. To increase muscular endurance, lighten the resistance and increase the repetitions.
4. Any increase in resistance should be applied gradually.
5. Students should successfully complete 20 repetitions (in good form) of an exercise before they are permitted to move on to the next progression.
6. Teach students the similarities and differences between strength and muscular endurance.
7. Give realistic, dynamic examples of strength and endurance (for example, strength of the arms and shoulder girdle allows one to pull up to the top of the tumbling table; the level of endurance of those same muscles will determine how long one can hand-travel on the horizontal ladder or how high one can climb up the climbing rope).
8. Emphasize the importance of always striving to perform as well or better than the last performance.
9. Give high frequencies of positive reinforcement to those students who demonstrate an all-out expenditure of effort.
10. Teach students the scientific and common names of the major muscle groups.
11. Teach proper breathing techniques (that is, the breath should not be held, but rather exhaled during exertion and inhaled during recovery).

12. All exercises should be repeated for six repetitions unless otherwise noted. Generally speaking, the number of repetitions can be increased by one every three days. Individual abilities, however, must be the true determiner of increased work load.

Planning Reminders for the Teacher
1. Postural development depends upon a balance of muscular strength/endurance and flexibility development.
2. Abdominal strength, psoas and hamstring flexibility, and back strength and flexibility are most critical for optimum postural development.
3. Adequate strength will enable students to perform fundamental skills with higher degrees of success.
4. Students with low levels of muscular strength and endurance are more apt to sustain injuries.
5. Isotonic (resistance against a moving muscle) exercises are most appropriate for students in Levels I and II.

LEGS

1. Partial Squats:
   Starting Position: standing, arms at sides
   Procedure: With torso leaning slightly forward and arms held out in front, sit on an imaginary stool (thighs parallel to the ground); hold position for a minimum of six seconds.

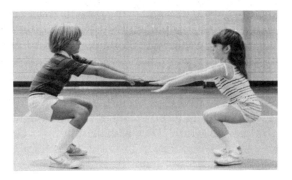

Figure 13–40

2. Heel Walks:
   Starting Position: standing
   Procedure: Walk on heels with legs straight throughout and toes pointed toward the ceiling; first attempt should be two sets of 10 yards each (see Figure 13–25).
3. Running for Speed:
   Starting Position: standing
   Procedure:
      a. Run short distances of up to 50 yards;
      b. Alternate running for speed with quick stops;
      c. Additional challenges can be obtained form Chapter 9, "Running."
4. Puppy Run:
   Starting Position: on hands and feet, knees slightly bent, head up
   Procedure: Run (scamper) about like a puppy, forward, backward, sideward.
5. Bear Walk:
   Starting Position: weight primarily on feet but with hands touching floor in front
   Procedure: Slowly travel forward by simultaneously moving the hand and foot on the same side; movements are slow, heavy, deliberate; nonsupporting arm and leg should be lifted high.
6. Jumping:
   Starting Position: standing
   Procedure:
      a. Jump repeatedly for height;
      b. Jump for distance;

      c. Jump into the air and click heels together (center, right, left);

      d. Additional challenges can be obtained from Chapter 9, "Jumping."

7. Jump to Run:

   Starting Position: supine or prone position

   Procedure: On signal, quickly get to feet and run to a designated area as fast as possible.

8. Skier's Sit:

   Starting Position: in a sitting position (thighs parallel to the floor with entire back against the wall; arms held crossed in front of body at shoulder height)

   Procedure: Have students sit in the isometric position for as long as possible.

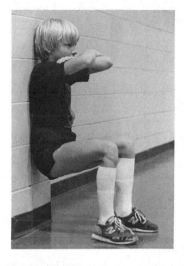

Figure 13-41

9. Chinese Get Up:

   Starting Position: children of equal size stand back-to-back with elbows hooked

   Procedure: Slowly sit down while backs press against one another.

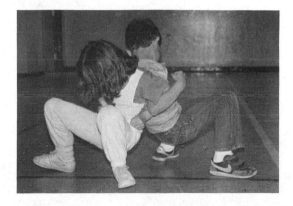

Figure 13-42

10. Partner Tug-of-War:

   Starting Position: (partners) holding on to opposite ends of an individual tug-o-rope, forward stride position

   Procedure: On signal, both students begin pulling against one another; pulling continues until one student is pulled across the line separating the two students.

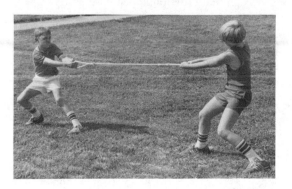

Figure 13-43

TRUNK

1. Curl-Ups:
   Starting Position: hook lying, arms folded across chest.
   Procedure: Lift head, chin on chest, lift shoulders; hold this curled position for a minimum of 6 seconds (exhale).

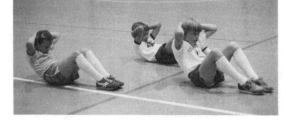

Figure 13-44

2. Crunchies:
   Starting Position: hook lying, arms folded across chest.
   Procedure: Lift head and shoulders from floor while simultaneously pressing the back against the floor and rolling pelvis backward; feet may come off the ground.

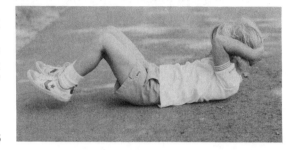

Figure 13-45

3. Reverse Curl-Ups:
   Starting Position: supine, arms held out to side
   Procedure: Bring legs to the chest and hug both knees tightly to chest; extend legs, repeat.

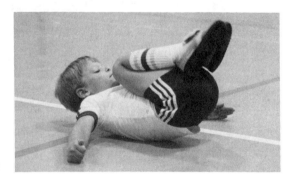

Figure 13-46

4. Back Press:
   Starting Position: hook lying, arms at sides
   Procedure: Inhale allowing abdomen to rise; exhale while pressing back flat against the floor. Continue pressing until all air is exhaled; repeat the procedure four to six times (see Figure 13-27; eliminate the initial pelvic tilt-arch).

5. Cocoon Hang:
   Starting Position: straight hang from a bar
   Procedure: Both legs are curled to chest and held for as long as possible; repeat as many times as possible.

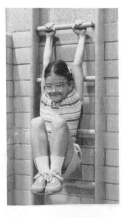

Figure 13-47

6. Prancing Ponies:
   Starting Position: standing, arms at sides
   Procedure: Rhythmically lift knees to hip level
   in a prancing fashion; alternate slow to fast
   speeds; various arm position can be used.

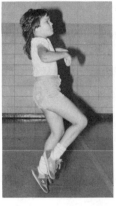

Figure 13-48

7. Swan Balance Variations:
   Starting Position: prone, arms at sides
   Procedure: Lift arms, head, hold a minimum
   of 6 seconds; with each repetition the arms
   move to a new position.

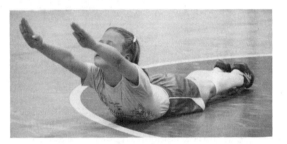

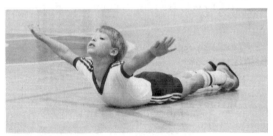

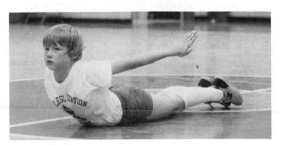

Figure 13-49

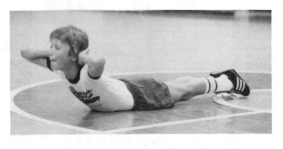

8. Prone Leg Lifts:
   Starting Position: prone, arms bent, hands under face
   Procedure: Alternate lifting straight legs, attempting to free thigh from the floor. Stronger students will be able to lift both legs from the floor simultaneously.

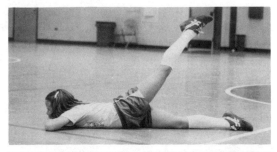
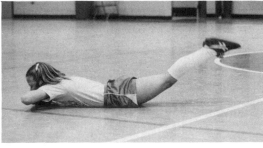

Figure 13-50a,b

9. Mad Cat:
   Starting Position: hands and knees, head up, back relaxed
   Procedure: Arch the back up by pulling the abdominals in, tightening the buttocks, lowering the head, and exhaling; hold until exhalation is completed then relax, letting the back sag while inhaling; repeat cycle rhythmically for six repetitions (see Fig. 13-28).

ARM AND SHOULDER GIRDLE

1. Birds and Butterflies:
   Starting Position: standing, arms out to sides
   Procedure: Flap wings (arms) up and down in large, vigorous (birds) or floating (butterfly)-type movements while moving, about quickly on tips of toes; encourage "vigorous flaps" for extended period of time.

2. Shoulder Shrugs:
   Starting Position: standing, arms at sides
   Procedure: Alternate shrugging shoulders 10 times each side; shrug both shoulders simultaneous 10 times.

3. Swimming:
   Starting Position: moderate straddle stand
   Procedure: Bend trunk forward, head up; make crawl-stroke movements with the arms; stand erect and make back-crawl movements with the arms. Do not lock the knees.

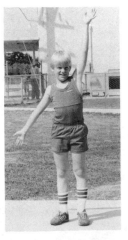

Figure 13-51

4. Sawing Wood:
   Starting Position: slight stride stand, holding hands with partner.
   Procedure: Arms make sawing movements back and forth; once movement is learned, encourage partners to offer mild resistance.

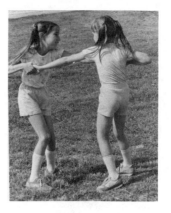

Figure 13-52

5. Flat Tire:
   Starting Position: hands and feet
   Procedure: While students move about on hands and feet (as an automobile), an occasional "flat (left/front, right/rear) tire" will be called out by the teacher or a student. All "autos" will simulate the flat tire as it is called and then lift up as tire inflates.

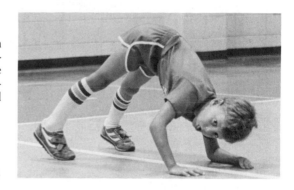

Figure 13-53

6. Front Leaning Rest Variations:
   Starting Position: front leaning rest
   Procedure:
   a. Hold firm, straight position, head up;
   b. Alternate lifting each hand (different heights for different abilities);

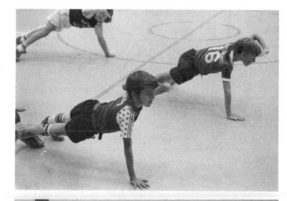

Figure 13-54

   c. Alternate lifting each foot;
   d. Alternate lifting one hand and one foot, and alternate slapping the chest with each hand in rhythm (marching tempo);

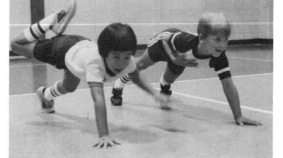

Figure 13-55

   e. Move forward, backward, and sideways while maintaining the firm-straight position.

7. Let-Downs:
Starting Position: front-leaning rest
Procedure: This is a reverse push-up. Slowly lower the body until it touches the ground, then immediately assume the front-leaning rest position again; child can use any movement necessary to get back into the starting position, including placing the knees on the floor. The object is to keep the arm and shoulder girdle muscle groups in a contracted state for the longest time possible; rather than fighting gravity from the ground up, this exercise allows the child to resist gravity from the top down.

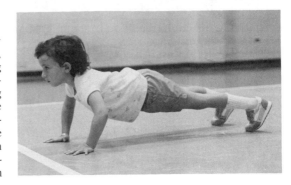

8. Elevator Ride:
Starting Position: front-leaning rest
Procedure: Teacher gives the "top floor" (starting position) a number and proceeds to call out the floors as the elevator moves down to ground level (lobby) and back up. If the elevator becomes stuck on a floor ("Oops, we're stuck on the second floor") the students must remain in that position until the teacher calls "repair completed"; while "stuck" on a floor, students can also sound the emergency bell (yell).

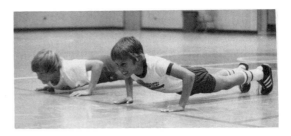

9. Wall Push-Ups:
Starting Position: standing 1 ½ to 2 feet from wall, hands on wall, shoulder height, elbows straight, feet slightly apart
Procedure: Bend arms to bring chest as close as possible to the wall, then return to starting position; body and knees kept straight, feet pointed straight ahead.

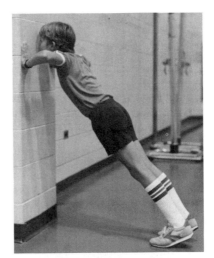

Figure 13-58

10. Mountain Climber:
Starting Position: front-leaning rest, head up
Procedure: Alternate drawing each leg up under the body; change speed from slow to fast.

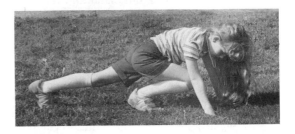

Figure 13-59

11. Seal Crawl:
Starting Position: front-leaning rest, tops of feet on floor
Procedure: Use the hands and arms to drag the stiff body forward; feet do not assist; strive for a distance of 15 feet. At first it is permissible to recline to prone position (and give seal grunts) if needed for intermittent rest.

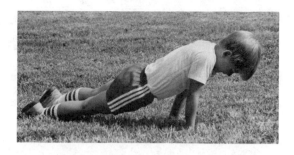

Figure 13-60

12. Elbow Crawl:
Starting Position: same as for seal crawl except weight is on elbows rather than hands
Procedure: Use the elbows and arms to drag the body forward.

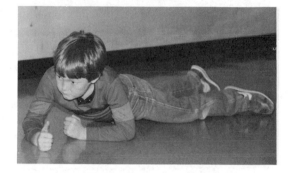

Figure 13-61

13. Crab Variations:
Starting Position: crab
Procedure: Alternate lifting each leg as high as possible; additional strength is required to lift an arm and leg in opposition.

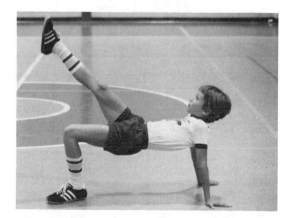

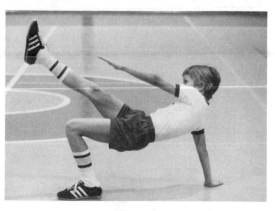

Figure 13-62a,b

14. Ball Squeeze:
Starting Position: moderate stride standing
Procedure: Hold playground ball at chest height between palms of hands, elbows out; attempt to squeeze the air from the ball. For this exercise and the variations to follow, the ball should be squeezed for a minimum of 6 seconds with each repetition; exhale while squeezing.

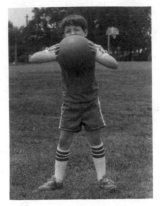

Figure 13-63

Hold playground ball between knees and attempt to squeeze air from ball; hold for minimum of 6 seconds.

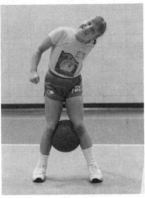

Figure 13-64

Hold ball between forearm and upper arm and attempt to squeeze air from ball; repeat with other arm.

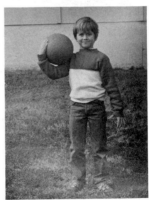

Figure 13-65

15. Crab-Tug:
Starting Position: crab position with one end of tug-o-rope looped around one foot; partners on either side of a line.
Procedure: Each student tries to pull opponent over the line.

Figure 13-66

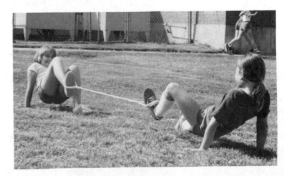

Rope can also be held in hands.

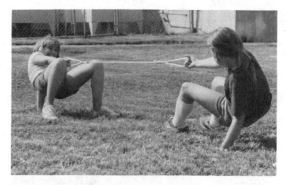

Figure 13–67

16. Partner Arm Tugs:
    Starting Position: partners facing, moderate stride standing; both hands hold one end of a tug-o-rope (or a jump rope or deflated 10-speed bicycle tube)
    Procedure: Partners alternate pulling and offering resistance to their partner's pulls; variations can include pulling with biceps only (upper arm held stationary), and pulling with a straight arm (downward, sideward, upward).

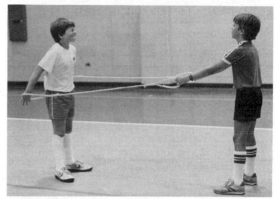

Figure 13–68

Partners can also position themselves back-to-back and pull over the shoulder and sideways.

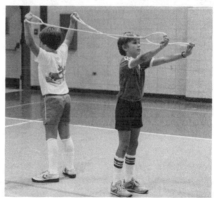

Figure 13–69

A triceps pull can also be used. Partners bend forward approximately 45°. Partner A will flex right arm as partner B extends left arm; their opposite arms will work in opposition at the same time; rhythmical pulling in this manner will result in a pumping-arm action similar to that found in running. Children should be reminded to keep abdominal muscles tight and thereby avoid low back strain. These exercises can also be executed from a sitting position.

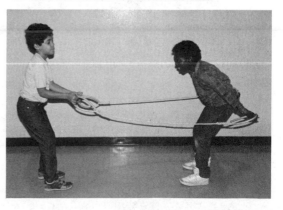

Figure 13–70

17. Partner Pull-Ups:
    Starting Position: supine with partner in straddle-stand, feet placed approximately midway along trunk
    Procedure: Partners assume double wrist grip; standing partner keeps trunk upright, tightens buttocks and abdominals, and flexes knees slightly to relieve pressure on back; supine partner pulls stiff body up; repeat 10 times.

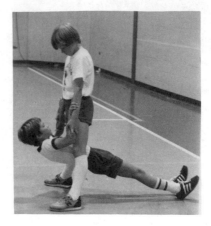

Figure 13–71

18. Rings, foam equipment, cargo nets, climbing ladders, and other apparatus provide excellent opportunities for strength development. Special attention should be given to the height of the apparatus (it is best that the children's feet be no more than 14″ from the ground and the landing surface not be pavement or concrete).

Calisthenic Routines to Music. These are specific calisthenics sequenced with little or no locomotor movement incorporated, and they are conducive to muscular strength/endurance development. A cadence is used initially until the sequence is performed to music, at which time the music provides the sequence. Students in Level III and above enjoy exercising to music and should be capable of performing with good form in rhythm to the music. The teacher is encouraged not to rely solely on the commercial exercise records. If these are used occasionally, the teachers should use the "talkie" side only to learn the routine so it can be taught to the children. Only if the teacher is incapacitated (for example, has laryngitis) should the "talkie" records be used in class. The conscientious teacher will want personally to give the cues for the routines to the children and thereby remain the teacher of the class!

CARDIORESPIRATORY ENDURANCE ACTIVITIES

One would think that cardiorespiratory endurance would surely be a natural product of the constant activity in which most children engage. However, research (Gilliam, 1982) has shown that even active elementary-grade children seldom attain heart rates greater than 160 beats/minute, and most often heart rates do not rise above 120 beats/minute. One could conclude that children are not as strenuously active as they appear to be. Clearly the 25 minutes to 60 minutes of physical education class time needs to provide ample opportunities for high-intensity aerobic activity and the necessary motivation for children who do not normally engage in high-intensity activity. (See Table 13–1, which lists recommended working heart rates for children.)

The recommended working heart rates should be maintained for at least 15 minutes, four days a week, if full benefit is to be realized. Naturally, this cannot happen in a 30-minute class where the development of motor skill is also important. In other words, a lesson on manipulative skills will not be as rigorous as a lesson on locomotor skills. However, teachers who are aware of this information will surely be further stimulated in their endeavors to plan and teach effectively so that children are engaged in maximum activity time and little or no waiting time. If the daily lesson begins with a fitness activity that stimulates the cardiorespiratory system and the rest of the lesson is paced so that there are frequent short demands of high-intensity work, heart rates are more apt to at least occasionally reach above the minimal 126 to 129 working heart range, which would indicate 60 percent of the maximum. Remember that other periods of the day such as before and after school, as well as recess (fitness breaks), are excellent times to incorporate this concept.

Teaching Hints:

1. Use locomotor movements in a variety of challenges and story plays to keep the children moving.
2. Teach children appropriate pacing techniques so they can "slow down and keep moving" rather than stop completely when they begin to fatigue.
3. Teach proper breathing techniques.
4. Motivate through stimulating visuals, current sports events, contests, and a variety of activities, equipment, methodologies, and reinforcement.
5. Gradually increase the time spent in endurance activities, for only when the cardiorespiratory system experiences an overload will it actually be strengthened.
6. Teach preschool and kindergarten children to be aware of their change in heart rate because of certain activities. They can discern this simply by feeling their heart beat through their chest wall before and after vigorous activity. Show older children how to take their heart rate at the carotid and/or brachial arteries.
7. Stress the use of proper footwear (socks and shoes).
8. If alternatives are available, avoid running on pavement and concrete.
9. Inspect the running area prior to children running on it.
10. Encourage participation in cardiorespiratory activities during recess.
11. Develop short-term and long-term fitness games that can be played outside of class yet recognized in class ("Jogging to Disneyland," to "Astroworld," to "Washington, D.C.," and so forth). Provide map with mileage between cities; let one jogged mile equal 10 miles, 3 continuous minutes of rope jumping equal 10 miles on the map).

Entire families can get involved with this activity. Different ratios can be given for older brothers and sisters and parents.

Aerobic Jumping Routines.   These routines are continuous jumps in which the arms, feet, and legs assume various positions. The jumps should be rhythmical (music is usually used) and the students are reminded of the proper landing techniques as discussed in Chapter 9. Each jump should be executed for 4, 8, or 16 repetitions (as determined by the music being used). Combinations of arm and leg variations can be developed from the following suggestions:

1. Scissor: From a forward and back stride position, the legs alternately land left-right foot in front (legs scissor); weight should be evenly distributed over both feet.

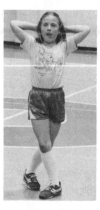

Figure 13-72

2. Straddle: As in jumping jacks, feet alternately land together and apart.

3. Ski Jumps: Feet held together and alternately land to the right and left sides of midline (may also land forward and back of center of gravity).

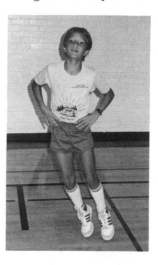

Figure 13-73

4. Jump Kicks: On the first count, both feet land on floor; on second count one leg kicks while weight is supported by other leg as it simultaneously hops. Cues might be "2, kick-R; 2, Kick-L" with the 2 signifying that both feet land on floor.
5. Pendulum Kicks: A double hop is taken on the right foot while the left leg swings (pendulum style) out to the left side and then back to center for a double hop while the right leg swings out the right side (cue: and-a-1 [L], and-a-2 [R], etc.) with the "and-a" signifying the double hop.

ARM VARIATIONS:

1. jogging position (clapping will add to the rhythm);
2. hands on hips;
3. hands clasped behind head, elbows out.

Rope Jumping can be used for a set number of jumps or a set length of time. Children are encouraged to pace themselves (stop the rope but continue walking in place) so that the full number of repetitions or duration of time can be completed.

Fartlek running is a technique of pacing that enables participants to vary their speed by alternating from high to low intensities of running/walking. An entire class can be active at one time with the teacher giving verbal or whistle signals to stimulate the children to jog, walk, run, or sprint. Interesting variations (run-knees high, walk on tiptoe, turn and sprint) may also enhance motivation. The children can also be encouraged to create their own routines, changing their pace as their bodies indicate the need for change.

Indian running is an activity whereby the students jog in a line (follow the leader) or in a large circular pattern. On signal, the last child in line must sprint to the front of the line and become the new leader. The rest of the line does not break the jogging pace, and when the new leader is in position he or she also resumes jogging. The "Indian" sprinting to the front may pass the line either to the outside of the circular path or to the inside. Children should be reminded that the outside path will require more effort than the inside path, and that they are encouraged to exert the strongest effort they can. As the sprinter moves up to the front, the remainder of the line can be encouraged to "holler," thereby causing a slightly additional oxygen demand on the body.

Tag games serve as excellent cardiorespiratory endurance activities. Recognition should be given to those who can finish the game without having to be "it" (those who avoid being tagged earn the title of "Super Dodger"). This will discourage low levels of movement in order to be tagged and win the opportunity to be center stage—"it".

Aerobic dance has become a very popular activity and is appropriate for children in Level III and up. Children in Levels I and II will exert more energy in activities that allow more freedom of movement. Aerobic dance routines incorporate both locomotor and nonlocomotor skills into simple dances, and they are usually composed of no more than three step patterns. They can be quickly learned and are very effective at keeping the heart rate elevated if children really dance vigorously. Large groups of children of varying fitness levels can participate at the same time as each can pace the level of exertion (that is, some will kick high and some will kick low).

Circuit training experiences are appropriate for Level II and above. It is best to plan for these students to rotate no more than four or five times (see Table 13–3). If the class is large, eight to ten stations might be set up, but the students would only need to rotate to four or five stations as the others would be duplicated. No matter which station a child starts at, four rotations will complete the circuit.

Outdoor circuits (for example, fitness trails, vita parcours) are excellent fitness-enhancing additions to the elementary school playground. They combine station tasks for muscular strength/endurance and flexibility and they provide room to run. Activities stimulating the skill-related fitness components of balance and agility are also often included. These outdoor fitness events will usually require more time to complete and are sometimes used as the major activity of the lesson on a once-a-week basis. During the remainder of the week the students participate at selected stations rather than all stations.

TABLE 13-3   Circuit Training Layout

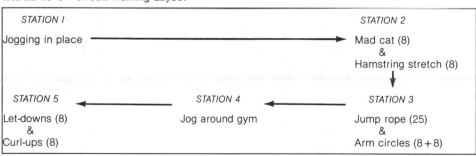

time/station = 1 min.   5 min
transition time = 10 secs   1 min
total time =   6 min

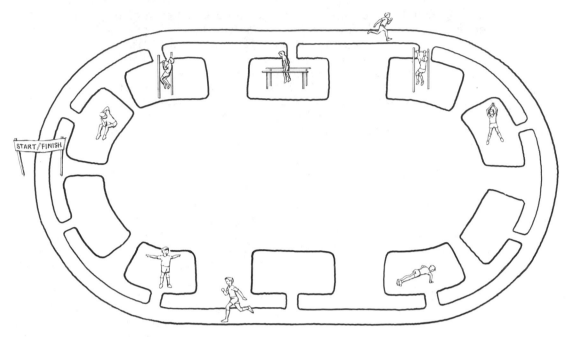

Figure 13-74

TEACHING HINTS FOR CIRCUIT TRAINING (INDOORS/OUTDOORS)

1. Arrange stations so that the same body area is not stressed consecutively.
2. Posters at each station should be concise and readable from 6 feet away. Colors with best visibility are black or blue on light-colored poster board. Red is acceptable on white posters only. Stick figures or other pictures are often helpful to students.
3. Only familiar exercises should be used, and a quick "tour" of the circuit will be necessary if this is the first presentation to students.
4. Once class is divided, each group will start at a different station. For example, a class of 30 would be divided into 5 groups of 6 students for a 5-station circuit.
5. Some exercises require more time to complete than others. The solution to this potential problem is either to increase the number of sets required (for example, 2 sets of 10 repetitions each) or require two different exercises at certain stations.
6. Taped music can serve both as an excellent motivator and as the signal for rotation between stations. By recording a whistle signal at timed intervals, you will let students know when to stop, replace equipment, run to the next station, and begin as the music resumes. By using a tape recorder, the teacher is free to provide more individual instruction and feedback to the children rather than be a timekeeper.
7. Most children operate best if they rotate according to a predetermined schedule and signal. This technique ensures that all children participate in all stations and also eliminates wasted time, due to slow rotation or bottlenecks at the stations.
8. As children become accustomed to the circuit procedures and more skilled with the exercises, the rotation time can often be shortened and the time spent at each station lengthened.
9. If the range of ability levels is widespread within the class, different difficulty requirements should be stated on each poster. For example, a poster for the strength/endurance station might look like the example presented in Table 13-4.
10. Frequently scan the entire area to notice any potential trouble spots caused by improper use of equipment (or procedures), inactivity, or lack of concentration.

TABLE 13-4 Circuit Training Station: Strength/Endurance

Push-ups/Let-downs
Level III 6 push-ups
Level II   6 sets of 4 stops (let-downs)
Level I   3 sets of 4 stops (let-downs)

Obstacle courses (challenge courses), which can be set up indoors or outside, offer challenging opportunities for fitness development. Children should move through the course as rapidly (and safely) as they can. If balance beams are used, it is best not to include rapid movements, for this poses a safety hazard. Specific stations may be designated for various levels of difficulty, thus promoting individualized instruction.

Table 13-5 presents a summary of general activity areas used to enhance specific fitness components. In addition to the activities suggested in this chapter, it is also recommended that game and gymnastic sources be reviewed for inclusion in the fitness phase of the lesson. Table 13-6 presents a partial listing of game and gymnastic activities that are appropriate for inclusion.

TABLE 13-5 General Fitness Development Activities

CARDIORESPIRATORY	FLEXIBILITY	MUSCULAR STRENGTH/ENDURANCE
Jogging/Running	Dance/Rhythms	Calisthenics
Fartlek (Change Speeds)	Body Part Stretching	Isometrics
Aerobic Dance	Shoulder	Playground Equipment
Jump Rope	Lower Back	Bars
Parachute	Quadriceps	Horizontal Ladders
	Hamstring	Vertical Pole
	Calf	Rope Climb
	Parachute	Parachute

TABLE 13-6 Partial Listing of Enhancement Activities

FITNESS COMPONENT	ACTIVITY	LEVEL
	Games	
Cardiorespiratory Endurance	Charlie Over the Water Jet Pilot Scarecrow and Cranes Whistle Stop	I&II
	Eyeglasses Wild Horse Roundup In the Creek Hop Tag Stickey Popcorn Indian Running	II&III
	Goal Tag Chain Tag	III
	Gymnastics (descriptions found in Chapter 16)	

(cont.)

TABLE 13-6 (continued)

Flexibility	Row Boat Inchworm Eggroll Wring the Washrag	I–III
	The Bridge	II&III
Muscular Strength/Endurance	Bouncing Ball Push the Donkey Pull the Donkey Partner Pullups	I–III
	Kangaroo Jump Crab Walk Turk Stand Crane Dive Coffee Grinder Rabbit Jump	II&III
	Toe Push Up-spring Single Squat Spanker	III

REFERENCE

GILLIAM, T., MacCONNIE, S. E., GEENEN, D. L.,
PELS III, A. E., & FREEDSON, P. S. (1982).
Exercise programs for children: A way to prevent. *The
Physician and Sportsmedicine, 10,* 96–106.

SUGGESTED READINGS

AAHPERD, (1979). *Implementation of aerobic programs.* Reston, VA: Author.

DAUER, V. & PANGRAZI, R. (1986). *Dynamic physical education for elementary school children.* (8th ed.)
Minneapolis: Burgess.

DAVIS, R. G. & ISSACS, L. D. (1973). *Elementary
physical education: Growing through movement* (2nd
ed.). Winston-Salem, N.C.: Hunter.

GETSELL, B. (1979). *Physical fitness: A way of life.*
New York: Wiley.

KIRCHNER, G. (1985). *Physical education for elementary school children* (6th ed.). Dubuque, Ia.: Wm. C.
Brown.

KUNTZLEMAN, C. T. (1971). *The physical fitness en-
cyclopedia.* Emmaus, Pa.: Rodale Books.

MILLER, D. K., & ALLEN, T. E. (1982). *Fitness—A
lifetime commitment.* Minneapolis: Burgess.

SHARKEY, B. J. (1979). *Physiology of fitness.* Champaign, IL: Human Kinetics.

SCHURR, E. L. (1980). *Movement experiences for children* (3rd ed.). Englewood Cliffs, NJ: Prentice-Hall.

SIEDENTOP, D., HERKOWITZ, T., & RINK, J.
(1984). *Elementary physical education methods.* Englewood Cliffs, N.J.: Prentice-Hall, Inc.

WOOD, D. A.   Aerobic dance for children: Resources
& recommendations. *The physician and sports medicine, 14,* 225–229.

SUGGESTED RECORDS

Chicken Fat 209 CF 1000 Merrbach Records

Rhythmic Rope Jumping, Elementary K 4001 Kimbo Records

And the Beat Goes On KEA 5010 Educational Activities

Jumpnastics Kea 6000 Educational Activities & Kimbo Records

Fitness for Everyone HPR-R-24 Kimbo Records

Sorenson's Aerobic Dancing, Elementary LP1110 Kimbo Educational Records

Hap Palmer Educational Activities

Ruth Evans Merrbach Record Service

Dancers Without Partners Educational Activities Album No. 32

14

GAMES

As we begin Section IV of this text, Chapters 14 through 16, the reader should note that the next three chapters not only present information related to methodology and the teaching of game, rhythm/dance, and gymnastic activities but that each chapter also contains material depicting (in developmental order with skill description) enhancement activities suggested in Chapters 9 through 12. We have also included recommendations for Level IV–VI selections and a reference list of activity sources, which complement each content area.

INTRODUCTION

Probably the most recognized, yet many times misused, aspects of children's physical education are *games*. Because games are motivating and fun, they are considered one of the easiest forms of physical activity to teach. Although some forms of games are quite simple and require little teacher intervention (perhaps another reason for their popularity), games can be as diverse and complex as any physical activity. As previously noted in the general philosophy of the "developmental theme approach," games should serve as vehicles for enhancing and utilizing the fundamental movement abilities of children rather than as the primary objective of the lesson.

DEVELOPMENTAL VALUE

Games that are carefully selected can be a valuable part of the physical education program by contributing to the total development of children. Games offer a multitude of opportunities that may add significantly not only in support of motor-skill enhancement but also to cognitive and affective development.

Many game-type activities (the types will be discussed in the next section of this chapter) offer acceptable enhancement to the motor-skill foundation and provide for the development and maintenance of physical fitness. Games have the potential to provide both of these assets along with a very effective element—fun!

The cognitive value of games is evident in several ways: (1) in many instances game complexity is not only related to skill but also to cognitive involvement (that is, understanding rules, responsibilities, options, and strategies); (2) when children are provided the opportunity to modify and create their own games, cognitive stimulation occurs; and (3) games may be utilized to teach and reinforce specific academic concepts (as discussed in Chapter 2).

Although games offer children an opportunity to enhance their skills, fitness, and cognitive abilities, such activities may also present a tremendous benefit to social and emotional development. Many physical educators cite the primary importance of games as a medium to enhance the child's affective development (the authors of this text would also add the enhancement of skills and fitness). The physical education setting is an excellent environment where children may learn such values as sportsmanship, leadership, self-discipline, self-worth, honesty, cooperation, patience, and respect for others.

GAMES: FORMS AND STRUCTURE

The structure and the diversity with which games may be presented are illustrated in Figure 14–1.

Conventional Games

Also referred to as *predesigned* or *structured* games, *conventional* games are activities that have been designed by others and are usually taught without modification. This form of game mandates the use of specific skills and is found in most elementary textbooks.

Figure 14–1 The structure and diversity of games.

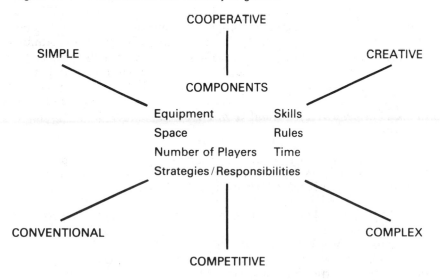

Typical of this form is a game hierarchy that ranges from games of low organization (for example, tag games and relays) to more complex, highly organized activities associated with sports and the Level IV–VI program. Most conventional games, especially of the low-organized variety, are easy to teach and require little planning or background skill or knowledge. Because of their structured form, however, conventional games must be carefully selected with regard to the specific movement abilities that a theme emphasizes. Although many conventional games can be used in their "intact" form, instances will arise when the activity needs to be "modified" to increase its developmental value. The items featured in the center of Figure 14–1 present the components of a game that can be modified to meet specific needs. Morris (1976) popularized the idea that games can be changed in a multitude of ways to accommodate lesson objectives and needs of children. Frequent modifications in the intact game include changing the number and/or organization of players, equipment used, rules, scoring contingencies, or, as presented in this text, altering the skill-utilization requirements to meet theme objectives.

Cooperative and Creative Games

As previously indicated, games may range on a continuum from simple to complex, cooperative to competitive, and also be conventional (predesigned) or created by individuals to fit specific needs and desires. In recent years a strong movement has brought attention to what many educators describe as the most important yet neglected contributions of games, namely opportunities for achieving a goal through a cooperative spirit, and development of the child's creative abilities. Along with the focus upon these characteristics of the game has emerged a philosophy of game value as well as the creation of new games and an understanding of how to change existing activities to accommodate program objectives.

Cooperative Games

Whereas some children love to challenge others because of their own competitive spirit, other youngsters prefer not to be placed in a competitive situation. Many physical educators believe that with our present game selections, too much competition has been emphasized at the expense of cooperation and other affective values. Perhaps the greatest criticism connected with children's sport programs has been the degree of competition and emotional stress generally associated with such programs. Although some degree of competition stimulates interest and motivation, practices such as emphasizing winning and focusing on the score rarely if ever contribute to a healthy learning environment. Cooperative games emphasize the cooperation and sharing of people to achieve a common goal.

Terry Orlick (1977, 1978, 1982), a leading authority on the subject and author of *The Cooperative Sports and Games Book,* describes the cooperative game concept thus:

People play with one another rather than against one another; they play to overcome challenges, not to overcome the person; and they are freed by the very structure of the game to enjoy the play experience itself. (Orlick, 1982, p. 4)

Through cooperative experiences, individuals learn to be considerate of others, to be more aware of an individual's feelings, to practice sharing, and to be willing to perform with another's interests in mind.

To better understand the cooperative game philosophy and its value toward development of the individual, one should examine the primary aspects of cooperative activities. These aspects, the structural components, separate cooperative games from other game-type activities. The exciting aspects of cooperative games are that they provide freedom from competition (*cooperation*), freedom to *create*, freedom to *choose,* and freedom *from exclusion.*

As previously mentioned, the cooperative component serves to have individuals play with rather than against each other. The primary goal is to confront a challenge through cooperative action with others. The freedom to *create* is stressed in the fact that cooperative games should never be so rigid that they are resistant to creative input from the participants.

Orlick (1982) points out that cooperative games and their multiple variations have grown out of many people's creative thought, which is the basis for the cooperative game philosophy. Another vital aspect to the cooperative concept is the provision of *choice.* When children are given the freedom to choose, to offer suggestions, and to make decisions, motivation is enhanced immensely. The act of choice usually begins on a realistic, limited basis, then progresses to a level where children have almost total responsibility.

Regarding *freedom from exclusion,* one of the worst game choices that the teacher could make is an activity that removes individuals from the game (that is, exclusion, elimination-type games). Cooperative games eliminate these possibilities and reject the general concept of having winners and losers. Each game is designed so that all participants are involved as much as practically possible. Participants are making a contribution as a part of the activity and everybody has fun.

Whereas some predesigned cooperative game suggestions can be found in textbooks, the concept can be easily incorporated into traditional activities by changing various structural components (refer to Fig. 14–1). Basically the structural change should elicit the four freedoms previously described (cooperation, creativity, choice, nonexclusion). Orlick describes three general game categories: games with no losers, collective score game, and reversal activities.

The *no-loser* concept is promoted by having the goal of the game a challenge against a standard rather than against other individuals. *Collective score* games involve scoring contingencies where points are awarded when a number of teams cooperate to achieve a common goal. The *reversal* concept is manifested by deemphasizing team membership. This may be accomplished by having team members systematically rotate from one team to another during the game. Orlick also suggests game structure change with traditional team sports to provide a "semicooperative" activity. In games such as basketball, hockey, and volleyball, for example, all participants would be required to handle the scoring object before a scoring attempt.

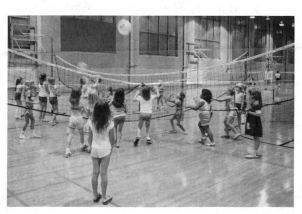

Cooperative games stress working together for a common goal.

Creative Games

Frequently teachers will use games in their intact form that derive from a source. However, because of specific characteristics of the class, (class size, skill level, equipment, objectives, and so forth) the teacher may be confronted with a need to modify the game or create a new activity to meet lesson objectives. As previously noted, the concept of changing games to meet lesson objectives was popularized by Morris (1976, 1980) and has become an integral part of the educational games program. Whether modifying an existing game or creating a new one, the elements that are generally used in structural change are the basic game components, which may be initiated by the student as well as the teacher.

Riley (1975) defines an original game as any structured activity that is the creation of the teacher, the teacher and children together, or the children alone. Riley (1977) also notes that creative activities should be used in balance with traditional games and that their contributions are not only toward meeting general lesson objectives, but also in challenging children cognitively in their own learning.

Creative games may be utilized in connection with any of the three phases of a lesson (fitness, skill development, and final activity). They may also stand on their own to develop basic skills (for example, activities to refine running, dodging, throwing, jumping) or be used to enhance a traditional game theme during the selection of a practice and final activity.

Creative games may be designed by: (1) the teacher, (2) the teacher/child, or (3) the child. The extent of change may vary from a simple component modification to a totally inventive activity. Although most game modifications are planned by the teacher to accommodate class needs and to facilitate skill development, occasions arise when modification of a predesigned activity does not seem adequate or the teacher wishes to stimulate the creative abilities of the children. This end of the game continuum enters the cognitive/creativity barrier associated with *exploration* (teaching style) as presented in this text and Muska Mosston's (1981) "Going Beyond." Many teachers feel more comfortable using a "guided" approach that does not deter the number and quality of responses, but rather controls the general area of discovery. This is accomplished by first presenting the problem and then setting practical limitations related to boundaries, equipment, safety, and time.

Teacher/child and child-designed games, to be effective, require a greater understanding of class characteristics than those activities modified and invented by the teacher alone. When the teacher and children work cooperatively to design a game, the teacher presents the general problem and limitations. The teacher and child then work together to determine specifics of the structured components (that is, rules, equipment, boundaries). Activities of this type generally evolve slowly and, as previously mentioned, require a different teaching style from most teacher-initiated activities. The teacher acting in a cooperative effort with the class serves as a facilitator who guides within general limitations but does not impose strong ideas concerning alternatives and discoveries. It is no easy task to manage the creative processes involved with children, at the same time holding to a preplanned set of teacher-directed objectives (even though they are general).

Child-designed games—those activities that may be identified in the spectrum of learning associated with creativity—present a new dimension not only to the child but also the teacher. At this level of game creation, it is common for a number of groups to be playing several games at the same time, rather than the entire class responding to the teacher en masse. The teacher's primary role is to interact with groups at the same time being sure not to "interfere" when not needed. This type of instruction requires an experienced and observant teacher, one who has an understanding of individual abilities in both the cognitive and motor-skill dimensions. Graham (1980) points out that child-designed games have some definite advantages:

1. Children in groups with similar skill ability are allowed to design activities that are interesting to them.
2. Children with little creative game experience are given the opportunity of time (which they manage) to develop the game-design process.

Graham (1977) has also suggested the following guidelines for helping students create their own games:

1. Begin gradually. More structure will be needed at the beginning; however, as students become more adept, the teacher should gradually lessen the imposed structure.
2. Limit your interference. If students are to learn to make significant decisions, they must be responsible for the consequences.
3. Always be aware of safety. Regardless of the level of decision making given the child, a safe environment is the teacher's responsibility. An unsafe situation is one of the few times that the teacher must interfere. When possible, unless the situation calls for an immediate change, make the students aware of the potential hazard and allow them to decide on an alternative.
4. Allow students to enforce their own rules. If students are given the opportunity to make rules, they should enforce them as well. Keep the control in their hands and act only as a facilitator.
5. Remind students of the creative concept—the only rule is that the game can always be changed. Be flexible; if you are unhappy or can create another aspect, do so!
6. Teacher—be patient! The creative process is at times time-consuming. The process is as important as the product. Once the general idea of game components and how to manipulate them is mastered, the quality of responses will increase.

One of the first organizations to develop written materials devoted to the "New Games" concept was the New Games Foundation,* which introduced *The New Games Book* in 1976, and *More New Games* in 1981. The philosophy behind the New Games concept emphasizes the adaptation of predesigned games and invention of new activities. A primary objective of this approach to games is *challenge* rather than competition. The focus is upon challenges that are meaningful to all players, so that the participants remain the central element of the game. New Games can also be considered cooperative activities because they attempt to temper the competitive spirit with a spirit of cooperation. Many New Games are designed to create and communicate a feeling of trust.

The New Games material, along with Terry Orlick's texts (see Suggested Readings) on cooperative activities, is a highly recommended source for the beginning (and experienced) teacher who wishes to establish a base for incorporating the creative and cooperative game philosophy into the game and sports curriculum.

Evaluation and Selection

Although the majority of the games presented in this and other texts are predesigned, it is stressed that teachers, when applicable, either create or modify game activities to meet the developmental needs of the children. With an understanding of game structure, teachers can learn to evaluate games by examining

*New Games Foundation, P. O. Box 7901, San Francisco, California 94120.

their various facets and, if needed, adapt new or modified activities. Davis (1983) supports the use of a "rating scale" with which a game receives a high of "5" to a low of "1" for its contribution to each of the three developmental areas: psychomotor, affective, and cognitive. After the teacher has examined the game and determined a rating, the basis for modification is set. It is also noted that games that are rated fairly low still have developmental value if used prudently, provided that they are fun—an important aspect in the development of a positive attitude toward physical education.

The following are general points to remember when selecting games. Games should:

1. Be fun;
2. Provide maximum activity for all children; circle and relay games generally fail to qualify in this area;
3. Enhance the development of specifically determined motor skills and/or develop and maintain fitness; to do this, maximum activity for all is crucial;
4. Promote inclusion and not elimination. Such games as dodgeball and musical chairs are basically elimination activities and need to be modified to provide inclusion.

Additional Considerations and Instructional Hints

1. Use progression, moving from partner activities to small and then team games.
2. When selecting games, progressively increase the number and complexity of rules and strategies required.
3. Use the game situation to evaluate and enhance affective behavior as well as motor-skill proficiency.
4. Safety should be a primary consideration; check for hazards and remind children of safety awareness factors. The teacher must study the game thoroughly to be aware of these possibilities.
5. Place the children into the formation (then allow them to sit) and make the instructions as brief as possible.
6. Although maximum participation is stressed, if children must be eliminated, it should be for one or two turns only; modify the game to accommodate this need. Avoid the situation that occurs where winners are more active than losers (they need more practice); a plan of rotation may help.
7. Avoid excessive emphasis on competition.

Developmental Activity Chart—Games: Level I–III (As suggested in Chapters 9-12)

NAME	SKILL(S)	LEVEL
Bridges	climb	I–III
Cat and Rat	auditory, directional, eye-hand, locomotor, spatial	
Circle Ball	catch, throw	
Circle Kick Ball	kick, trap	
Command Cards	directional, locomotor	
Clothespin Drop	eye-hand, visual	
Follow the Leader	locomotor, nonlocomotor	
Finding Different Objects	visual	
Go Touch It	auditory	
Hopscotch	balance, hop, leap	
American		
Italian		
French		
Kick the Pin	kick	
Kitty, Kitty	auditory	
Leap Frog Relay	leap	
Moon Soccer	kick	
Old Man/Old Lady	locomotor	
Peripheral Vision	visual	
Over the Brook	balance, hop, jump, leap, spatial	
Prui	auditory	
Round Stones	roll	
Skin the Snake	body awareness, stretch/bend, twist/turn	
Spoon and Ball Relay	balance	
The Feely Bag (or Mystery Bag)	tactile	
What's Missing?	visual	
Ball Race	bounce/dribble	I–II
Beach Ball Nerfs	strike	
Beanbag Ring Throw	throw	
Bean in a Can Relay	eye-hand	
Birds and Cats	dodge, run	
Bounce Ball	bounce/dribble	
Broomstick Relay	gallop	
Brownies and Fairies	eye-hand, locomotor, spatial	

NAME	SKILL(S)	LEVEL
Cars	directional, locomotor	I–III
Catch the Witch	directional, locomotor	
Charlie Over the Water	body awareness, locomotor, spatial	
Circle Beanbag Relay	eye-hand	
Cut the Pie	dodge, spatial	
Freight Train Relay	walk	
Gardener and Scamp	locomotor, spatial	
Giants, Dwarfs, and Men	auditory	
Hoop-Hop	balance, eye-foot, body awareness, hop, jump, leap, spatial	
Hot Rolls	strike	
I Don't Want It	throw	
Jet Pilot	run, spatial	
Just Now	auditory	
Kneeling Tag	balance, eye-hand, run, walk	
Letter Race	visual	I–II
Man from Mars	dodge, locomotor, spatial	
Marching Ponies	locomotor	
Nuts and Bolts	visual	
Partner Tag	directional, dodge, stretch/bend, tactile, twist/turn	
Rat Poison	ball rolling	
Red Light	walk, run	
Ring the Tire	throw	
Scarecrows and Cranes	direction	
Seven Dwarfs	dodge, eye-hand, spatial	
Slow Pok	jump, locomotor	
Squirrels in the Trees	direction, run, spatial, walk	
Throw and Go	eye-hand	
Toss-Jump-Pick	jump	
Traffic Cop	eye-foot	
Train Station	eye-foot, hop, jump	
Walking Robot	walk	
Whistle Stop	balance	

(cont.)

Level I–III (continued)

NAME	SKILL(S)	LEVEL
Ball Toss	catch, throw	
Call a Guard	ball rolling	
Gap Ball	throw	
Individual Dodgeball	throw	
Kick the Beast Relay	eye-foot	
Popcorn	stretch/bend	
Potatoe Race	eye-foot	
"Sock" It-to-Me Ball	throw	
Twenty-Five Throws	catch	
Agents and Spies	eye-hand	II–III
All-Up Relay	locomotor	
Attention Relay	auditory, locomotor	
B-B Ball	eye-hand	
Back to Back	balance, direction, dodge, stretch/bend, tactile	
Ball and Stick Relay	eye-hand, strike	
Bat Ball	catch, strike	
Beat Ball	catch, throw	
Beater Goes Round	directional, locomotor	
Boundary Ball	eye-foot, kick, trap	
Bowling Relay	ball rolling	
Call Ball	bounce/dribble, catch, strike	
Can-Can	throw	
Canoes and Rapids	locomotor, throw	
Chinese Hurdle	body awareness, hop, jump, leap	
Circle Stride Ball	catch, eye-hand	
Club Guard	throw	
Colors	auditory, locomotor	
Come Along	locomotor	
Count Three Tag	locomotor	
Cross Over	catch, throw	
Crossover Dodgeball	nonlocomotor	
Deep Freeze	balance, body awareness, hop, jump, leap	
Eyeglasses	hop, jump, leap, spatial	II–III
Finger Toss	eye-hand	
Fire Engine	dodge, run, walk	
Fire on the Mountain	run	

NAME	SKILL(S)	LEVEL
Fly Trap	run, stretch/bend	II
Formation Jumping	eye-foot	
Frog in the Pond	jump, leap, run, spatial	
Frozen Beanbag	balance, body awareness, jump	
Guard the Toys	directional, nonlocomotor	
Here to There	direction, hop, jump, leap	
Hit the Pins	ball rolling	
Hop Tag	directional, nonlocomotor	
Human Tangles	twist/turn	
Hurdle Race	leap	II–III
In and Out	directional, stretch/bend, twist/turn	
Indian Chief	auditory	
Indian Running	directional, locomotor	
In the Creek	balance, body awareness, hop, jump, leap, spatial	
Islands	balance, directional, hop, jump, leap, spatial	
Jump the Clubs Race	hop, jump, leap	
Jump the Shot (or Pole)	eye-foot, jump, spatial	
Kangaroo Relay	balance, hop, jump	
Knock, Knock	auditory	
Little Red Fox	auditory	
Magic Wand	eye-hand	
Memory Ball	tactile	
Mousetrap	directional, dodge, locomotor	
Newcomb	catch	
Octopus	nonlocomotor	
O'Leary	auditory	
One Step	catch	
Over and Over	eye-hand	
Parachute Play	locomotor, nonlocomotor	
Pass and Duck	catch	
Pebble Flip	eye-hand	
Ping-Pong Bounce	visual	
Place Kickball	kick	
Poison Circle	nonlocomotor, throw	
Put in Order	tactile	II–III
Race Around the Bases (Relay)	directional, run	

Level I-III (continued)

NAME	SKILL(S)	LEVEL
Rattlesnake	spatial	II–III
Rescue Relay	nonlocomotor, spatial	
Run for Your Supper	locomotor	
Sack Relay	jump	
Sandpaper, Numbers, Letters	tactile	
Ship Wreck	directional	
Shoe Twister	twist/turn	
Skeet Ball	throw	
Soccer Steal	eye-foot	
Sticky Popcorn	hop, jump	
Stool Hurdle Relay	hop, jump, leap	
Thread the Needle	locomotor	II–III
Top Hat Tag	eye-hand	
Toppleball	strike	
Tug-of-War	push/pull	
Two Square	bounce/dribble, strike	
Up the Field	catch	
Wagon Wheels	roll	
Weathervane	jump	
Wild Horse Round-Up	dodge, gallop, run	
Balance Dodgeball	balance, dodge, stretch/bend	III
Battle Ball	kick, trap	
Beanbags	body awareness, catch	
Blue and Gold	dodge, eye-hand, locomotor	
Bucket Ball	bounce/dribble	
Catch Up	throw/catch	
Chain Tag	dodge, stretch/bend	
Chase the Bulldog	dodge	

NAME	SKILL(S)	LEVEL
Circle of Friends	push/pull	
Circle Soccer	kick, trap	
Crab Soccer	eye-foot, kick, trap	
End Zone Ball	catch	
Exchange Dodgeball	directional, nonlocomotor	
Fistball	strike	
Freeze Ball	balance, catch, dodge	
Goal Tag	directional, dodge, stretch/bend, twist/turn	
Hand Grenade III	throw	
Hoop Activities	catch	
Hot Ball	directional, body awareness, catch, eye-foot, kick, trap	
I Pass These Scissors to You	visual	
Jacks	eye-hand	
Long Ball	catch	
Math Merriment	auditory	
My Ball	eye-hand	
Overtake Ball	catch	
Par Three	eye-hand	
Pull the Tail	push/pull	
Roll Dodgeball	ball rolling, directional, nonlocomotor	
Scoot the Hoop	eye-hand	
Snake Catcher	nonlocomotor	
Soccer Dodgeball	kick, trap	
Snow Ball	dodge, throw	
Stealing Sticks	dodge	
Sweep Up Relay	eye-hand	
Tetherball	strike	
Wall Ball (Handball)	bounce/dribble	

Developmental Activity Chart—Games: Level IV-VI (Recommended activities for skilled children)

It is suggested that the reader refer to Table 5–11 in Chapter 5 ("Curriculum and Planning") for activity recommendations under the categories of individual/partner and team games. The following recommendations are of the low-organization (simple group games) variety.

NAME	SKILL(S)	LEVEL	NAME	SKILL(S)	LEVEL
Newcomb	catch, throw	IV–VI	Bombardment	catch, throw	IV–V
Box Ball	ball handling, run		Long Base	run, strike	
Chain Tag	dodge, run		Grabbing Sticks	dodge, run	
Pirate's Gold	dodge, run		Running Dodgeball	run, throw	
Tug-O-War	pull		Catch the Dragon's Tail	eye-hand	
Protect Me Tag	dodge		Star Wars	run	
Triangle Dodgeball	catch, dodge, throw		Whistle Ball	catch, pass	
Balloon Ball	eye-hand				
Busy Ball	catch, throw				
Basket Baseball	catch, run, throw, shoot baskets				
Crab Soccer	kick		Circle Tug-O-War	pull, push	V–VI
Alaska Baseball	ball handling, kick, run, strike		Borden Ball	catch, throw	
Nine Lives	dodge, throw		California Kickball	catch, kick, run, throw	
Trees	dodge, run		Ricochet	throw	
Steal the Treasure	dodge, run, tag		Capture the Flag	dodge, run	
Pig in the Middle	catch, run, throw		Football Goal Catch	catch, throw	
Running Score	eye-hand		Machine-Gun Run	dodge, run, throw	
			Battle Ball	dodge, throw	

REFERENCES

DAVIS, R. G. & ISAACS, L. D. (1983). *Elementary physical education: Growing through movement.* Winston-Salem, NC: Hunter.

GAMES TEACHING. *Journal of Physical Education and Recreation.* Special feature on games for elementary school children. September 1977, 17–35. (Authors include: Graham, Morris, Barret, Riley, Orlick.)

GRAHAM, G., HOLT/HALE, S. A., MCEWEN, T., & PARKER, M. (1980). *Children moving: A reflective approach to teaching physical education.* Palo Alto, Calif.: Mayfield.

MORRIS, G. S. D. (1976). *How to change the games children play.* Minneapolis: Burgess.

MORRIS, G. S. D. (1980). *How to change the games children play* (2nd ed.). Minneapolis: Burgess.

MOSSTON, M. (1981). *Teaching physical education.* Columbus, OH: Chas. E. Merrill.

NEW GAMES FOUNDATION. (1976). *The new games book.* Garden City, NY: Doubleday.

NEW GAMES FOUNDATION. (1981). *More new games.* Garden City, NY: Doubleday.

ORLICK, T. (1977). *Winning through cooperation: Competitive insanity: Cooperative alternatives.* Washington, DC: Hawkins & Associates.

ORLICK, T. (1978). *The cooperative sports and games book.* New York: Pantheon.

ORLICK, T. *The second cooperative sports and games book.* New York: Pantheon.

RILEY, M. (1975, February). Games and humanism. *Journal of Physical Education and Recreation.* 46:46–49.

SUGGESTED ACTIVITY SOURCES

AMERICAN ALLIANCE FOR HEALTH, PHYSICAL EDUCATION, RECREATION AND DANCE. (1976). *ICHPER book of worldwide games and dances.* Reston, VA: Author.

ARNOLD, A. (1972). *The world book of children's games.* New York: World Publishing.

BLAKE, O. (1964). *Lead-up games to team sports.* Englewood Cliffs, NJ: Prentice-Hall.

COCHRAN, N., WILKINSON, L. C., & FURLOW, J. J., (1982). *A teacher's guide to elementary school physical education* (4th ed.). Dubuque IA: Kendall/Hunt.

DAUER, V., & PANGRAZI, R. (1986). *Dynamic physical education for elementary school children* (8th ed.). Minneapolis: Burgess.

FARINA, A. (1981). *Developmental games and rhythms for children.* Springfield, IL: Chas. C. Thomas.

KIRCHNER, G. (1985). *Physical education for elementary school children* (6th ed.). Dubuque, IA: Wm. C. Brown.

RICHARDSON, A. (1951). *Games for the elementary school grades.* Minneapolis: Burgess.

SCHURR, E. (1980). *Movement experiences for children* (3rd. ed.). Englewood Cliffs, NJ: Prentice-Hall.

SIEDENTOP, D., HERKOWITZ, J., & RINK, J. (1984). *Elementary physical education methods.* Englewood Cliffs, NJ: Prentice-Hall.

SUGGESTED READINGS

LOGSDON, B. J., BARRETT, K. R., AMMONS, M., BROER, M. R., HALVERSON, L. E., MCGEE, R., & ROBERTSON, M. H. (1984). *Physical education for children: A focus on the teaching process,* (2nd ed.). Philadelphia: Lea & Febiger.

MAULDON, E. & REDFERN, H. B. (1981). *Games teaching* (2nd ed.). London: Macdonald & Evans.

MORRIS, G. S. DON. (1980). *Elementary physical education: Toward inclusion.* Salt Lake City: Brighton.

ORLICK, T. & BOTTERRILL, C. (1975). *Every child can win.* Chicago: Nelson-Hall.

PAULSON, W. (1980). *Coaching cooperative youth sports.* LaGrange, IL: Youth Sport Press.

WERNER, P. (1979). *A movement approach to games for children.* St. Louis: C. V. Mosby.

15

RHYTHMS AND DANCE

The dance and rhythmic activities found in this chapter will serve as excellent enhancement activities for children in the process of building their movement foundation. The child's urge for self-expression through movement can be well served if the teacher presents appropriate dance activities in a manner that frees the child to express thoughts and feelings through movement. Through dance, the child is given the opportunity to use the entire body in a very individualistic manner that is satisfying to both the child and the teacher.

The many forms of dance range from elementary creative (expressive) dance to the more structured aerobic, folk, square, and social dance and even further to complex modern dance. This chapter primarily offers methodology related to the teaching of dance and activities for the enhancement of fundamental skills and movement awarenesses. Additional information associated with the teaching of fundamental rhythmic activities may be found in the "Rhythmic Awareness" section in Chapter 12.

PROGRESSIONS

The *progressions* found in dance closely parallel the progressive psychomotor, cognitive, and affective development characteristics of children. In other words, the egocentric child will find pleasure in using the developing fundamental movement skills in simple combinations that allow freedom of expression and are not encumbered by the encroachment of a partner. With increased development, children in Levels IV–VI can concentrate on the refinement of fundamental skills; therefore, dances become more structured, creative challenges more complex, and synchronization with a partner more feasible.

The following progressions are offered as flexible guidelines for the teacher (Levels I–III).

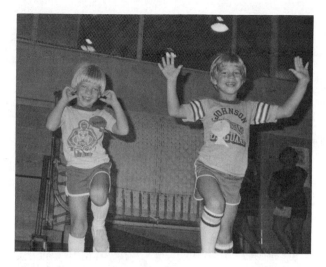

Opportunities for creative expression are numerous in dance.

Level I

Rhythm knowledge to be learned by students at this level include underlying beat, tempo, and simple accents. If the school supports a good school music curriculum, the physical educator and the music educator could coordinate many of their lessons.

Rhythmical movement using fundamental locomotor and nonlocomotor skills to move expressively with an accompaniment (for example, percussion, records, singing, rhymes). Locomotor movement receives the strongest focus.

Creative dance in which feelings and/or thoughts are expressed with accompaniment (percussion, records, story plays, and other imaginative instrumentation) are centered around the use of fundamental skills, as in rhythmical movement.

Finger plays in which manipulating the hands and fingers to accompanying songs reinforce the child's rhythmic awareness and finger dexterity. These skills are continued at this level from preschool experiences.

Structured dance in which students learn simple choreographed dances with accompaniment (singing nursery rhymes, chants).

Level II

Rhythm knowledge to be learned includes accents, even and uneven rhythms, measures, and simple rhythmic patterns.

Rhythmical movement focuses on locomotor and nonlocomotor skills and simple sequences of both. Variability of space, time, force, and relationship is stressed. Specific dance steps include the step-hop and slide.

Creative dance for this level continues to focus on the child's interpretation of stimuli provided by the teacher. The creation of short movement sequences is also introduced.

Structured dances are longer and sometimes involve more movements in the sequence. Suggested formations for Levels I and II are scattered, single, and double circles.

Level III

Rhythm knowledge to be learned includes rhythmic patterns, phrasing, and note values.

Rhythmical movement will focus on quality of movement as movement combinations are continued and variations are increased. Exercise and jump-rope routines are presented as are simple ball, hoop, and streamer routines. Specific dance steps include the schottische, draw, and polka (see section on "Hopping" in Chapter 9 for further explanation of these steps). Creative dance for this level focuses on more specific problem solving and increased variability of improvisation. Children should also be challenged more frequently with abstract stimuli.

Structured dance includes the additions of small groups, double lines, quadrilles, and squares. Simple dance positions such as the promenade and open position are introduced as are simple figures (honor, elbow, and two-hand turn; reel, do-si-do, grand right and left, allemande, and promenade). Dance steps include the two-step, grapevine, waltz, and mazurka.

CREATIVE DANCE

Generally, creative dance lessons for Levels I and II should contain activities that allow for individualization and require the use of fundamental skills (hop, skip, for example) with simple variability being introduced through the use of space, time, force, and relationship variables. Creative dance and dance challenges (that is, movement dramatization of the rhyme or story play) offer excellent opportunities for the child to use large movements involving the total body. Naturally, the main objective for using a dance-enhancement activity is to provide opportunities for the development of a sense of rhythm as it is expressed through movement. The child moves from an inner stimuli (rhythmic awareness) to an external stimuli (record, drum, song, rhyme) and tries to control body movement so that there is harmony between body and stimuli. Creative dance provides children with the following advantages:

1. Provides a gradual progression from moving to an internal beat to responding to an external beat.
2. The lack of rigid structure (as found in aerobic and folk dance) encourages the development of an attitude of freedom.
3. Children can use a familiar movement vocabulary (fundamental skills) rather than having to learn new moves. New challenges can be experienced as these familiar fundamental skills are sequenced in many different ways.

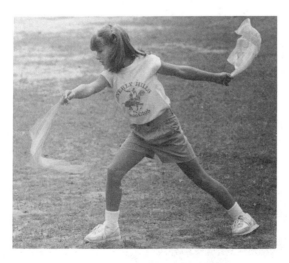

Scarfs and appropriate music encourage full extensions.

4. Promotes creativity and a sense of success.
5. The possibility for individualization makes it more efficient for classes with diversified skill levels.
6. Offers a natural outlet for the many feelings that are naturally felt by children. They will feel encouraged to develop their power of creative thinking.

Teaching Styles

Crucial to the success of any lesson are the teachers' decisions regarding teaching strategies for each lesson. Exploration, guided discovery, and problem solving offer the best teaching style for the creative dance activities found at Levels I–III (and Levels IV–VI).

Class Organization

The most efficient formation for creative dance is a scattered arrangement in which each child occupies enough "self-space" to feel free to move with abandonment. Some of the dances require a circular formation, and students can assume this position rather quickly by clustering into a group and then moving backwards (that is, "Everyone take eight big steps backward") until the circle becomes the appropriate size.

Stimuli for Creative Dance

Poems, being rhythmical in structure, offer a good beginning for creative dance. Begin with poems that contain a moving character or familiar object (for example, nursery rhymes). The teacher may choose to have the children "act out" the poem as it is read or the poem can be read to the class before hand, discussed, and then the children can describe the poem through movement.

Music (tapes and records) provides an excellent stimulus, and many very fine records are on the market at this time. Choose music that has meaning to the children, and make sure the rhythm pattern is simple (marches are a good choice). Some of today's contemporary music contains too many different sounds for the young child to hear clearly the underlying beat.

Percussion instruments (drums, tambourines, finger spoon, sticks) are a favorite of children. The teacher should begin by providing the percussion and gradually allowing students to manipulate the instruments.

Color is an exciting stimulus for creative dance in which the students demonstrate through movement the feeling that each color elicits. The teacher should remember that these responses may not follow a norm (that is, to some, red may signal danger or anger, and to others happiness or excitement).

Stories provide very appropriate outlets for dramatization. Children should be encouraged to use exaggerated movements to express the emotions of the story rather than simply pantomime the actions suggested by the story. Children at Levels I and II should be allowed to interpret the story line by line. Older children, however, can usually perform in phrases.

Everyday life and "real people" offer opportunities for the teacher to observe the perceptions children have about the police officer, teacher, sanitation worker, physician, doughnut maker, and others.

Nature offers both simple and complex challenges as a child responds to challenges involving animals to more abstract things (sunbeams, moonlight, lightning).

Sensory stimuli provide abstract stimuli for the Level-III student who is able, for example, to demonstrate an individual perception of what the sound of a drippy faucet might *look* like.

Word pictures are perhaps the most elementary of abstract stimuli. Children must know the meaning of the words that are used. For example, a child could demonstrate individual perceptions of such words as short, tall, snappy, gooey, straight, crooked, happy, sad, young, and old.

Teaching Hints

1. Remember *not* to evaluate "good" and "bad" movement; rather, encourage exploration.
2. Reinforce expressions of freedom, variety, honesty.
3. Allow for considerable exploration prior to problem-solving challenges.
4. Show enthusiasm for efforts in a way children can understand (children think a teacher is really "with it" when the teacher is able to get excited about what happens in the class; in other words, it's okay for the teacher occasionally to seem hyper with excitement over the children's performance).
5. Begin with individuals, then partners, and finally small groups for those who are ready.
6. Allow for time to practice (repetition) and refine movements.
7. If time permits, allow those who want to share their creative dance with the class to do so.
8. After a presentation by individuals or groups, be prepared to offer an evaluation. Begin with the positives and move on to areas for improvement (for example, "Mark, you certainly moved well at the medium level. Can you think of a nifty and smooth way to also move at the low and high levels?").
9. Remember that the *process* is often more important than the *product*. Thus provide ample time for rhythmical exploration through movement.
10. If the term "dance" seems to affect the children negatively, call it something else (rhythmic play, musical moves).
11. Begin with rather well-known stimuli (nursery rhymes, animals, holidays, birthdays).
12. Use props (streamers, lummi sticks, drums, etc.) to help children expand feelings and thoughts beyond themselves.
13. Use variability of space, time, force, and relationships during the dance activity to help challenge and stimulate excitement in the students.
14. Observe the children carefully and use their movement as a stimulus to become more creative in planning.

STRUCTURED DANCE

Structured dances (for example, singing dances, folk dances, aerobic dances) are available for all levels of students. The teacher should select carefully the dance most appropriate for the motor, cognitive, and emotional needs of the children at each level. Structured dances are comprised of specific patterns and sequences and are often handed down as part of different cultures. Physical educators should, whenever possible, teach folk dances in conjunction with the social studies and music curricula.

The objectives of the structured dance program include the following:

Psychomotor: motor control, balance, agility, coordination, muscular strength and endurance, and cardiorespiratory endurance (if danced vigorously over an extended period of time).

Cognitive: sequence, synchronization of movement to accompaniment, understanding of different cultures.

Affective: cooperative effort with others; personal expression of movement.

Teaching Styles

The command style is more appropriate for the teaching of structured dance. In all lessons the teacher must carefully present the material in an appropriately sequenced manner so the child will feel secure in moving to the music.

Class Organization

Generally, children should learn each dance within two lessons, and if this is not achieved the teacher should seriously question the appropriateness of the dance that the students are being taught. Remember, learning in small doses with frequent successes is an important key to motivation. Children will feel joyful and proud to be able to perform simple dances well and with flair, whereas inappropriately difficult dances will elicit feelings of frustration and trigger avoidance behaviors to dance in general.

Unlike the freedom of creative dance, structured dance generally requires a strict adherence to specific formations and synchronization with a partner or a small or large group.

The following terms, to be taught as the dances require, are appropriate for children at all levels.

Positions

Open—Girl usually on right of boy; inside hands are joined.

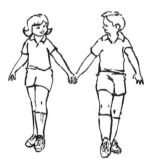

Figure 15-1 Open position.

Two-hand—Partners face and join both hands.

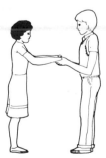

Figure 15-2 Two-hand position

Skating or *promenade*—Partners are side by side facing same direction; girl is on boy's right, right hands held above, left hands under right hands.

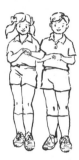

Figure 15-3   Skating or promenade position.

Directions:

Clockwise (C)—Face same direction as a clock hand moves.
Counterclockwise (CW)—The direction most often used in structured dances.

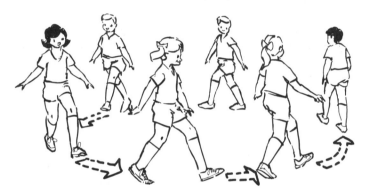

Figure 15-4   Counterclockwise circle formation.

Formations:

Scattered—Individuals, couples, or small groups at random in the area.
Single circle—All stand facing the same direction (center, out, clockwise, counterclockwise).
Double circle—One circle inside another. If in boy-girl couples, the boy is on the inside. Partners may face one another, both same direction (C or CW), or one may face C and one CW.

Figure 15-5   Double circle formation.

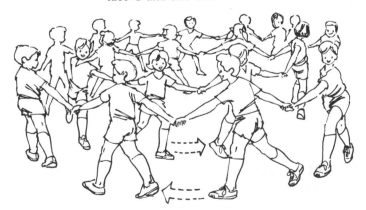

Contra or *Longways*—Line of couples with partners facing one another.

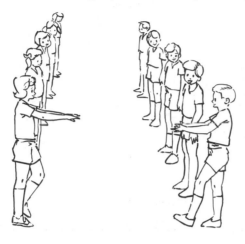

Figure 15-6   Contra or longways formation.

Figures:

Turns—Walking or skipping full or half turn may be made while hooking elbows, or holding both hands of partner.

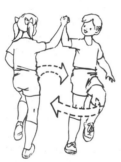

Figure 15-7   Turns.

Swings—While running or walking, partners hook elbows, single or both arms, to turn one another twice around quickly.

Figure 15-8   Swings.

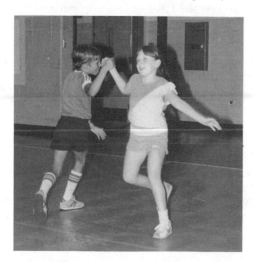

Buzz—Same hand/arm position; one foot is planted while the other foot pushes the couple into a pivoting turn. Movement in turns and swings is usually clockwise.

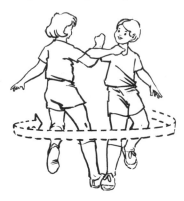

Figure 15-9   Buzz.

STEPS IN TEACHING DANCE

Step 1: Setting the Stage

Children are naturally curious, so a brief statement about any interesting cultural information concerning the dance will oftentimes pique their interest in the new dance. Naturally, the name of the dance should be repeated several times during this phase. The teacher's innate enthusiasm for the dance will also stimulate the children's interest. If the dance is to be among those performed at the upcoming open house, this is the time to make the fact known as this information will also serve to motivate rapid learning.

Step 2: Demonstration

The children's first view of the dance should be as close to the desired finished product as possible, and this includes dancing to the music at correct tempo. If the dance involves a partner it is best for the teacher to have one of the more alert students be a part of the demonstration; however, if this is not possible, simply demonstrating (with the music) the steps that will be used will suffice. The teacher should dance for about one minute, calling attention to the step pattern and how it fits to the music. Simple cues can be called out as the step pattern is performed.

Step 3: Listening to the Music

Listening to the music for about one minute acquaints the children with the tempo. Clapping out the rhythm is helpful, as is clapping the step pattern while the teacher continues to demonstrate and give verbal cues. Children should be encouraged to chant these verbal cues as they clap the music and/or perform the step pattern in their own personal space.

Step 4: Learning and Practicing the Steps

Regardless of the formation called for in the dance, the children should be in scattered- or multiple-line formation to complete the initial learning of the steps. The teacher must make sure everyone can see. Depending on the complexity of the step, the teacher may choose to face the class or face away. It is often easier on the children perceptually if they are behind the teacher's back. However, if the

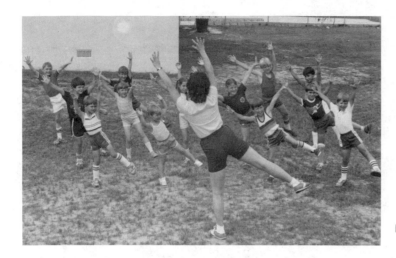

Figure 15-10 Teaching in opposition.

step does not involve a turn, it is permissible for the teacher to face the class. In this case the teacher must teach in opposition (that is, call "step right, close left" but actually demonstrate moving to the left and closing right), thereby providing a mirror image for the child to imitate (Fig. 15-10). Cues must be very clear, concise, and timely. It is a good idea also to have students verbalize the cues as this will enhance their memorization of the step patterns. When the class can call the cues as it practices, the teacher is free to move about and give individual help. Liberal use of praise and corrective feedback during this stage is very important.

Step 5: Music

As soon as most of the class is familiar with the step pattern, begin using the music. The music should be used as soon as the *step pattern* (for example, schottische) can be executed rather than waiting until part or all of the dance (for example, Buggy Schottische) can be executed. As new steps or phases of the dance are being taught, the music should be removed. Music not only keeps the children interested but it also facilitates learning the dance (that is, the music stimulates the appropriate rhythm). Students should continue giving the verbal cues, but now they can state them quietly to themselves as they learn to coordinate their movements with the music. As early in the learning process as is appropriate, the children should be encouraged to depend on the phrasing of the music for their cues. The teacher should continue to move freely about the class giving individual help unless the teacher's image is needed by most of the class, in which case it is best to remain dancing at the front of the class. As soon as several children are successfully performing the steps to the music, they can come to the front of the class and lead with their backs to the class. Leadership opportunities such as this should be rotated among all of the students.

Step 6: Formations

When most of the students are reasonably comfortable with both the steps and the music, the class should assume the required formation of the dance. If this formation is a circle, the teacher becomes a part of the circle (Fig. 15-11) while talking to the class. The teacher should switch positions in the circle several times

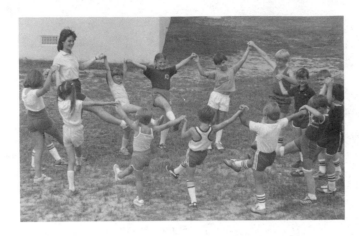

Figure 15-11 Teaching in circle formation.

so that all of the children have the opportunity to view the teacher's movement. Generally it is a good idea to have a "trial run" without the music and at a slightly reduced pace so students become familiar with the circular movement. It is important to remind the children not to watch others directly across from them in the circle as they may become confused when right and left moves are made. If an image is needed it is best to watch the dancers to either side rather than across the circle. The best place for the teacher to be to help an unsure dancer is to either side of that dancer, or, if necessary, directly in front of the performer.

Have a definite procedure for the selection of partners if boy/girl partners are necessary. For example, have the boys form an inner circle and the girls an outer circle. Each circle moves in opposite directions, and when the music stops the circles face each other with partners being directly across. Whenever possible it is best for children to form partners without reference to sex, in which case the two circles would be mixed.

During this phase, extra practice may be needed on the transitions from one step to the next. Also, the ending of the dance should be practiced several times. A strong ending makes the dancers feel good even if parts of the dance are still rough.

Step 7: Dance the Entire Dance

The first time the dance is attempted in its entirety may require playing the music at a slightly reduced tempo (a variable-speed record player is really a must!) so students will experience early success. However, if in the previous periods the music has been at full operational speed and the class has been successful, then reducing the tempo is not necessary. During this phase the teacher should be free to observe the dancers and make note of the students having difficulty with rhythm, step pattern, or motivation. Sometimes the teacher can correct this by becoming a part of the dance and offering additional instruction to each student. If several students demonstrate a lack of readiness for this phase it is best to arrange them into a separate group for additional practice with the teacher. This practice can be scheduled for the end of the class period or the beginning of class the next day. The students who know the dance can be performing at the same time in their separate groups.

It is important to remember that a class should complete steps 1 through 7 within two class periods. At all times, the teacher should strive enthusiastically to promote learning the dance. Positive reinforcement is often the most effective teaching tool.

Step 8: Refinement

Once the students can perform the steps of the dance in rhythm to the music, they should perform the dance often so it can become a permanent part of their dance schema. Each time they perform the dance the teacher should be alert for ways in which to refine their movement (that is, body carriage, styling of moves, and so forth). It is during this stage of relaxed performance that the children will demonstrate their gracefulness (or lack of it). Oftentimes this phase is omitted, which robs the children of an integral part of the total dance experience—relaxed, graceful, expressive movement.

Teaching Hints

1. Approach each dance with enthusiasm.
2. Do not hesitate to withdraw a dance that turns out to be too difficult (that is, cannot be learned in two class meetings).
3. Place students who have rhythmical difficulties between students who do not.
4. If at all possible, secure a variable-speed record player.
5. Prior to performing a previously taught dance, have the students listen to the music and call cues, or dance in place.
6. Keep directions short and clear.
7. Use the music as early in the learning process as possible.
8. Maintain the same cues and sequence of cues for each individual dance.
9. Occasionally use vigorous dances that are well-known by the children for fitness activities.
10. Use the questioning technique to test students' knowledge of terms, dance names, and cultural information.
11. Whenever possible coordinate the use of dance enhancement activities with related information being learned in other classes like social studies, art, and English.
12. Teach in phrases and repeat previous phrases where progress is shown.

Additional Hints for the Level IV–VI Program

Generally, the methodology presented for the Level I–III program also applies to teaching children having higher levels of skill. Activities for the Level IV–VI program should include more complex folk dances, aerobic dancing, tinikling, jumping rope to music, marching, and square dances. More sophisticated dance steps such as the schottische, two-step, polka, and waltz should be refined through developmentally selected dance activities. Dance is an excellent medium for the refinement of fundamental skills, cooperative behaviors, and development of coordination. A major asset in using dance is its progressive nature. Dance activities range from simple to extremely complex; thus the teacher can accommodate varying ability levels and challenge even the highly skilled child. Because of the progressive nature of dance, the categorization of activities into levels of difficulty and charting of individual and group progress can be determined with relative ease.

Developmental Activity Chart—Rhythms and Dance: Level I-III (As Suggested in Chapters 9–12)

RHYTHMS AND RHYMES

NAME	SKILL(S)	LEVEL
Rhythmic Games		
Crazy Clock	rhythmic	I–III
Levels	rhythmic	
Orchestra Leader	directional, rhythmic	
Jack, the Giant Killer	climb, rhythmic	I & II
Morse Code	eye-hand	II & III
Lummi Sticks	eye-hand, rhythmic	
Names in a Rhythm	eye-hand, rhythmic	
Rhythmic Echo	eye-hand, rhythmic	
Threes and Sevens	rhythmic	III
Reverse Ranks	rhythmic	
Line or Circle Clap	rhythmic	
Finger Plays		
Row, Row, Row	auditory, eye-hand, rhythmic	I–III
Where Is Thumbkin?	body awareness	I
Dig a Little Hole	eye-hand, rhythmic	I & II
If I Were a Bird	auditory, eye-hand	
Flowers	rhythmic	
Here Is the Beehive	eye-hand, rhythmic	
I'm a Little Teapot	auditory, eye-hand	
Itsy Bitsy Spider	eye-hand, rhythmic	
Over the Hills	rhythmic	
Ten Fingers	body awareness, rhythmic	
Little Fish	rhythmic	
Left and Right	rhythmic	
Three Little Monkeys	rhythmic	
The Little Clown	eye-hand, rhythmic	
Singing Rhythms		
Right hand, Left hand	directional	I–III
Rest Rhyme	body awareness	
You Can	rhythmic	
Little Miss Muffet	rhythmic	I
Look, See	rhythmic	

NAME	SKILL(S)	LEVEL
Teddy Bear	rhythmic	I & II
Tall and Small	body awareness	
Reach to the Skies	body awareness	
Two Little	body awareness	
My Hands	body awareness	
This Is the Circle, That Is My Head	body awareness	
Head, Shoulders, Knees, and Toes	body awareness	
Make a Fist		
Muffin Man	spatial, skip	II & III
Keep It Moving	rhythmic	
Hinges	rhythmic	
Clap Your Hands	rhythmic	III
Hobby Horse	gallop, rhythmic	
Rope-Jump Rhymes		
I Love Coffee	jump, eye-foot, rhythmic	II & III
Vote, Vote	"	
Mama, Mama	"	
Birthday	"	
Tick, Tock	"	
Bubble Gum	"	
Ice Cream Soda	"	
Hippity Hop	"	
Bulldog	"	
Lady, Lady	"	
All Together	"	
Teddie Bear, Teddie Bear	"	
One, Two, Buckle My Shoe	"	
Ask Mother	"	
Be Nimble, Be Quick	"	
Down in the Valley	"	
Charlie McCarthy	"	
Blind Man	"	
Chickety Chop	"	
Bobby, Bobby	"	
Mabel, Mabel	"	
Fudge, Fudge	"	
Apple, Apple	"	
Hokey-Pokey	"	

Level I–III (continued)

| | | DANCE | | | |
NAME	LEVEL	ORIGIN	SKILL(S)	FORMATION	RECORD
A Hunting We Will Go	I–III	England	slide, skip, visual, rhythmic	Line (P)	FK 1191; RCA 45–5064, 22759
Marching		England	eye-foot, rhythmic	Scattered at first	Any marching record
Baa, Baa Black Sheep	I&II	England	rhythmic, skip, slide, walk	Circle (P)	FK 1191
Bluebird		USA	walk, spatial	Circle	FK 1180
Butterfly		USA	rhythmic		"It's Toddler Time," KIM–0815
Chimes of Dunkirk		France	auditory, directional, slide, skip, spatial	Circle (P)	FK 1187; WFD 1624
Did You Ever See a Lassie?		Scotland	auditory, kick, rhythmic, skip, spatial, visual, walk	Circle	FK 1183; RCA Victor 45–5066
Farmer in the Dell		England/USA	auditory, rhythmic, spatial, walk	Circle	FK 1182; RCA Victor 41–6152
Hickory Dickory Dock		England	rhythmic, run, swing/sway	Circle	Childhood Rhythms Series 7, No. 702,
Hokey Pokey		USA	auditory, body awareness, kick rhythmic, balance spatial, stretch/bend	Circle	Capitol 2427, 6026
I See You		USA	rhythmic	Line (P)	FK 1197
Jack in the Box		England	directional	Scattered	"It's Toddler Time," KIM 0815
London Bridge		England	rhythmic, walk	Circle	RCA Victor 20806
Looby Loo		England	locomotor, kick, movement awareness	Circle	FK 1184; RCA Victor 45–6153
Muffin Man		England	skip	Circle	FK 1188
Mulberry Bush		England	rhythmic, walk	Circle	FK 1183
Oats, Peas, Beans, and Barley		England	rhythmic, skip, walk	Circle	FK 1182 RCA Victor 45–5067
Sally Go Round The Moon		England	gallop, rhythmic, run, slide, skip, walk	Circle	FK 1198; RCA Victor 45–5064
Sing a Song of Sixpence		England	rhythmic, walk	Circle	FK 1180; RCA Victor 22706
Spinning Tops		USA	rhythmic	Scattered	"It's Toddler Time," Kim 0815
The Little Green Frogs		USA	rhythmic	Scattered	"It's Toddler Time," Kim 0815
The Snail		USA	walk	Circle	RCA Victor 45–5064

(cont.)

Level I–III (continued)

NAME	LEVEL	ORIGIN	DANCE SKILL(S)	FORMATION	RECORD
Toot the Flute	I & III	USA	rhythmic	Scattered	"It's Toddler Time," KIM 0815
Top of the Morning		USA	rhythmic	Scattered	"It's Toddler Time," KIM 0815
Turn the Glasses Over		USA	directional, spatial, twist/turn	Circle	WOF–M112
Up, Down, Turn Around		USA	rhythmic	Scattered	"It's Toddler Time," KIM 0815
How Do You Do, my Partner	II	USA	rhythmic	Circle (P)	FK 1190; Pioneer 3012
Ten Little Indians		USA	auditory, hop, jump, rhythmic, skip, walk	Circle	FK 1197
Ach Ja	II & III	Germany	rhythmic, slide, walk	Circle (P)	Ruth Evans' Childhood Rhythm Series VII FK 1189
Bow Belinda		USA	hop, skip	Line (P)	WFD RCA 1622
Come Let Us Be Joyful		Germany	walk	Trios/circle	FD 1187; WFD RCA 1625
Dance of Greeting		Denmark	eye-hand, rhythmic, run	Circle	
Hansel and Gretel		Germany	jump, kick, rhythmic, skip, twist/turn	Circle (P)	FK 1193; WFD RCA 1124
Jolly Is the Miller		USA	rhythmic, skip, visual walk	Circle (P)	FK 1192; RCA 45–5067
Jump Jim Joe		USA	jump, rhythmic, run, slide	Circle (P)	FK 1180, Bowmar Album 3
Kinderpolka		Germany	rhythmic, slide, spatial	Circle	FK 1181; WFD RCA 1625; RCA Victor 45–6179
Limbo		West Indian	balance, rhythmic, stretch/bend	Line	Hoctor Dance Records 1608B
Maypole Dance		USA	rhythmic, skip	Circle	FK 1178, EA–20

Level I–III (continued)

NAME	LEVEL	ORIGIN	DANCE SKILL(S)	FORMATION	RECORD
Paw-Paw Patch		USA	gallop, rhythmic, slide, skip, visual, walk	Longways (P)	FK 1181
Pease Porridge Hot		England	eye-hand, gallop, rhythmic, run, slide, skip, twist/turn	Circle (P)	FK 1190
Round and Round the Village		England	directional, rhythmic, skip	Circle	FK 1191; WFD RCA 1625
Seven Jumps		Denmark	balance, jump, kick, rhythmic, skip, spatial	Circle	FK 1163; WFD RCA 1623
Shoo Fly		USA	rhythmic, skip, swing/sway, visual, walk	Circle (P)	FK 1102 and 1185; Decca 18222
This Old Man		USA	hop, rhythmic, run, skip	Circle	Russell 705
The Popcorn Man	II & III	USA	jump, rhythmic skip	Circle	FK 1180
The Wheat		Czechos-lovakia	rhythmic, skip, walk	Sets of 3	RCA Victor 1625
Badger Gavotte	III	USA	rhythmic	Circle (P)	FK 1094
Bingo		USA	auditory, rhythmic, walk	Circle	FK 1189; RCA Victor 45–6711
Bleking		Sweden	hop, jump, rhythmic	Circle (P)	FK 1188
Carousel		Sweden	slide, skip	Circle (P)	FK 1183; RCA 1625
Cat's Meow		USA	step-close, step-swing, balance, pivot	Line	EA 32 DWP
Crested Hen		Denmark	hop, rhythmic, spatial	Sets of 3	FK 1194; RCA 45–6176
Danish Scottische		Denmark	rhythmic	Circle (P)	RCA 1622
Easter Parade		USA	directional, spatial, walk	Circle (P)	White I–2, EA–20
Glowworm		USA	rhythmic, walk	Circle (P)	McGregor 310–B; Windsor 4613–B
Grand March		USA	rhythmic, skip, spatial, walk	Line	Any march or square-dance record
Greensleeves		England	directional, rhythmic, spatial, walk	Circle (P)	WFD 1624
Gustaf's Skoal		Sweden	rhythmic, skip, walk	Square (P)	FK 1175; Victor 20988
Horah		Israel	hop, kick, rhythmic, step	Circle	FK 1110

(cont.)

Level I-III (continued)

| | | | DANCE | | |
NAME	LEVEL	ORIGIN	SKILL(S)	FORMATION	RECORD
Klapptanz		Sweden	auditory, rhythmic, twist/turn	Circle (P)	WOF M-114(7)
Little Brown Jug		USA	rhythmic, skip, slide	Circle (P)	FK 1304-A; Columbia 52007
Lummi Sticks		USA	eye-hand, rhythmic, spatial		FK 1186; RCA 45-6178
Oh Susanna		USA	rhythmic	Circle (P)	
Pop Goes the Weasle		USA	skip, walk	Circle (P)	FK 1329; WOF M104; Columbia A 3078
Schottische		Scotland	hop, rhythmic	Circle	RCA Victor 4131
Skip to My Lou		USA	rhythmic, skip, spatial, swing/sway, walk	Circle (P)	FK 1192-A
Zip Code 001		USA	balance, jump, heel-toe, two-step	Line	EA 32 DWF

Developmental Activity Chart—Rhythms and Dance: Level IV-VI (Recommended activities for skilled children)

NAME	LEVEL	ORIGIN	SKILL(S)	FORMATION	RECORD
Duchess Hustle	IV-VI	USA	heel-toe, stomp, turn	Scattered	MH-39
Grand March		USA	walk, two-step	Line	Any marching record
Horah		Israel	step, swing, hop	Circle	WFD 1623; RCA-EPA-4140; FK 1110
Hopp Mor Annika		Sweden	step hop, skip, polka	Circle (P)	WFD 1624
Kalvelis		Lithuania	polka	Circle (P)	WOF M101, W-Vol. 3
La Raspa		Mexico	bleking	Free/Circle (P)	WOF M106;(6) WFD 1623
Limbo		West Indian	balance, various movements while moving under a pole	Line	Any "Jamaican" music
Mexican Clap Dance		USA	waltz	Circle	DWP EA 32
Mayim! Mayim!		Israel	walk, hop, grapevine	Circle	WOF M119; (6) FK 1108
Sicilian Circle		USA	chain, right/left hand star, do-si-do	Circle (P)	FK 1115; WOF M104
Ten Pretty Girls		USA	walk, point, kick, stamp	Line/Circle	WFD 1624, WOF 113
The Bird Dance		Europe	walk, skip, elbow-swing, star	Circle or scattered, partners or solo	Avia Disk AD-831-A

Level IV–VI (continued)

| | | | DANCE | | |
NAME	LEVEL	ORIGIN	SKILL(S)	FORMATION	RECORD
Uno, Dos, Tres		USA	bleking	Line	DWP EA 32
Ace of Diamonds	IV	Denmark	back to back polka, elbow swing	Circle (P)	WFD 1622; WOF M102
Heads and Sides		USA	honor, do-si-do, swing, promenade	Square	EA–1
Norwegian Mountain March		Norway	waltz, run, turn	Sets of 3	WFD 1622; FK 1177
Oh Susanna		USA	slide, skip, right and left	Grand Circle (P)	WFD 1623; FK 1186; RCA EPA 4140
Patty Cake Polka		USA	heel-toe, slide, skip	Circle (P)	FK 1260; WOF M107; WFD 1625
Tantoli		Sweden	heel-toe, polka, step-hop	Circle (P)	WFD 1621
Turnaround		USA	walk, heel touch, kick	Scattered	MH–39
Zip Code 001		USA	heel-toe, two step	Lines	DWP EA 32
Cshebogar	IV & V	Hungary	walk, skip, slide, Hungarian turn, buzz	Circle (P)	WFD 1624, WOF M101
Teton Mountain Stomp Mixer		USA	walk, two-step	Circle (P)	FK 1482
Virginia Reel		USA	walk, skip, swing, cast-off, do-si-do, slide	Longways set	WFD 1623; RCA EPA 4138; WOF M103
All-American Promenade	V–VI	USA	walk, balance	Circle	FK 1061
Black Nag		England	run, slide, do-si-do, skip	Longways set of 3 couples	W Vol. 2
Cherkassiya		Israel	grapevine, step-hop	Circle	RCA EPA 4140; WFD 1623
Cotton Eyed Joe		USA	heel-toe polka, two-step, chug	Free or Line (P)	WOF 118; WFD 1621
Heel and Toe Polka		USA	heel-toe polka, slide, two-step	Free (P)	
Little Man in a Fix		Denmark	waltz, run, turn, drawstep	Sets of 2 couples	WOF M121

(cont.)

Level VI (continued)

NAME	LEVEL	ORIGIN	DANCE		
			SKILL(S)	FORMATION	RECORD
Lott lst Tod		Sweden	slide, face-to-face and back-to-back polka	Circle (P)	WFD 1622
Put Your Little Foot		USA	sweep step, point, walk	Circle (P)	FK 1165; WOF M107
Road to the Isles		Scotland	walk, schottische	Free (P)	FK 1095; WOF M110
Romunsko Kolo		Yugoslavia	schottische, rock, step-hop	Circle	FK 1402; W Vol. 3
Susan's Gavotte		USA	walk, slide, step swing, two-step	Circle (P)	WOF M113
The Boogie Beat		USA	step, kick, two-step	Scattered	MH-39
Tinikling		Philippines	tinikling steps over tinikling poles	3/2 poles	WFD 1619
Turkey in the Oven		USA	grand right and left	Circle	EA 20
Wearing o' the Green		Irish	allemande, do-si-do, promenade	Square/circle	EA 20
Brown-Eyed Mary	VI	USA	walk, skip, promenade	Circle (P)	WOF M117 or any lively polka
El Bale		Guam	walking, two-step, hitting sticks	Couples	Any recording of "Narcissa Queen"
Highland Schottische		Scotland	Highland fling, schottische	Circle (P)	CFD–RCA–4133; WFD 1621
Irish Washerwoman		Ireland	grand right and left, allemande left, promenade	Square (P)	RCA EPA 4140; WFD 1623
Korobushka		Russia	schottische, balance, 3-step turn	Free (P)	WOF M108; FK 1170
Miserlou		Greece	step point, grapevine pivot, walk	Line/circle	WFD 1620; W Vol. 5
Nine Pin Reel		Scotland	slide, buzz, polka, shuffle	Square (P)	Any reel music
Oh Johnny		USA	walk, swing, allemande, do-si-do	Square (P)	FK 1037
Poi-Poi		Polynesia	two-step, eye-hand coordination, promenade, allemande	Free	Twinson
Rye Waltz		USA	slide, waltz, walk, skip	Circle (P)	FK 1103
Waves of Tory		Ireland	waves, whirlpools, whitecaps	Longways set (P)	WOF M102
Kool Kat		USA	walk, skip, turn	Varsou-vienne (P)	MH-39

FK, Folkraft; WFD, World of Folk Dance; Kim, Kimbo; DWP, Dances Without Partners; EA, Educational Activities; WOF, World of Fun (Records); MH, Melody House; W, White, Rhythms Productions; (P), denotes Partners required.

SUGGESTED ACTIVITY SOURCES

COCHRAN, N., WILKINSON, L. C., & FURLOW, J. J. (1982). *A teacher's guide to elementary school physical education.* Dubuque, IA: Kendall/Hunt.

DIMONDSTEIN, G. (1971). *Children dance in the classroom.* New York: Macmillan.

FARINA, A. (1980). *Developmental games and rhythms for children.* Springfield, IL: Chas. C. Thomas.

HARRIS, J., PITMAN, A. M., & WALLER, M. S. (1978). *Dance a while.* Minneapolis: Burgess.

KIRCHNER, G. (1985). *Physical education for elementary school children* (6th ed.). Dubuque, IA: Wm. C. Brown.

KRAUS, R. A. (1966). *Pocket guide of folk and square dances and singing games.* Englewood Cliffs, NJ: Prentice-Hall.

LATCHAW, M., & PYATT, J. (1966). *Folk and square dances and singing games.* Englewood Cliffs, NJ: Prentice-Hall.

MURRY, R. L. (1975). *Dance in elementary education.* New York: Harper & Row.

SIEDENTOP, D., HERKOWITZ, J., & RINK, J. (1984). *Elementary physical education methods.* Englewood Cliffs, NJ: Prentice-Hall.

VICK, M., & MCLAUGHLIN, C. R. (1970). *A Collection of dances for children* (card file). Minneapolis: Burgess.

RECORD SOURCES

Bowmar Records
622 Rodier Drive
Glendale, CA 91201

Bridges
310 West Jefferson
Dallas, TX 75208

Burns Record Co.
755 Chickadee Lane
Stratford, CT 06075

Childhood Rhythms
326 East Forest Park Ave.
Springfield, MA

Children's Music Center
5373 West Pico Boulevard
Los Angeles, CA 90019

Columbia Records
1473 Barnum Ave.
Bridgeport, CT 06605

Dance Record Center
1161 Broad Street
Newark, NJ 07114

Dances Without Partners
(See Educational Activities)

Educational Activities, Inc.
P.O. Box 392
Freeport, NY 11520

Educational Recordings of America, Inc.
P.O. Box 231
Monroe, CT 06468

Folk Dancer
Box 201
Flushing, NY 11363

Folkraft Records
P. O. Box 1363
San Antonio, TX 78295–1363

Freda Miller Records for Dance
Department J, Box 383
Northport, Long Island, NY 11768

Hoctor Educational Records, Inc.
Waldwick, New Jersey, 07463

Imperial Records
137 North Western Avenue
Los Angeles, CA

Kimbo—USA Records
Box 55
Deal, NJ 07723

McGregor Records
729 South Western Ave.
Hollywood, CA

Master Record Service
708 East Garfield
Phoenix, AZ 85006

Melody House Publishing Co.
819 NW 92nd Street
Oklahoma City, OK 73114

Merrbach Record Service
P.O. Box 7308
323 W. 14th Street
Houston, TX 77008

RCA Victor Education Dept. J
155 East 24th Street
New York, NY 10010

Record Center
2581 Piedmont Road NE
Atlanta, GA 30324

Rhythm Record Co.
9203 Nichols Road
Oklahoma City, OK 73120

Rhythm Productions Records
Dept. J., Box 34485
Los Angeles, CA 90034

Russell Records Co.
P.O. Box 3318
Ventura, CA 93003

Square Dance
Box 689
Santa Barbara, CA 93102

Twinson Co.
433 La Prende Road
Los Altos, CA

Windsor Records
5530 North Rosemead Blvd.
Temple City, CA 91780

World of Folk Dance
(See RCA Victor)

World of Fun Records
1908 Grand Avenue
P.O. Box 189
Nashville, TN 37202

World of Fun Records
Cokesbury Regional Service Center
1600 Queen Anne Road
Teaneck, NJ 07666

White
(See Rhythm Productions)

SUGGESTED READINGS

ANDREWS, G. (1976).   Creative rhythmic movement for children. Englewood Cliffs, NJ: Prentice-Hall.

BARLIN, A. (1979).   *Teaching your wings to fly*. Santa Monica, CA: Goodyear.

BRUCE, V. R. (1970).   *Movement in silence and sounds*. London: G. Bell & Sons.

DIMONDSTEIN, G. (1971).   *Children dance in the classroom*. New York: Macmillan.

HARRIS, J., Pitman, A. M., & Waller, M. S. (1978). *Dance a while*. Minneapolis: Burgess.

JOYCE, M. (1980).   *First steps in teaching creative dance to children*. Palo Alto, CA: Mayfield.

JOYCE, M. (1984).   *Dance technique for children*. Palo Alto, CA: Mayfield.

KIRCHNER, G. (1985).   *Physical education for elementary school children* (6th ed.). Dubuque, IA: Wm. C. Brown.

LOGSDON, B., BARRETT, K., AMMONS, M., BROER, M. R., HALVERSON, L. E., MCGEE, R., & ROBERTON, M. A. (1984).   *Physical education for children* (Educational dance, Chapter 6.) Philadelphia: Lea & Febiger.

MURRY, R. L. (1975).   *Dance in elementary education*. New York: Harper & Row.

SCHURR, E. L. (1980).   *Movement experiences for children* (3rd ed.). Englewood Cliffs, NJ: Prentice-Hall.

16

GYMNASTICS

Gymnastic activities are fun and inherently challenging across all skill levels. Such activities provide children with enjoyable opportunities to self-test emerging abilities, while allowing for immediate feedback. Gymnastics also provide children with opportunities to create movements that defy gravity and enhance the development of several health- and skill-related fitness components (flexibility, muscular endurance, balance, coordination, among others). These activities offer an excellent vehicle for developing an understanding of the laws of motion and fostering cooperation among students.

As children learn to transfer and support their weight on various body parts, unique and satisfying movements occur. Children learn to trust in their abilities and determine individually just how far to go, and how difficult a task to attempt. The child is generally the best judge of when to progress to a more difficult challenge. Consequently, it is the teacher's task to establish an environment that is safe, challenging, and provides for maximum participation.

Bearing in mind the fact that no two children in a class will perform the same stunt at the same time with an equal degree of proficiency, the teacher can use various teaching styles and types of class organization to create a learning environment that is safe and challenging for all children. The following section outlines specific considerations for planning these self-testing gymnastic activities.

SAFETY

For the teacher to establish a safe environment where youngsters can learn gymnastic skills, children must have certain responsibilities, and it is imperative that they are aware of what those responsibilities entail. Rules for conduct need to be established and posted where everyone can see them. Rules for conduct should include:

1. *Proper attire:* No loose or bulky clothes, jewelry, belts, or clothing that could catch on equipment or individuals.
2. *Proper conduct in the gymnasium:* No horseplay, unsupervised activity, or gum chewing.
3. *Proper use of spotters:* Children as spotters should only try to break a fall and should not be expected or be encouraged to carry or lift another student through a stunt.

Other rules may be added according to need; however, the list should be kept simple so that children can easily remember the rules. Table 16–1 presents an example of a gymnastics rules poster.

The fitness activity before gymnastic skills are presented should include general flexibility exercises that move all parts of the body, including the head and neck, through a complete range of motion, and strength exercises specific to the activities (see Chapter 13, "Physical Fitness Activities," for exercise suggestions).

The teacher is responsible for presenting activities that are commensurate with the child's abilities and that follow an accepted progression. The activities listed in this chapter are grouped according to suggested levels and categories of skills; however, most classes are not homogeneous in abilities. Consequently, the teacher must assume responsibility for determining which activities are appropriate for the students' varying skill levels and which also enhance the theme being developed.

As previously noted in the description of this curricular model, Level I–III activities should be used primarily as enhancements to skill themes, whereas Level IV–VI activities are themes (skills) to be introduced in the skill-development portion of the lesson.

The focus of the primary gymnastics program (Level I–III) is on developing movement awareness and the self-confidence necessary for performance. Variations in movement patterns are highly encouraged as children move to discover the multitude of possible patterns within each skill theme being explored. The enhancement activities are presented as logical extensions of the skills being perfected. Within each skill theme, a variety of enhancements should be used. For diversity, the activities can be divided into the following categories:

Animal movements	Partner balances
Individual stunts	Pyramids
Partner stunts	Small-equipment activities
Individual balance stunts	Large-equipment activities
Tumbling and inverted balance	

Activities within each category should be chosen to enhance each theme.

Table 16-1   Gymnasium Rules for Gymnastics

1. Move only when the teacher is in the gym.
2. Wear clothes that are not loose and bulky but enable you to move freely; NO JEANS!
3. Take off belts and jewelry; spit out gum.
4. Always have a partner to help break a fall.
5. Do not bug each other while you are working.
6. Only go one at a time on equipment unless otherwise directed.

At Level IV–VI, the same categories exist as the skills become more complex and attention to detail more rigorous. During these phases, students are encouraged to refine movements mechanically, aesthetically, and to combine various skills into sequences and routines.

At both the foundation and refinement levels, the child's readiness for specifically prescribed movements is determined by individual levels of strength, flexibility, vestibular awareness, and experience. Students should be required to demonstrate proficiency at less difficult skills before being permitted to attempt the more demanding and complex activities. Checklists and task sheets are extremely effective for keeping track of individual levels of proficiency in order to determine appropriate activities for each child (refer to Chapter 8, "Evaluation," and Chapter 6, "Organization and Instruction," for more detailed information on formulating task sheets). Generally, a progression that consists of performing alone on the floor, to working with a partner, to using small manipulative equipment, and finally trying skills on apparatus, is acceptable.

The incorporation of small manipulative equipment such as beanbags, hoops, and wands into the theme increases task complexity and serves to increase interest during the repetitive practice necessary to refine the skills. For example, when practicing the forward roll, the progression of activities might be:

1. Forward roll in tuck position, from one foot, a straddle or a pike position;
2. Forward roll to a straddle, one foot or straight leg landing;
3. Forward roll with a partner, holding hands, starting back to back, or in a circle;
4. Forward roll over a beanbag, wand, or hoop;
5. Forward roll and catch a ball tossed by a partner;
6. Roll a hoop and forward roll next to it, stopping it at the completion of the roll;
7. Forward roll across a padded vaulting box;
8. Forward roll across a bench;
9. Forward roll across a padded vaulting box through a hoop held by a partner.

There are many more options to this forward-roll progression. A thorough examination of time, space, force, and relationship variations will turn up a multitude of possibilities. The important concept to remember is that within each activity described or outlined in this chapter, there are many possibilities for variability. The following pieces of small manipulative equipment may be successfully used with gymnastics activities:

Balls—playground (small size), yarn, nerf	Indian clubs
Hoops	Ropes—jump ropes and stretch ropes
Wands	Cones
Beanbags	Parachute

The teacher's attitude about gymnastics is perhaps one of the most important factors in establishing a safe environment for learning. Students should always be encouraged for their efforts and not be expected to compete with classmates, but rather, with themselves. The teacher needs to remember that obstacle courses and relay races utilizing newly learned skills may not be conducive to initial skill acquisition and may be extremely unsafe. An atmosphere of trust and responsibility must be established.

TEACHING STYLE

The teaching style chosen for any particular lesson must by necessity establish a safe and controlled environment while at the same time enabling children to work at their own pace. The greatest success will be achieved by using a variety of teaching styles and frequently more than one within a particular lesson.

The command style and demonstrations should be used for making specific skill points on complex stunts and also for establishing a controlled atmosphere. Frequently gymnastics lessons need to be highly structured so that children perform only when they are signaled to do so and do only what they are told to do. Structuring lessons for control helps to show children how to take turns and directs their performance toward a specific goal.

As children demonstrate more responsible behavior (that is, taking turns, proper spotting, and directed practice habits), the guided discovery, problem solving, and exploration teaching styles should become more prevalent. Guided discovery is very useful in developing quality performance as well as teaching the laws of motion. Through guided-discovery techniques the child develops the much desired concept and movement schema associated with control in varying positions, at the same time allowing the teacher more control of the outcome (that is, specific objectives are predetermined).

The problem-solving style offers the greatest reward in terms of individualizing and self-pacing as the child chooses his or her own movement solutions to such problems as: "How many ways can you balance on one body part?" and "Show me how to move across the floor touching three different body parts as you go." As children move, they develop ideas, with and from each other, and they self-perpetuate activity. The movements that emerge will greatly resemble the patterns described in this section, except that the children will have the satisfaction of discovery and will have learned about the uniqueness of their own movements. This approach to gymnastics is often referred to as *educational gymnastics*, and it plays an important role in the total gymnastics program. The themes most applicable to educational gymnastics (goals of good body awareness off and on equipment) are jumping and landing, rolling (Chapter 9); bending/stretching, swinging/swaying (Chapter 10); body, spatial, and vestibular awareness (Chapter 12).

A second way of using the problem-solving style is to expand on the specific skills described in this chapter by introducing movement variability as proficiency develops. For example, the child who has refined the basic handstand would be encouraged to try different ways of getting into the position, different ways of getting out of the position, and various body shapes while in the balanced position, thus expanding on the basic pattern. In this way children put movements together to form, first, sequences and eventually routines linking the various categories of stunts together. It is the ultimate goal of the gymnastics program to produce quality movement sequences at each level. To this end, the problem-solving approach may be quite effective.

For a more detailed discussion of teaching styles, refer to Chapter 6, "Organization and Instruction."

CLASS ORGANIZATION

The organization of the class into formations for the most effective teaching will be determined primarily by the equipment available and the activity. Individual mats or large carpet squares can be utilized effectively for a variety of activities,

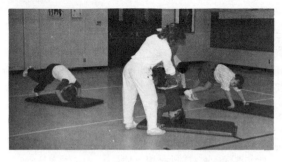

Figure 16-1 Scattered on individual mats.

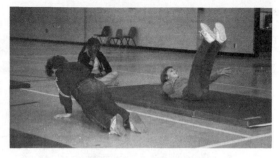

Figure 16-2 Mats in rows and children doing return activities beside them.

especially those that are nonlocomotive. A scattered formation (Fig. 16–1) may be utilized with each child working on an individual mat. Proper spacing should be encouraged along with reminders about self-space. Strip-tumbling-type mats may be linked together to form one long mat or separated into individual sections and used for activities that require locomotion or soft padding.

If the mats are separated, the children may need to share in groups; therefore, some type of traffic pattern and return activity for the floor space between the mats should be planned to maximize activity. For example, a forward roll may be done on the mat and a seal walk done between the mats as a return activity. Figure 16–3 illustrates a suggested formation.

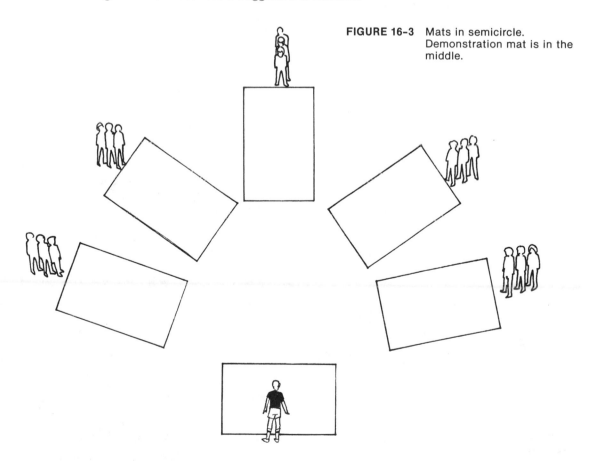

FIGURE 16-3 Mats in semicircle. Demonstration mat is in the middle.

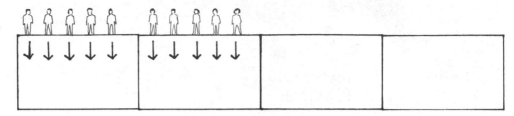

Figure 16-4 Mats hooked together with the children working widthwise across them provides more activity.

The mats can also be linked together with velcro strips and utilized as one long piece with the children working individually across the width of the mat as illustrated in Figure 16-4.

Those activities which demand movement from one end of a mat to the other should be well organized. Children can be lined up on one side of a large activity mat, for example, and a "wave plan" used to allow turns (Fig. 16-5), or they can be lined up in groups at one side and move across in turn ("line plan"), waiting at the opposite side for return activities (Fig. 16-6). Children should never be allowed to walk across the mats, but should be trained to go around in all activities to prevent collisions with performers.

Wave plan: Each child begins movement as the child to the left completes one movement of a series across the mat.

Line plan: Each row completes a turn across the mat at one time, then the next row takes a turn.

Generally, a station or group organization works best for utilizing available mats and equipment. In a group, children can be rotated among stations on a signal from the teacher, or individually they can progress according to their accomplishment of certain tasks. The teacher will find the use of station cards or posters that outline suggested problems or activities to be very helpful. Task sheets are very appropriate and desirable as a technique for facilitating station work (see Chapter

Figure 16-5 Wave plan.

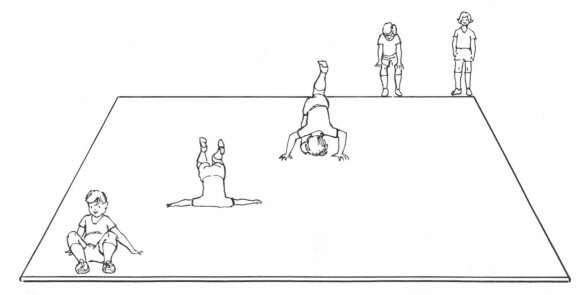

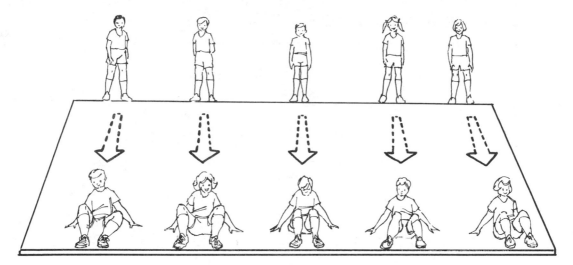

Figure 16-6 Line plan.

6, "Organization and Instruction," for details concerning organization and class formations). When using stations, remember that the teacher should be safety conscious and not allow potentially dangerous activities (stations) to be unsupervised.

SMALL EQUIPMENT

In order to incorporate small manipulative equipment into gymnastic activities, one should examine the basics of movement variability. A progression of complexity can then be established. The following list reveals the possibilities of movements in relationship to equipment and the suggested progression for incorporation with the activities:

1. Equipment stationary (for example, use prescribed movement to move over, around, through, and under the equipment);
2. Equipment carried or balanced on the body (use prescribed movement while carrying or balancing equipment in hands, under arms, on head, on shoulders, on knees, between legs, knees, ankles);
3. Equipment moving (roll ball and roll self next to it, or roll hoop and frog-hop through it);
4. Equipment manipulated before or after start (that is, throwing, catching, rolling, striking, kicking before or after stunt);
5. Equipment manipulated during stunt (throwing, catching, rolling, striking, kicking as stunt is performed). Not all skills will be adaptable to this variation.

LARGE EQUIPMENT

Most schools do not have sufficient numbers of apparatus (for example, vault, large beam) to allow the teacher effectively to involve all the students in the same activity at the same time. For example, it would not be a good idea to require 30 children to wait a turn to cross one of two balance beams. Therefore, the teacher must be creative in organizing apparatus activities and using an appropriate teach-

TABLE 16-2   Gymnastic Station Plan

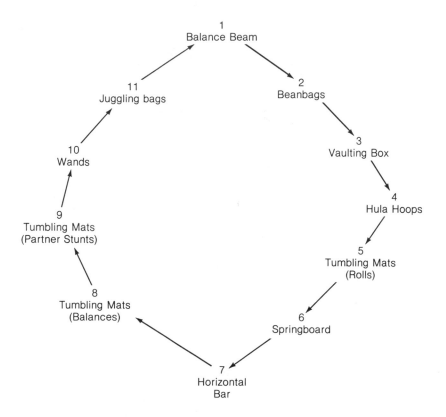

ing style. The teacher can use a variety of equipment and mats in one lesson to maximize activity or first have children use the floor and imitate the activity to be done on the apparatus. Lines on the floor serve well as practice balance beams and stations help provide for maximum participation on available equipment. The teacher should endeavor to set up creative arrangements of apparatus and mats to stimulate and challenge the children's capabilities. An example of one gymnasium organization is provided in Table 16-2. Whether the children rotate on a signal or at their own pace will be determined by the teaching style employed. If they rotate as a group, there must be enough stations so that there are no more than three or four students at each station. To increase the number of stations, the teacher can add small manipulative activities to the plan.

Whatever the equipment used, the teacher must be sure that sufficient ground padding is provided (in relationship to the height of the apparatus) and that the equipment is well spaced in the gymnasium or play area. Taking turns and spacing between students participating and students waiting will be a key consideration when choosing the teaching style and class organization.

For Levels IV–VI, specific skills are recommended for the various pieces of equipment. Large-equipment activities for Levels I–III are incorporated into the skill themes under the additional movement variations sections. Movement variations with large equipment should be reviewed with Level IV–VI children before progressing to the skills outlined in this chapter.

RHYTHMIC GYMNASTICS

The current rise in popularity of *rhythmic gymnastics* in the United States warrants its inclusion in this chapter for Level III (and above) students. The key concept in rhythmic gymnastics is that specifically prescribed movement skills are performed in time to music. Children will derive great pleasure from practicing and finally mastering these skills because they are challenging and offer a great deal of task complexity. Chosen for inclusion in this chapter are beginning progressions for rhythmic ball, hoop, wand, and ribbon gymnastics. As children develop proficiency in these skills, they should be encouraged to put movements together into simple routines.

Teachers will find that the inclusion of rhythmic gymnastics into their programs expands the possibilities for challenging skill development. Some basic suggestions to enhance success include:

1. Use music in 3/4 time.
2. Always practice with music.
3. Use a variety of music to encourage creativity and interest.
4. Space children so that there is no danger of a tossed and missed implement striking another child.
5. Stress giving with arms and knees simultaneously as objects are caught.
6. Practice all skills on both sides of the body.
7. Allow children to create their own skills and routines.
8. Allow children the opportunity to perform their routines for others.

PROGRESSION

The most important concept to adhere to in the teaching of gymnastic activities is *proper progression*. The following general progression outline is provided to assist the teacher in choosing activities wisely.

1. Animal Walks and Movements (for example, bunny hop, measuring worm, bouncing ball, rocker). These simple movements should stress placing part of the body weight on the hands; the more weight, the more difficult the stunt. A further importance of these stunts is in their development of flexibility and abdominal strength, necessary for more advanced activities.
2. Individual and Partner Stunts (for example, coffee grinder, double walk, Chinese get-up). These serve to increase flexibility and strength, and they demand coordination of movements between two children.
3. Individual Balance Stunts (for example, balance stand, thread the needle, turk stand, rooster hop, crane stand). These stunts enable children to practice balancing in a variety of positions; the more complicated the position and the narrower the base of support, the more difficult the stunt.

The previously described categories of stunts should be worked on simultaneously, choosing the simplest stunts in each category and gradually progressing to the more difficult. Follow the same procedure for the next three categories.

4. Tumbling and Inverted Balance (forward roll, headstand, handstand). Each of these stunts may be performed in a variety of positions, each of which changes the difficulty of the stunt. For example, a forward roll from a tuck position is simpler to perform than a forward roll from a pike position. Generally, the more force received in the transfer of weight the more difficult the stunt (that is, the farther from the ground at the start of the movement).

5. Partner Balances and Combatives (for example, angel balance, sitting balance, rooster fight, hand wrestling). These stunts demand considerable strength on the part of both performers, and they should not be attempted without due consideration. Partners should be paired according to similar height and weight for maximum safety.

6. Pyramid Building demands careful adjustments to other children and varying amounts of strength, depending on the various positions; therefore, some pyramids (those that don't involve children balancing on top of each other) are appropriate for Level I children. However, most should be reserved for Level II through Level VI, and then only when children have demonstrated proficiency at partner balancing.

7. Large Apparatus. Once proficiency on the floor is established, certain stunts may be attempted on apparatus. The following pieces of apparatus provide gradually increasing difficulty, and the child should progress only as proficiency is established on each piece. Many activities done on the floor can be tried on equipment, and specific skills for each piece can be taught. For Levels I–III, review the following skill themes for specific large-equipment activities.

Jumping and Landing	(Chapter 9)
Rolling	(Chapter 9)
Climbing	(Chapter 9)
Swinging and Swaying	(Chapter 10)
Vestibular Awareness	(Chapter 12)

Specific skills on large equipment are listed in the section for skilled children (in a later part of this chapter). The following basic pieces of large apparatus are recommended for use in the program:

Low padded box (2 ft.).
Low bench
Incline board (wide)
Low balance board (on the ground)
Ladder on the ground
Incline board (narrow)
Incline ladder
High horizontal ladder (3 ft. to 5 ft. from the floor)
High balance beam (1 ft. to 2 ft. from the floor)
Low horizontal bar
Climbing rope (single)
Double ropes

TEACHING HINTS

1. Use task sheets extensively to determine student readiness and progress.
2. Maximize activity by increasing the number of stations and using small manipulative equipment with large equipment.
3. Establish a responsible atmosphere, with a supportive attitude and specific safety rules.
4. Use relay races with extreme caution. Animal walks are most appropriate because of the relatively simple nature of the skills involved. More complicated skills should not be used for racing. Skills where the head and neck are involved and balance skills are the most dangerous (for example, forward rolls and balance beam).
5. Children should be encouraged to sequence skills and formulate routines utilizing their knowledge of space, time, and force variables.

6. Stress transferring body weight smoothly using a variety of body parts (that is, not just hands to feet and feet to hands).

7. Lessons should flow smoothly from skill-development to enhancement activities, and frequently these parts may be indistinguishable. Large apparatus work may encompass both these parts of the lesson.

8. Combine locomotor-type stunts with balance and agility stunts at each level to maintain interest and offer the most diverse program possible.

9. Encourage responsible behavior by having children work in pairs. Spotting habits should be stressed and children should be taught where to stand in order to break or prevent a child's fall on the floor or on large equipment.

10. Use small equipment to increase the complexity of specific skills and maintain interest.

11. Remember that gymnastics is a developmental activity with increases in strength and flexibility resulting directly in more successful performance.

GYMNASTICS ACTIVITIES

SEAL WALK

DESCRIPTION: The seal walk is started in a lying position, stomach down, with the legs held straight. The arms are held as straight as possible and used to move the body with the legs dragging.

PUSH AND CLAP

DESCRIPTION: Partners stand 3 feet apart facing each other with feet spread slightly. On the "go" signal, raise both hands, clap them to partner's hands, then push them against hands in an attempt to push partner off balance. When one partner moves a foot, the contest is over.

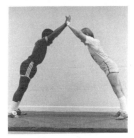

Figure 16-7

ROW YOUR BOAT

DESCRIPTION: Partners sit facing each other with legs spread and soles of feet touching. One person leans forward and the other leans backward pulling gently on each other; reverse. Try this with legs crossed.

Figure 16-8

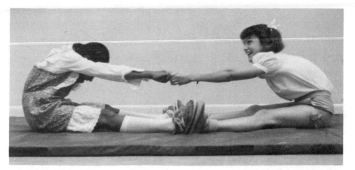

PULL–PUSH THE WAND

DESCRIPTION: Grasp the wand near the center with hands about 6 inches apart. Extend the arms and maintain a tight grip, then slowly pull the hands apart. Use different grips (overhand, underhand, crossed). Reverse the procedure and push the hands together. (Equipment: one wand per child.)

OVER THE HEAD—PLOUGH

DESCRIPTION: Lie on back with arms at side and hands flat on the floor. Bend knees bringing the legs to the chest and extend the legs over the head to touch the toes to the floor. This should be done slowly, and the extreme position should be held for 5 to 10 seconds before returning to the original position.

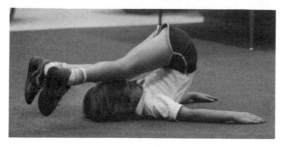

Figure 16-9

SEAT CIRCLE

DESCRIPTION: Sit on the floor with knees bent and hands placed behind the seat. Push with the hands and lift the feet off the floor and spin in a circle. Do this both ways, then try to hold a beanbag between the knees or toes and spin without dropping it.

LONG STRETCH

DESCRIPTION: Stand with feet together behind a line. With a piece of chalk in one hand, squat down and place free hand on the floor. Walk forward on hands as far as possible and mark distance with the chalk. Return to squat position and stand. (Equipment: chalk.)

EGG SIT

DESCRIPTION: Sit in a tuck position and grasp right toes with right hand and left toes with left hand. Then rock back on seat and straighten legs without letting go of the toes. Balance in this "V-sit" position without grasping the toes.

RAG DOLL

DESCRIPTION: Stand with feet together and arms at sides. Count 1, bend head forward to touch chin to chest; count 2, rotate head sideward to position above right shoulder; count 3, rotate head backward to look at ceiling; count 4, rotate head sideward to position above left shoulder.

TOE REACH

DESCRIPTION: Stand with feet together and arms at side. Count 1, bend forward and reach toward the toes with hands; count 2, stand erect. Keep legs straight throughout the exercise. Relax the neck muscles and allow the head to drop and the shoulders and upper body to aid in this bending position.

STOOP AND STRETCH

DESCRIPTION: Squat with feet shoulder-width apart. First, reach back between the legs and stretch without losing balance. Next, reach around and through the legs from the back to the front. Then lower to the squat position, grasping a beanbag in the right hand, reach around the right leg, and toss the beanbag forward. Throw as far as possible this way.

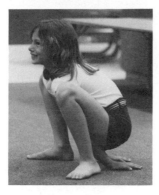

Figure 16-10

GIRAFFE WALK

DESCRIPTION: Extend arms straight up along side ears and hook thumbs over head. Bend hands at the wrist to make the giraffe's head. Without bending the knees, walk on tiptoes. Bend slowly forward to take a drink of water.

WALKING CHAIR

DESCRIPTION: Positioned one behind the other (two or three children may engage), holding onto the hips of the one in front, all sit back so the legs touch the thighs of the one behind. In unison, all move in the desired direction (initially forward).

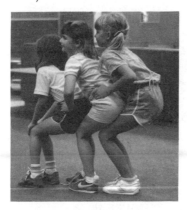

Figure 16-11

CLOWN TRICK

DESCRIPTION: Lie on back on the floor; place beanbag on the forehead. Get up to a standing position and return to a lying position without touching or dropping the beanbag.

ROPE STUNTS

DESCRIPTION: All involve various arrangements and designated forms of jumping or hopping (or both).

LAZY ROPE

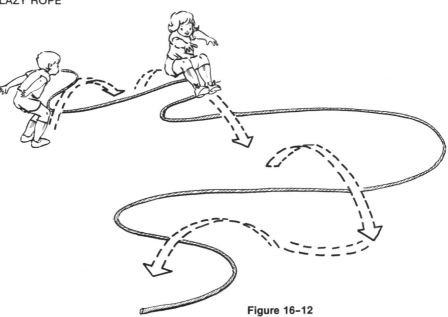

Figure 16-12

SNAKE ROPE

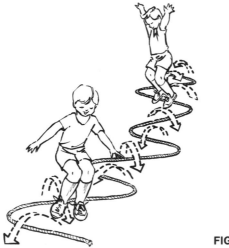

FIGURE 16-13

CIRCLE ROPE

DESCRIPTION: (Also a game.) One person stands outside the circle, the other inside. As the outside person jumps in, the inside person jumps out.

STRAIGHT ROPE

DESCRIPTION: (Also a game.) One partner stands on each side of a straight rope (or a line) holding one ankle and stretching the free hand with palm open toward opponent. Hop on one foot and try to push each other off balance.

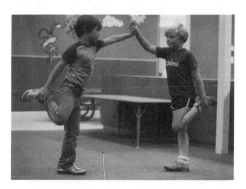

FIGURE 16-14

V-ROPE

DESCRIPTION: Jump (or hop) over "V" at various widths. As a game, divide "V" into sections and assign point-value to each.

FIGURE 16-15

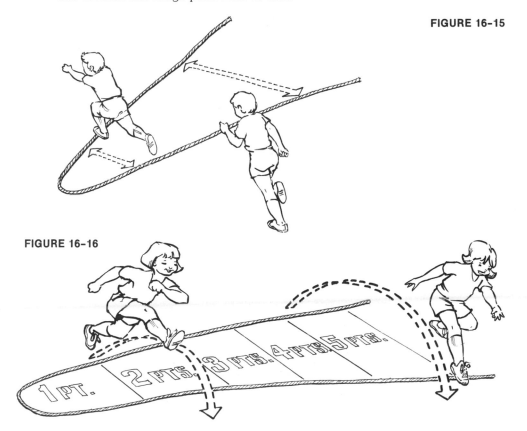

FIGURE 16-16

ROPE RINGS

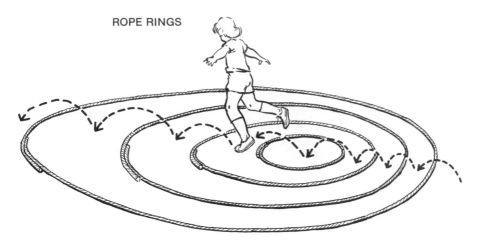

FIGURE 16–17

FROG JUMP

DESCRIPTION: Squat down with hands on the floor (leaning over) and arms between the knees. Jump forward by pushing equally with the hands and feet. The
landing should be on both feet and then the hands.

BEAR WALK

DESCRIPTION: Bending over to the "all fours" position, move in the desired direction trying to keep the legs and arms stiff and head up.

DUCK WALK

DESCRIPTION: Squatting down with knees turned out wide, and hands under the
armpits, move in the desired direction by swinging each foot wide to the side while
flapping the wings.

ANKLE WALK

DESCRIPTION: While grasping the ankles and keeping the head up, walk slowly in
various directions.

CAMEL WALK

DESCRIPTION: With one foot placed in front of the other and the body bent over
at the waist, lock hands behind back (the camel's hump) and walk slowly, raising the
head and chest with each step.

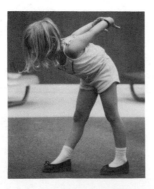

FIGURE 16–18

LAME–PUPPY WALK

DESCRIPTION: The lame-puppy position begins by placing both hands and one foot on the floor. Then walk on "all threes" optionally changing direction and hand position (close, wide, one hand in front of the other).

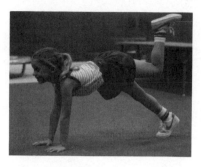

FIGURE 16–19

INCHWORM

DESCRIPTION: Beginning in a push-up position (without moving the arms), take short steps with the feet until the feet come as close to the hands as possible. Then, without moving the feet, take small steps with the hands until the body returns to the push-up position. The sequence of these movements may be reversed (that is, hand movements first).

GORILLA WALK

DESCRIPTION: The knees are bent and the trunk slumped forward. While moving in the desired direction (forward, backward, or sideward), the person's fingers should periodically touch or drag across the floor.

ELEPHANT WALK

DESCRIPTION: Begin by bending forward at the waist and clasping the hands together to simulate an elephant trunk. While moving, the trunk swings side to side like a pendulum. The trunk may also be used to imitate an elephant drinking water, eating, or washing.

CROCODILE CRAWL

DESCRIPTION: Move along the ground on the stomach by advancing same arm and leg, then do with opposite arm and leg, and finally on the back with hands bent and placed alongside the body.

ANIMAL WALK MOVEMENT COURSE

DESCRIPTION: Design a movement course that challenges the children to remember and use various animal walks they have learned. Tape signs on the floor with the animal's picture or name. As the children move through the course, they change movements according to instructions. (Equipment: signs/pictures or names of animals, tape.)

DIRECTIONAL WALK

DESCRIPTION: Standing with side toward the desired direction and arms at sides, take a sidestep in the desired direction (right or left), simultaneously lifting the arm and pointing in the direction of movement. At the same time, the head is turned in the direction of movement; sound off the direction. The sidestep is completed by closing with the other foot, dropping the arm to the side, and turning the head back to normal position. The movements should be definite and forceful, and the directional command should be called out crisply. After a number of sidesteps in one direction, reverse.

BLOW UP THE BALLOON

DESCRIPTION: Stand with feet shoulder-width apart, then squat and place hands on the floor in front of the feet. Keeping the hands flat on the floor, straighten the legs slowly by raising the hips upward and tightening the abdominals. To let the air out of the balloon, slowly return to the original position.

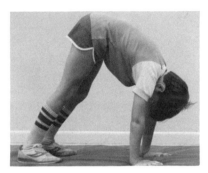

FIGURE 16-20

PICK THE GRASS

DESCRIPTION: Stand with feet in a wide straddle. Count 1, bend over and touch the ground in front of the feet; count 2, touch the ground between the feet; count 3, touch the ground behind the feet; count 4, return to a straight standing position.

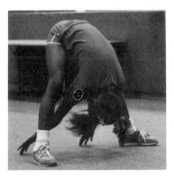

FIGURE 16-21

JACK IN THE BOX

DESCRIPTION: Squat with all fours on the floor (leaning over) using the fingers for balance. When the signal is given (drum, whistle), jump up and extend the arms and legs. Variation: Use different sounds but only one is the signal to jump. (Equipment: drum, sticks, or whistle for signal.)

MISSILE MAN

DESCRIPTION: Cross the arms over the chest and move down into a squat position. On signal (blast off!), jump up into the air and then land with the feet in various positions (for example, one leg extended in front, to the side, alternate extended foot, or on two feet).

POGO STICK

DESCRIPTION: With the hands positioned in front of the body as though grasping a pogo stick, jump up and down using only the toes and feet to exert force. The rest of the body is held stiff with the knees bending as little as possible.

KNEE WALKS

DESCRIPTION: Beginning in a kneeling position, reach back and grasp the ankles or feet. The weight is shifted to one side and the first step taken with the opposite-side knee. After forward movement is accomplished, move sideward and backward. The folded-leg knee begins by taking the left foot and placing it as high as possible against the right thigh. The right leg is crossed over the left and placed high on the left thigh. The arms may be folded or extended to the sides for balance. To move, rise to a kneeling position and proceed forward.

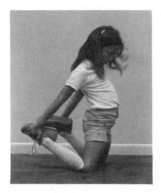

FIGURE 16-22

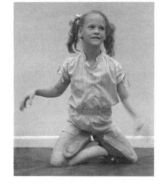

FIGURE 16-23

INVERSE TWISTER

DESCRIPTION: Partners stand back to back, bend over, reach with right hands between the legs, and hold hands. Maintaining the hand grip, one partner leans to the right and lifts the left leg over partner's back. Reverse the movement to return to the original position. Try this holding left hands also.

FIGURE 16-24a,b

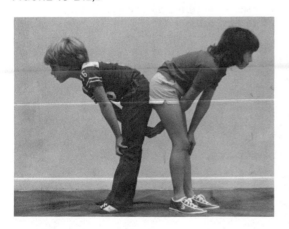
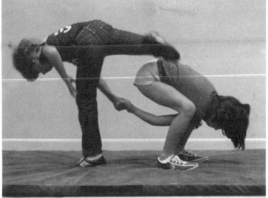

PARTNER PULL-UP

DESCRIPTION: Partners sit facing each other with legs in front and toes touching. Grasp hands, bending knees if necessary, then pull together until standing. Then try to return to sitting position. This can also be done in groups.

STAND-UP

DESCRIPTION: Partners sit on the ground back to back with knees bent and elbows locked. Partners push against each other and try to stand up without letting go of each other. If successful, add one more person. Try four, five, six, even more. See how many can get up successfully.

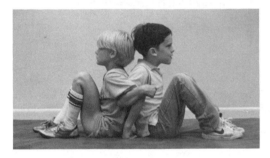

FIGURE 16-25

GOING DOWN

DESCRIPTION: Partners sit side by side with arms linked. On the "go" signal, try to force the other person to roll backwards without touching the free hand to the floor.

PUSH 'EM INTO BALANCE

DESCRIPTION: Partners begin standing and facing with palms of hands together. Take one step or several, depending on challenge needed, and lean on each other for balance. On the "go" signal, try to push each other back into balance without moving feet. Be sure feet are secure on the floor to avoid slipping. When executed properly, this looks like a standing push-up done on a mirror.

WRING THE DISHRAG

DESCRIPTION: Partners face each other, holding hands. Raise one arm on the same side (right arm for one and left for the other) and turn back to back. Continue around by repeating with the other arm and return to the original position. This may also be done by grasping a wand.

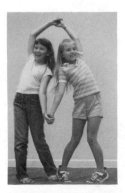

FIGURE 16-26

FLOOR TOUCH

DESCRIPTION: Partners sit cross-legged facing each other and grasp a wand with the palms facing down and arms extended. The wand is parallel to the floor. On the "go" signal, try to touch the wand to the floor on the right side. Change sides and grips on the wand. (Equipment: one wand per pair.)

TWIST AWAY

DESCRIPTION: Partners face each other with feet comfortably apart and grasp a wand with palms down. Try to twist to the right, forcing the other person to loose grip. The contest begins again when one partner has released the grip. Use different grips and body positions.

GRAPEVINE

DESCRIPTION: Hold the wand with an overhand grip near the ends. Bring right foot through both arms and step over the wand. Duck head under the wand and pass it over the head and right shoulder until standing erect with the wand between the legs. Reverse, and use left leg.

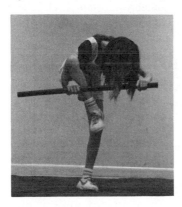

FIGURE 16-27

BACK SCRATCHER

DESCRIPTION: Grasp the wand with an underhand grip and arms crossed in front. Bring the wand over and behind head, then pass the wand over and behind head and down the body from the shoulders to heels without letting go.

FIGURE 16-28

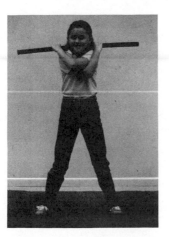

WAND WHIRL

DESCRIPTION: Stand the wand up in front of the body. Let go, and turn around once and catch the wand before it falls. Try turning twice. Now move around the wand once and catch it before it falls.

TWIST UNDER

DESCRIPTION: Hold the wand upright with either right or left hand; twist under the arm without letting go or lifting the wand off the floor. Do not touch knee to the floor while performing this stunt.

SLAVE TWIST

DESCRIPTION: Place the wand behind head and drape arms over it from behind. Very slowly, rotate the body to the right or left and touch the opposite knee with the end of the wand.

CORKSCREW

DESCRIPTION: Stand with feet shoulder-width apart; place left arm behind back. Place right arm across body and behind left knee and touch the toes of the right foot by bending the knees and balancing on the toes. Use the left arm.

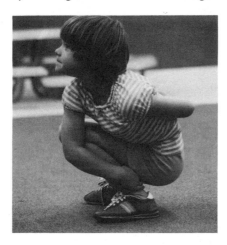

FIGURE 16-29

CRAZY WALK

DESCRIPTION: Try to walk forward by bringing one foot behind and around the other. Do this going backwards, bringing the foot in front each time.

RISING SUN

DESCRIPTION: Start by lying on back with arms over head to represent the sun. Slowly rise to a standing position by bending the knees, placing feet on the floor, and then raising the arms, head, shoulders, and trunk, pushing to a standing position.

CRANE TWIST

DESCRIPTION: Stand on a line 2 feet from the wall and facing it. Then place forehead carefully on the wall and try to turn completely around without taking head from the wall. Try to turn both ways.

THE BRIDGE

DESCRIPTION: Start by lying on back with knees bent, heels against the seat. Bend the elbows and place hands on mat next to ears, fingers pointing toward shoulders. Once in this position, push up slowly, arching the back and relaxing the neck to let the head drop behind arms. Feet should stay flat on the mat.

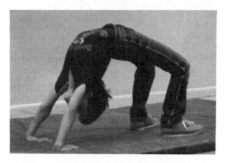

FIGURE 16-30

WHO'S BEHIND?

DESCRIPTION: Choose a partner; one stands behind the other. On the "go" signal from the teacher, the persons standing behind change places quietly. The person in front tries to determine "who's behind?" by bending straight backwards and looking behind.

GREET THE TOE

DESCRIPTION: Stand on one leg and try to raise the toes of the opposite foot to touch forehead, using arms to grasp the foot.

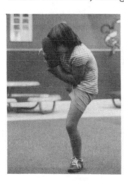

FIGURE 16-31

STRADDLE SEAT

DESCRIPTION: Sit in straddle position with legs straight. Bend over and slide hands out in front and see how far they can go without straining. Stretch slowly and continuously to reach for an object placed in front of the body. Stretch over each leg and try to touch toes.

HUMAN SPRING

DESCRIPTION: Fold arms across the chest and squat down. Spring up as high as possible, landing with the majority of weight on the heels and toes. Variations: Arm position may vary, such as at the sides, straight out in front, or at the side and then up (as in the long jump).

CHURN THE BUTTER

DESCRIPTION: Partners of similar size stand back to back and lock elbows. One partner bends forward at the hips; the other partner gently springs from the floor, leans back, and lifts up his or her feet. Repeat by changing roles.

KNEE SLAPPER

DESCRIPTION: Jump upward, drawing the knees toward the chest. As the knees are moved upward, the legs are slapped with the hands near the knees. Variations: Slap one knee at a time; double time on both knees; cross-slap each knee; perform an "ankle slapper."

TOE TOUCH

DESCRIPTION: While jumping upward, the legs are extended forward and upward with the feet apart. At the height of the jump, touch the toes while trying to maintain a vertical back position. The landing should be on both feet. (Equipment: mini-tramp—optional.)

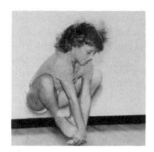

FIGURE 16-32

KANGAROO JUMP

DESCRIPTION: Begin in a squat position with the arms folded across the chest. The body weight should be over the toes. Jump up and forward, land on the toes, and lower the body to starting position.

BOUNCING BALL

DESCRIPTION: Starting in a bent-knee position (squatting), begin with a jump that is high and then lower each jump to simulate a bouncing ball that loses height with each bounce. Variations: Partners pretend to bounce (or dribble) to each other. Bounce to music. Bounce next to a real bouncing ball.

TOP

DESCRIPTION: With hands at the side, squat down and jump into space, trying a half, quarter, or full turn. The landing should be as the start, with hands at the side. This may also be executed with the arms in various starting positions (for example, folded, straight out, or extended to the side).

LEAP FROG

DESCRIPTION: The formation should be two single-file lines with 4 to 6 feet between each person. Leap frog consists of two units: the base and the frog. The base bends forward into a stationary creeping, knees-and-hands position. The head should be tucked down. The frog runs, places its hands on the base's back and pushes off with the legs straddled and extended to the sides. The landing is on two feet with knees slightly bent. The activity may be performed as a relay or singular activity.

TIGHTROPE WALKER

DESCRIPTION: Using a line drawn on the floor, with one foot in front of the other, walk (forward or backward) placing the toe and then heel on the line. Initially, the arms should be extended sideward; however, variability in arm position may be practiced. (Equipment: floor tape or chalk.)

CRAB WALK

DESCRIPTION: Beginning in the sitting position, lift the seat off the floor, transferring body weight support to the hands and feet. The back should be held fairly straight. The direction of movement may be either forward, backward, or sideward.

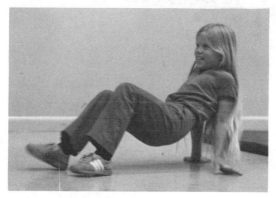

FIGURE 16–33

JUMPING SWAN

DESCRIPTION: While jumping upward, the person's arms are pulled high overhead and the body is arched. The hips are moved forward, and the head and shoulders pulled back hard with the legs extended to the rear. The landing should be on both feet with body vertical.

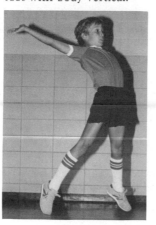

FIGURE 16–34

TUCK JUMP

DESCRIPTION: Jump upward, drawing the knees to the chest while grasping the shins (tuck). The back should remain as vertical as possible and the landing should be on both feet.

RABBIT JUMP

DESCRIPTION: Start in a squatting position, back straight, body weight over the toes. Jump forward, bringing the seat high; land on the hands and then both feet. Variations: Backwards; click heels together; kick feet out as a donkey.

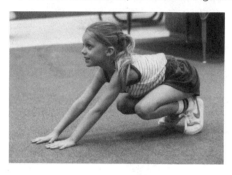

FIGURE 16-35

KNEE JUMP

DESCRIPTION: Start in a standing position with knees slightly bent. Jump upward, pulling the knees to the chest while placing the hands on the knees. The landing should be made with the knees bent.

ELEVATOR

DESCRIPTION: Start in a squatting position, then slowly straighten legs to a tall stretched position like an elevator going up. Return slowly to a squat position like an elevator going down.

PUSH THE DONKEY

DESCRIPTION: In pairs, one in front of the other, on the teacher's signal the person in back tries to push the front person over a designated line. Partner in front resists by pushing backward.

ELBOW WRESTLING

DESCRIPTION: Kneel facing partner; place right elbows on the mat and left forearms on the mat. On the "go" signal, try to push the other person's hands to the mat without moving the person's elbows from the mat.

PULL THE DONKEY

DESCRIPTION: In pairs facing each other, on the "go" signal the person in front tries to pull the other over a designated line by grasping hands only.

HEEL SLAP

DESCRIPTION: Starting in a relaxed, standing position, jump up, kicking the legs back behind the body, bending them at the knee. Slap the hands to the soles of the feet. Before landing, straighten the leg but allow a slight bend to cushion the shock. Variation: Jump up and touch hands to toes, extended in front of the body.

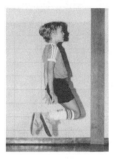

FIGURE 16–36

HEEL CLICK

DESCRIPTION: Stand with feet comfortably apart and ready to jump. Jump into the air and click feet together while in flight. Upon landing, bend the knees slightly to cushion the shock.

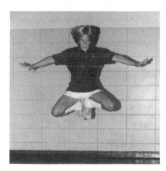

FIGURE 16–37

TUMMY BALANCE

DESCRIPTION: Lie on stomach, keeping arms and legs straight. Raise arms, legs, head, and chest off the floor and balance on tummy.

ROCKING HORSE

DESCRIPTION: Partners sit on each other's toes facing; grasp forearms. One partner leans back, and raises the other off the floor. The partner being raised straightens the legs, sits back, and raises the other partner off the floor. A rhythmic rocking should be the goal.

FIGURE 16–38

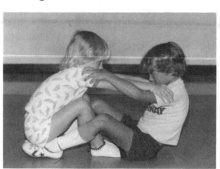

TWISTER

DESCRIPTION: Join right hands with a partner. Partner 1 brings right leg over joined hand; partner 2 brings left leg over. Then partner 1 brings left leg over, and partner 2 brings right leg over to finish in original position.

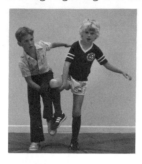

FIGURE 16-39

BLIND TOUCH

DESCRIPTION: From a standing position, reach behind back and grasp one wrist with the other hand. Keeping the elbows straight, slowly bend the knees and look straight ahead; touch the free hand to the floor. Return to a standing position. Switch hands.

DOUBLE KNEE BALANCE

DESCRIPTION: On knees, grasp right foot with right hand and hold it off the floor. Then repeat with the left foot and hand. Try raising both feet off the floor at the same time maintaining balance on the knees.

CRANE DIVE

DESCRIPTION: Take a front-scale position and slowly lean forward as far as possible without losing balance. Change the position of the arms; then attempt to pick up an object off the floor.

HUMAN BRIDGE

DESCRIPTION: Sit on the floor with hands behind; place heels on the edge of a chair with toes pointing toward the back of the chair. Raise the seat up until trunk and legs form a straight line. (Equipment: 1 chair per child.)

SIDE BALANCE

DESCRIPTION: Lie across a chair on side, and place the bottom hand on the floor. Simultaneously, raise the top arm and leg. Be sure to have the chair support the hips. (Equipment: 1 chair per child.)

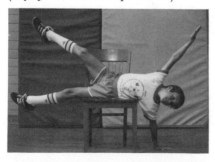

FIGURE 16-40

PEOPLE PYRAMIDS

DESCRIPTION: Children should be encouraged to design their own balance structures, first working in pairs, then threes, fours, fives, etc. A few safety precautions need to be observed:

1. Place weight over a firmly supported base, never in the small of the back or at a joint.
2. Form pyramids carefully by climbing to high positions; do not jump onto another person.
3. Have one child responsible for signaling to "squash" or dismantle the pyramid. To squash a pyramid, all children should lift arms forward and legs back at the same time.
4. Always use mats.

Pyramids can be formed using a variety of balance stunts and shapes as the focus.

TURK STAND

DESCRIPTION: With arms folded across the chest, sit cross-legged on the floor. Stand without using hands or changing position of the feet.

TRIPOD

DESCRIPTION: Squat position; place hands flat on mat; place crown of head at hair line about one foot in front of hands so the three points form a triangular base; lift body weight, resting knees on bent elbows. Maintain this position. (See Fig. 16–41.)

UP-SPRING

DESCRIPTION: Kneel with toes pointed and ankles extended; swing the arms backward and then forward creating lift, while simultaneously pushing the feet. The result should be an upswing to the standing position.

BEAR DANCE

DESCRIPTION: Squat on one heel, extend the other foot forward. Draw extended foot under body and shoot other foot out to front. Arms are folded across the chest. (See Fig. 16–42.)

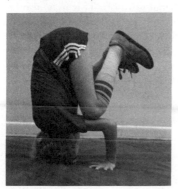

FIGURE 16–41

FIGURE 16–42

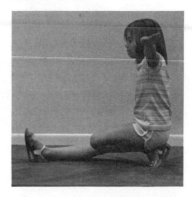

MULE KICK

DESCRIPTION: Place both hands on the mat; bend knees, and kick one leg at a time into the air. Return to the floor, and stand.

BALANCE STAND—FRONT SCALE

DESCRIPTION: Stand on either foot, bend forward at the waist to form a right angle, and extend free leg behind and arms out to the side.

HAND WRESTLING

DESCRIPTION: Partners face each other and join right hands; each raises one foot behind. On signal, attempt to cause the other to touch either free hand or foot to floor. (See Fig. 16–43.)

WHEELBARROW

DESCRIPTION: One person grasps legs of other at knees and walks as if guiding a wheelbarrow. The front wheel walks on hands and keeps back straight.

FROG SQUAT

DESCRIPTION: Children should squat, keeping their backs straight and folding their arms across their chests. They should hop on their left foot and extend their right leg to the side. They should hop again on their left foot and draw their right leg under their body and extend their left leg to the side.

DOUBLE WALK

DESCRIPTION: Partners face and grasp upper arms. One person steps diagonally across insteps of the other, who walks forward. The person on top shifts weight as the other walks.

THREAD THE NEEDLE

DESCRIPTION: Standing, grasp hands or hold wand in front of body. Bend forward and step over hands or wand one foot at a time and finish with hands still clasped behind. Reverse, and return to original position. This may also be done from a back-lying position with the knees bent by passing the feet up and under the hands or wand without touching them, then returning to the original position. (See Fig. 16–44.)

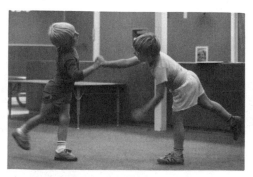

FIGURE 16-43

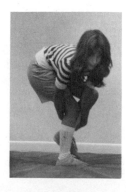

FIGURE 16-44

COFFEE GRINDER

DESCRIPTION: Place one hand on the floor, extend other arm up and legs out. Keeping arms straight, walk around the stationary hand using it as a pivot point.

JUMPING TUBES

DESCRIPTION: In circles of three to six around inner tubes that are scattered, one at a time jump onto and rebound off the surface of the tube, landing in the same starting space. Explore turning, twisting, and various positions. (Equipment: large car or truck inflated inner tubes.)

TOE PUSH

DESCRIPTION: Partners sit facing, raise legs in a V-sit position, and clasp hands under knees. On the "go" signal, try to force each other off balance by pushing against the other's feet with toes.

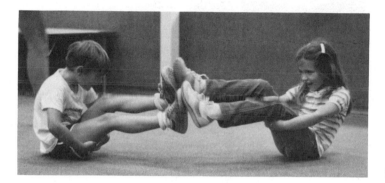

FIGURE 16–45

PUSH WAR

DESCRIPTION: Partners stand opposite each other across the center line and place hands on the other's shoulders. On the "go" signal, attempt to push opponent back over the end line. (Equipment: draw three lines 20 to 30 feet apart.)

SHOULDER WRESTLING

DESCRIPTION: Start in a kneeling position side by side with partner's shoulders touching and hands locked behind back. On the "go" signal, partners attempt to push each other off balance without losing contact with shoulders.

FIGURE 16–46

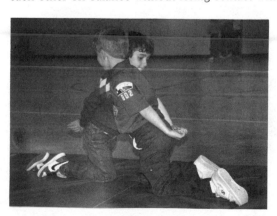

LEG WRESTLING

DESCRIPTION: Partners start by lying on backs side by side and facing opposite directions. On the "go" signal, both raise inside legs so that knees cross. In this position push opponent's legs down to the mat.

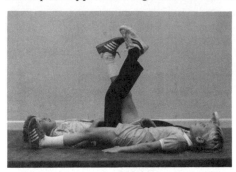

FIGURE 16-47

ROOSTER FIGHT

DESCRIPTION: Partners stand on one leg opposite each other with arms folded across the chest. On the "go" signal, attempt to push the other off balance; do not hit. When one partner touches the floor with the free leg, the other partner is declared the winner.

SEAL SLAP

DESCRIPTION: Start in a front-lying position with hands directly under the shoulders and toes on the mat. Push off from the hands and toes, and at the same time, clap hands in the air. Then return to the starting position.

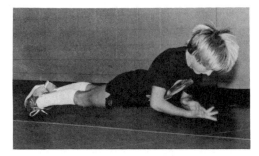

FIGURE 16-48

CRAB FIGHT

DESCRIPTION: Partners sit side by side facing opposite directions in the crab-walk position so that one's knees are opposite the other's shoulders and hips are adjacent. On the "go" signal, attempt to push the other off balance using hips.

FOOT PUSH

DESCRIPTION: Partners sit facing, placing the balls of feet together. Hands, seat, and feet are the base of support. On the "go" signal, push against the soles of each other's feet and try to force the other out of position.

FROG STAND, TIP-UP

DESCRIPTION: Squat down, place hands on floor about shoulder-width apart, and bend elbows out away from the midline of the body. Place inside of knees on elbows and raise feet from floor to balance. (See Fig. 16–49.)

SITTING BALANCE

DESCRIPTION: Base (bottom person) lies on mat with legs raised and knees slightly bent. Top sits on base's feet and extends arms back, grasping base's hands. Base straightens legs and releases top's hands, who extends arms to sides to help maintain balance. (See Fig. 16–50.)

HORIZONTAL STAND

DESCRIPTION: Base lies on back with knees bent. Top stands with feet just behind base's head and hands on the base's knees. Base grasps ankles of top. As top springs up and shifts weight to hands, base raises arms perpendicular to floor. (See Fig. 16–51.)

FIGURE 16-49

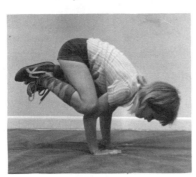

FIGURE 16-50

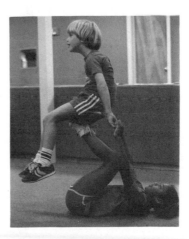

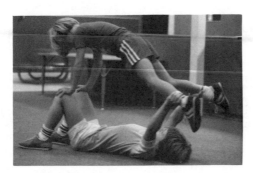

FIGURE 16-51

ANGEL BALANCE

DESCRIPTION: Base lies on back with legs raised, knees slightly bent, and feet placed diagonally alongside top's pelvic bones. Base takes top's hands and slowly raises top into a balanced position. Hands are let go, and top balances with arms out to side. On signal, base bends knees and lowers top to floor where top returns to standing position.

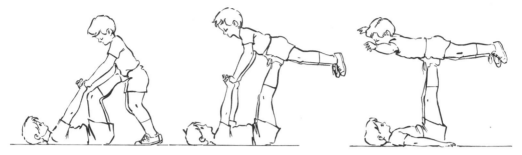

FIGURE 16-52

FOREARM BALANCE—TIGER STAND

DESCRIPTION: Kneeling position with forearms on mat. Palms down, index fingers and thumbs touching, head is placed between them; extend right leg and swing it up overhead. At the same time, spring off the left leg and bring both legs into straight balanced position.

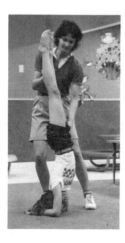

FIGURE 16-53

THIGH BALANCE

DESCRIPTION: The base stands directly behind the top in a semisquat position with back straight and feet about shoulder-width apart. The top places one foot on the thigh of the base, and the base grasps the leg at the knee. Then the top places the other foot on the other leg while the base grasps other knee. The top should lean forward and straighten up to form a balanced position. To return to the ground, the top jumps down, and the base lets go of the legs. Partners should be of equal weight, or the base can be heavier.

HEADSTAND

DESCRIPTION: Take tripod position and extend legs over head, keeping legs straight and toes pointed. Maintain balance. To come down, bend knees and let body weight come down into squat position. A partner may stand beside and hold arm across and behind other person so legs can be stopped from flying over too far. (Partner should not lift legs.)

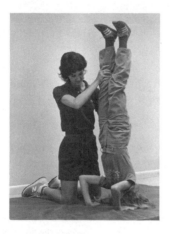

FIGURE 16-54

HANDSTAND

DESCRIPTION: Extend arms straight up beside the ears; place one leg in front of the other. Step on front leg, and kick back leg up placing hands on the floor and maintaining the head between the arms' position. Bring second leg to first, point toes, and tighten abdomen and buttocks to maintain a straight body position. Bend one leg at a time, and step back to original position. A partner may assist by standing beside the performer and extending an arm behind the legs to prevent overbalancing. The spotter should never lift the legs.

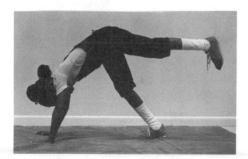

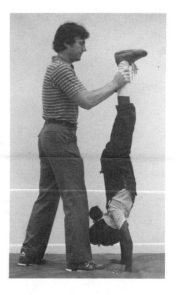

FIGURE 16-55

SPLIT JUMP

DESCRIPTION: Jump upward, spreading the arms overhead and feet as wide as possible. Land with feet together.

JACKNIFE

DESCRIPTION: Similar to Toe Touch except that while the legs are extended forward and upward during the upward movement, the feet are together (not apart) to touch toes. (See Fig. 16–56.)

BENT KNEE HOP

DESCRIPTION: Squat and take a tuck position (arms and hands wrapped around knees). Proceed to hop (2 feet) on balls of feet.

JUMP FOOT

DESCRIPTION: Stand with one foot against wall, about 12 inches from floor and in front of inside leg. Spring from inside foot, and jump over leg.

STIFF KNEE PICK UP

DESCRIPTION: Stand with feet together; bend forward, and pick up article placed 3 inches in front of toes without bending knees.

FREE STANDING

DESCRIPTION: Lie on back on mat with arms folded across chest. Come to standing position without unfolding arms or using elbows.

SINGLE SQUAT

DESCRIPTION: Stand on mat and raise arms to side for balance. Raise one leg in front, keeping knee straight. Squat, keeping weight well over supporting leg. Return to standing position without losing balance.

SPANKER

DESCRIPTION: Take position as for Crab Walk. Raise both feet in the air, and slap seat with right hand, then left hand. Advanced: Hop, extend right leg, and spank with left hand; hop, extend left leg, and spank with right hand. (See Fig. 16–57.)

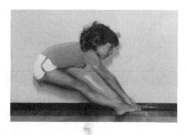

FIGURE 16-56

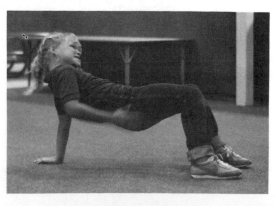

FIGURE 16-57

CARTWHEEL

DESCRIPTION: (cartwheel to the right side) Stand sideways to the direction one is going. Raise both arms straight overhead, shoulder-distance apart; raise right leg and step onto it, placing right hand on the floor as the left leg is kicked overhead. The left hand is then placed on the floor as both legs come overhead and are split in the air. Land on the left foot followed by the right foot facing the original position. There should be an even 4-count rhythm to this movement (that is, right hand count 1, left hand count 2, left foot count 3, right foot count 4).

RHYTHMIC GYMNASTICS—BALLS

Area:	Participants:
Classroom, Gymnasium	Class
Equipment:	**Formation:**
Music with a 3/4 time signature; 6-inch diameter playball	Lines or scattered

Description:

Use the following basic techniques for manipulating the ball (rolling, swinging, bouncing, and throwing patterns are used):

1. Rest the ball on the hand and avoid grasping it for most rhythmic ball activities.
2. Toss the ball using motion from the shoulders rather than the arms when executing rhythmic ball activities.
3. Catch the ball with the fingertips and let it settle into the palm when receiving the ball.
4. Swing and roll the ball by holding the ball with a wrist grasp (ball lies between the palm and forearm).

The following progression is suggested for beginning ball-gymnastics activities. Skills can be made more complex by varying and adding the different arm and leg movements and turning to catch.

1. Standing, roll the ball along the floor from a right-hand wrist grasp to a left-hand wrist grasp.
2. In a V-sit, roll ball under legs from right- to left-hand wrist grasp.
3. Sit with legs extended and roll ball from right hand around legs to left hand and continue around back to finish in right hand.
4. Standing, extend arms in front and grasp ball in both wrists; lift arms to roll ball toward chest, then separate arms and allow ball to bounce once and catch with both hands.
5. Standing, with ball in right wrist grasp, swing arm across body and transfer to left hand and reverse.
6. Standing, with ball in right hand, bounce in front and catch in left hand (palms up). Try bouncing under a leg. Bend knees with each bounce.
7. Standing, with ball in right hand, throw ball up overhead and catch in both hands. Try from the left. Try tossing right to left catch.

RHYTHMIC GYMNASTICS—WANDS

Area: Participants:

Classroom, Gymnasium   Class

Equipment: Formation:

Music in 3/4 time;   Lines or scattered (well spaced)
  3 ft. or shorter wand

Description:

Grasp wand with hands either shoulder-width apart or at the ends, depending on the movements to be attempted. The following progression is suggested for beginning skills. Children should be encouraged to create their own patterns.

1. Standing, grasp wand at ends and jump over forward then backward.
2. Standing, grasp wand at the ends and drop it to bounce on one end and catch it. Try bouncing and catching one-handed.
3. Standing, grasp wand at ends and toss and catch it. Try tossing and catching one-handed.
4. Standing, grasp wand in right hand at one end, arms out to the side, and swing wand across body and catch with left hand. Try swinging behind body.
5. Standing, hold wand with one hand, swing one leg over and catch wand before it falls.
6. Standing, hold wand with one hand, release, run around it once and catch before it drops.
7. Squatting, hold wand on end with both hands and turn so that back faces the wand, then complete turn to end in starting position.
8. Try using various locomotor movements with above activities.

RHYTHMIC GYMNASTICS—HOOPS

Area: Participants:

Classroom, Gymnasium   Class

Equipment: Formation:

Music in 3/4 time; hoops 20 in.   Lines or scattered
  to 27 in. diameter
  (smaller for smaller children)

Description:

Grasp hoop with either an under-grip (palm up) or over-grip (palm down) for hoop activities. Use the entire body to move with the hoop. The following are suggested skills to try:

1. Using an under-grip in one hand at a time, swing hoop up and back down. Try changing hands at the top.
2. Grasp hoop with both hands in an under-grip, arms extended in front of body. Swing hoop from right to left, switch to an over-grip and continue around behind body.

3. Hold the hoop on the ground with one hand and push it with the other so that it rolls. Run a few steps and catch it.

4. Grasp hoop in an under-grip. Swing out and release hoop, pulling hard toward body to put backspin on the hoop so that it returns rolling on the ground.

5. Hold hoop on ground vertically and turn hoop with fingers to spin and catch.

6. Hold hoop in an under-grip out to the side and circle hoop once around the hand. Hold in front and circle with one hand; change to the other hand and repeat.

7. Hold hoop in under-grip out to the side and toss over head and catch on the other side.

8. Hold hoop in an over-grip and bounce from one side to the other.

9. Hold hoop in both hands (over-grip) in front, jump over, and swing around head and repeat, like jumping rope.

RHYTHMIC GYMNASTICS—RIBBONS

Area:	Participants:
Classroom, Gymnasium	Class

Equipment:	Formation:
Music in 3/4 time; ribbons 10 ft. to 15 ft. long	Scattered

Description:

Maintain a rhythmic flow with ribbon to avoid its collapse while exploring various ways of manipulating it. Try these set patterns:

1. Swing ribbon from one side of the body to the other in front in an arc pattern.
2. Swing ribbon in an arc on one side of the body.
3. Swing ribbon in a horizontal wave pattern at high and low levels.
4. Swing ribbon in a full circle in front of the body.
5. Swing ribbon in a figure-8 pattern in front of body.
6. Swing ribbon in a spiral pattern in front of body.
7. Do all activities using both hands.
8. Combine activities with locomotor skills.

Developmental Activity Chart—Gymnastics: Level I-III (As suggested in Chapters 9-12)

NAME	TYPE	LEVEL
Seal Walk Giraffe Walk Frog Walk Bear Walk Duck Walk Camel Walk Lame Puppy Walk Inchworm Gorilla Walk Elephant Walk Crocodile Crawl	Animal Movement	I-III
Animal Walk Movement Course	Animal Movement	I-II
Kangaroo Jump Crab Walk Rabbit Jump Bear Dance	Animal Movement	II-III
Push and Clap Over the Head Seat Circle Long Stretch Egg Sit Rag Doll Toe Reach Stoop and Stretch Clown Trick Ankle Walk	Individual Stunt	I-III
Directional Walk Blow up the Balloon Pick the Grass Jack in the Box Missile Man	Individual Stunt	I-II
Pogo Stick Knee Walks Corkscrew Crazy Walk Rising Sun Crane Twist The Bridge	Individual Stunt	II-III

NAME	TYPE	LEVEL
Straddle Seat Human Spring Knee Slapper Toe Touch Top Jumping Swan Tuck Jump Knee Jump Elevator Heel Slap Heel and Click Blind Touch Turk Stand Up Spring Frog Squat Thread the Needle		
Seal Slap Split Jump Jackknife Bent Knee Hop Jump Foot Stiff Knee Pick Up Free Standing Single Squat Spanker	Individual Stunt	III
Row Your Boat Walking Chair Inverse Twister Partner Pull-up Stand-up Going Down Push 'em into Balance Wring the Washrag Twist Away Who's Behind? Churn the Butter Bouncing Ball Leap Frog Push the Donkey Elbow Wrestling Pull the Donkey	Partner Stunt	I-III

Level I–III (continued)

NAME	TYPE	LEVEL
Rocking Horse	Partner Balance Stunts	II–III
Twister		
Hand Wrestling		
Wheelbarrow		
Double Walk		
Coffee Grinder		II–III
Toe Push		III
Push War		
Shoulder Wrestling		
Leg Wrestling		
Rooster Fight		
Crab Fight		
Foot Push		
Greet the Toe	Individual Balance Stunt	II–III
Tightrope Walker		
Tummy Balance		
Double Knee Balance		
Crane Dive		
Human Bridge		
Side Balance		
Balance Stand-Front Scale		
Log Roll	Tumbling and Inverted Balance	I–III
Side Roll		
Egg Roll		
Human Ball		II–III
Step Jump Roll		
Reach Over Roll		
Back Roll		
Tripod		
Mule Kick		
Frog Stand Tip Up		
Headstand		
Back Roll		
Dive Roll		III
Handstand		
Cartwheel		
Forearm Balance-Tiger Stand		

NAME	TYPE	LEVEL
People Pyramids	Partner Balance Stunts	II–III
Sitting Balance		
Horizontal Balance		
Angel Balance		
Thigh Balance		
Rope Stunts:	Small-Equipment Skills	I–III
Lazy Rope		
Snake Rope		
Circle Rope		
Straight Rope		
V-Rope		
Rope Rings		
Wands:		II–III
Push the Wand		
Floor Touch		II–III
Grapevine		
Back Scratcher		
Wand Whirl		
Twist Under		
Slave Twist		
Rhythmic Gymnastics:		III
Balls		
Wands		
Hoops		
Ribbons		
Rope Jumping:		I–III
Two Step		
Alternate Foot		
Swing Step		II–III
One-Foot Hop		
Rocker		
Stride		
Cross Leg		
Side Shuffle		III
Crossing Arms		
Vaulting: (Jumping)	Large-Equipment Skills	I–III
Squat		
Flank		

NAME	TYPE	LEVEL
Straddle		II–III
Head		III
Horizontal Bar: (Swing and Sway)		I–III
One-Foot Touch		
Swing Back		
Swing Back and Catch		
Drop to Basket		
Front Support Variations		II–III
Skin the Cat		
Basket		
Pull-Over Progression		
Balance Beam: (Vestibular Awareness):		I–III
Locomotor Movements		
Manipulative Movements		II–III
Tires (Vestibular Awareness)		I–III
Jumping Tubes		II–III
Balance Board: (Vestibular Awareness)		
Individual Variations		I–III
Manipulative Movements		II–III
Trampoline: (Vestibular Awareness)		
Jumping Variations (turns)		I–III
Jumping Rope		II–III
Manipulative Movements		II–III
Horizontal Ladder on Ground: (Vestibular Awareness)		
Locomotor Variations		I–III
Manipulative Movements		II–III

Developmental Activity Chart—Gymnastics: Level IV–VI (Recommended activities for skilled children)

NAME	TYPE	LEVEL
Double Lame Dog	Animal Movement	IV–VI
Turtle		
Walrus Walk and Slap		V–VI
Donkey Kick		
Knee Drop	Individual Stunts	IV–VI
Front Drop		
Front to Back		
(Rolling the Log)		
Dead Fall		V–VI
Skier's Sit		
Walk and Jump Through		
Bounce Pretzel		
Single Leg Circle		VI
Backbend Down and Up		
Balance Jump	Individual Balance Stunts	IV–VI
Fish Hawk Dive		V–VI
V-Up		
Toe Jump		VI
Front Seat Support		
Elbow Balance		
Judo Roll	Tumbling and Inverted Balance	IV–VI
Forward Roll Variations		
Backward Roll Variations		
Backward Extension Roll		
Headstand Variations		
Handstand Variations		V–VI
Neck Spring		
Cartwheel Variations		
Round-off		
Headspring		
Handspring		VI
Wheelbarrow Variations–Partner Stunts		IV–VI
Dromedary Walk		
Centipede		
Double Scooter		

Level IV–VI (continued)

NAME	TYPE	LEVEL
Eskimo or Double Roll Tandem Bicycle Circle High Jump Triple Roll (Monkey Roll)		V–VI
Double Bear Front Sit Back Layout Stand on Partner's Knees	Partner Balance	IV–VI
Handstand Hip Support Chest Stand		V–VI
Handstand on Thighs or Knees Knee and Shoulder Stand People Pyramids (Advanced)		
Rhythmic Gymnastics: Balls Wands Hoops Ribbons	Small-Equipment Skills	IV–VI
Rope Jumping: Combine primary individual rope skills into routines		IV–VI
Double Dutch Long Rope		V–VI
Juggling: Bags Balls Scarves		IV–VI
Clubs		VI
Single Hanging Rope: Supported Pull-Up Climbing Swing and Jump Straight Hang	Large Equipment Skills	IV–VI
L-Hang Inverted Hang		V–VI
Double Hanging Ropes: Straight Arm Hang Tuck Hang L-Hang		IV–VI

NAME	TYPE	LEVEL
Tuck Hang L-Hang Skin the Cat Inverted Hangs Climbing		V–VI
Balance Beam: Locomotor Movements Manipulative Movements Individual Balance Stunts Animal Movements		IV–VI
Tumbling Skills (rolls, etc.)		V–VI
Vaulting: Squat Flank Wolf Straddle Head		IV–VI
Handspring		V–VI
Trampoline: Seat Drop Hands and Knees Drop Knee Drop		IV–VI
Front Drop Combine with Turns		V–VI
Horizontal Bar: Monkey Hang Pull-Ups Skin the Cat Scramble Over Pull Over Knee Swing Penny Drop		IV–VI
Horizontal Ladder: Chinning Swing and Drop Single Rung Travel Double Rung Travel Side Rail Travel Rung Travel Sideways		IV–VI

SUGGESTED ACTIVITY SOURCES

BAILIE, S. & BAILIE, A. (1969). *Elementary school gymnastics.* St. Louis: Atlas Athletic Equipment Co.

BALEY, J. A. (1968). *An illustrated guide to tumbling.* Boston: Allyn & Bacon.

DAUER, V. & PANGRAZI, R. (1986). *Dynamic physical education for elementary school children* (8th ed.). Minneapolis: Burgess.

KIRCHNER, G. (1985). *Physical education for elementary school children* (6th ed.). Dubuque, IA: Wm. C. Brown.

LOKEN, N., & WILLOUGHBY, R. (1977). *Complete book of gymnastics* (3rd ed.). Englewood Cliffs, NJ: Prentice-Hall.

O'QUINN, G. (1967). *Gymnastics for elementary school children.* Dubuque, IA: Wm. C. Brown.

RYER, O. E. & BROWN, J. R. (1980). *A manual for tumbling and apparatus stunts* (7th ed.). Dubuque, IA: Wm. C. Brown.

SIEDENTOP, D., HERKOWITZ, J., & RINK, J. (1984). *Elementary physical education methods.* Englewood Cliff, NJ: Prentice-Hall.

SKOLNIK, P. L. (1974). *Jump Rope.* New York: W. P. Workman.

SZYPULA, G. (1968). *Tumbling and balancing for all* (2nd ed.). Dubuque, IA: Wm. C. Brown.

SUGGESTED READINGS

BOUCHER, A. (1978, September). Educational gymnastics is for everyone. *Journal of Physical Education and Recreation,* 48–50.

KIRCHNER, G., CUNNINGHAM, J., & WARREL, E. (1970). *Introduction to movement education* (1st ed.). Dubuque, IA: Wm. C. Brown.

MAULDON, E. & LAYSON, J. (1965). *Teaching gymnastics.* London: MacDonald and Evans.

O'QUINN, G. (1978). *Developmental gymnastics.* Austin: University of Texas Press.

PARENT, S. (ed.). (1978, September). Educational gymnastics. *Journal of Physical Education and Recreation,* 31–50.

Appendix A

PROCEDURES AND NORMS FOR THE AAHPERD HEALTH-RELATED PHYSICAL FITNESS TEST

DISTANCE RUNS (CARDIORESPIRATORY ENDURANCE)

Equipment and Facilities. Either of the two distance-run tests can be administered on a 440-yard or 400-meter track or on any other flat, measured area. Examples of appropriately measured areas are the 110-yard or 100-meter straightaway, other outside fields, or an indoor court area (Fig. A–1).

Description. Standardized procedures and norms are provided for two optional distance-run tests: the 1-mile run for time and the 9-minute run for distance.* The decision as to which of the two tests to administer should be based on facilities, equipment, time limitations, administrative considerations, and personal preference of the teacher.

One-mile run: Students are instructed to run one mile in the fastest possible time. The students begin on the signal "ready, start." As they cross the finish line, runners' elapsed time should be called to the participants (or to their partners). Walking is permitted, but the objective is to cover the distance in the shortest possible time.

Nine-minute run: Students are instructed to run as far as possible in nine minutes. The students begin on the signal "ready, start." Participants continue to run until a whistle is blown at nine minutes. Walking is permitted, but the objective is to cover as much distance as possible during the nine minutes.

Scoring: The mile and 1.5-mile runs are scored to the nearest second. The 9-minute and 12-minute runs are scored to the nearest 10 yards or 10 meters.

*From the AAHPERD Health-Related Physical Fitness Test Manual, with permission of the American Alliance for Health, Physical Education, Recreation and Dance, 1900 Association Dr., Reston, VA 22091.

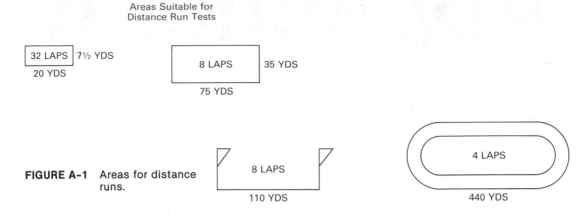

Areas Suitable for
Distance Run Tests

FIGURE A-1 Areas for distance
runs.

SUM OF SKINFOLDS (BODY COMPOSITION)

Equipment: The Harpenden (Quinton Instrument Company, Seattle, WA) and Lange (Cambridge Scientific Industries, Cambridge, MD) skinfold calipers are recommended for obtaining these measures. Characteristics of these skinfold calipers include accurate calibration capability and a constant pressure of 10 gm/mm² throughout the range of skinfold thickness. Care needs to be taken to ensure that the instrument is properly calibrated and that when in the closed position it registers zero. If the calipers recommended above are not currently available to the teacher, several inexpensive calipers are commercially available and may serve as a suitable temporary substitute.

Description: In a number of regions of the body, the subcutaneous adipose (fat) tissue may be lifted with the fingers to form a skinfold. The skinfold fat measure consists of a double layer of subcutaneous fat and skin the thickness of which may be measured with a skinfold–fat caliper (Fig. A–2). Two skinfold–fat sites (triceps and subscapular) have been chosen for this test because they are easily measured and are highly correlated with total body fat.

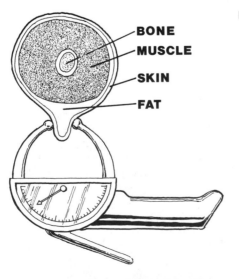

FIGURE A-2 Skin fold caliper pinch and
underlying subcutaneous fat.

BONE

MUSCLE

SKIN

FAT

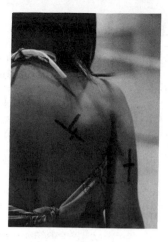

FIGURE A-3 Subscapular and triceps skin fold sites.

The triceps skinfold is measured over the triceps muscle of the right arm halfway between the elbow and the acromion process of the scapula with the skin-fold parallel to the longitudinal axis of the upper arm (Fig. A-3). The subscapular site (right side of body) is 1 cm (½ inch) below the inferior angle of the scapula in line with the natural cleavage lines of the skin (Fig. A-3).

The proper method for measuring these skinfolds is shown in Figure A-4a, b. The recommended testing procedure is:

1. Firmly grasp the skinfold between the thumb and forefinger and lift up.
2. Place the contact surfaces of the caliper 1 cm (½ inch) above or below the finger.
3. Slowly release the grip on the calipers, thus enabling them to exert their full tension on the skinfold.
4. Read skinfold to nearest 0.5 mm after needle stops (1 to 2 seconds after releasing grip on caliper).

In measuring the subscapular skinfold in the female, it is recommended that the individual being tested wear a loose-fitting T-shirt or similar garment. The shirt can be raised in back to allow access to the skinfold site. If the person tested is wearing a bra, the strap need only be pushed upward 2 or 3 inches to allow the measurement. It might also be possible to have the female subject wear a halter or swimsuit top.

FIGURE A-4 (a) Subscapular skinfold; (b) triceps skinfold.

(a)   (b)

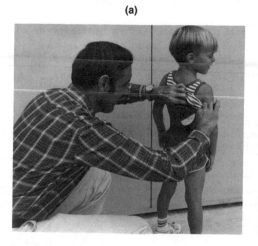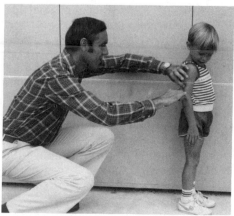

Suggestions.   The skin should be lifted by grasping the fold between the thumb and forefinger. This should be a firm grasp, but not so firm that the student experiences pain. One is cautioned not to place the calipers at the base of the skinfold, for this will give a reading that does not reflect the true thickness and will be too large. The correct distance from the crest is the point on the fold that true double thickness of skinfold fat exists; this is approximately midway between the crest and base of the skinfold. The caliper should be placed about 1 centimeter (slightly less than ½ inch) from the point where the skinfold is held. This is shown in Figure A–4.

For testers who have not used calipers before, it is advisable to practice locating the sites and measuring them on several children. When a reproducibility from 1 to 2 mm or less is consistently achieved, then the tester can begin evaluating skinfolds on school children. On occasion, consecutive measurements will differ by more than 2 mm, especially in obese children, even with experienced testers. If this is the case, it is recommended that an additional set of three measurements be taken. Record the average of the two middle scores.

Skinfold thickness should be measured separately for each child without comment or display. Each child has the right to share or withhold the results of this test. In all cases, interpretation of the measurements should be individually given.

For location of the triceps site, it is essential to locate the measurement at the midpoint of the back of the upper arm and avoid measuring above, below, or to either side of the midpoint as described in Figure A–3 and Figure A–4.

Whenever possible, it is recommended that the same tester administer the skinfold–fat test on the same persons on subsequent testing periods. Intertester error is common and may make the interpretation of subsequent measurements confusing and misleading.

Scoring.   The skinfold measurement is registered on the dial of the caliper. Each measurement should be taken three consecutive times with the recorded score being the median (middle) of the three scores. To illustrate: If the three readings were 18, 15, and 16 mm, the score recorded would be 16. Each reading should be recorded to the nearest 0.5 mm. Norms are provided (Tables A–5 to A–8) to interpret the skinfold measures. The recommended procedure is to use the sum of the two skinfolds; however, if it is possible to secure just one skinfold, the triceps should be the selected site. Separate tables are included for both the sum of the two skinfolds and the triceps site as a single measurement.

Interpretation of Skinfolds.   The exact relation of skinfold fat to body fatness in children has not yet been fully documented. Therefore, while skinfolds are known to be related to body fatness in children, the absolute amount of body fat cannot be determined with certainty. Further, as children advance in maturity, the relation of skinfold fat to body fatness changes with sex and age. Thus, a given thickness does not correspond to the same body fat content for 7-year-olds as for 17-year-olds.

At the present time the national percentile norms provide the best frame of reference for interpretation of skinfold–fat results. The criterion for a desired level of fatness for children is above the 50th percentile. When children are below the 50th percentile but above the 25th percentile, it is recommended that their weight be maintained at the same level for the current year. For those below the 25th percentile, strong encouragement needs to be given to reduce body fatness until their skinfold–fat data reach a more desired level. An increase in the daily physical activity together with a reduction in food intake is recommended for weight control and fat reduction. To illustrate, for a boy aged 14, the desired range of body fatness would be below 14 mm for the sum of triceps and subscapular (for triceps alone the value would be below 8 mm). When the sum of the two skinfolds for a 14-year-old boy is 20 mm or more, the need for weight control and fat reduction is indicated (12 mm for triceps alone).

Skinfold measurements greater than the 90th percentile represent exceptional leanness. Above this level, reduction in weight may involve tissues other than fat (for example, muscle) and may have both short- and long-range undesirable consequences for health, performance, and growth and development. To attempt further weight reduction in children who are already at the 90th percentile is not a desirable goal.

MODIFIED SIT-UPS (ABDOMINAL MUSCULAR STRENGTH AND ENDURANCE)

Equipment and facilities. Mats or other comfortable surfaces are recommended. A stopwatch or sweep-second hand on a wristwatch or clock may be used for timing.

Description. To assume the starting position, the student lies on the back with knees flexed, feet on the floor, with the heels between 12 and 18 inches from the buttocks. The arms are crossed on the chest with the hands on the opposite shoulders. The feet are held by partners to keep them in contact with the testing surface. The student, by tightening his or her abdominal muscles, curls to the sitting position. Arm contact with the chest must be maintained. The chin should remain tucked on the chest. The sit-up is completed when the elbows touch the thighs. To complete the sit-up the student returns to the down position until the midback makes contact with the testing surface (Fig. A–5).

The timer gives the signal "ready, go," and the sit-up performance is started on the word "go." Performance is stopped on the word "stop." The number of correctly executed sit-ups performed in 60 seconds shall be the score. Rest between sit-ups is allowed, and the student should be aware of this before initiating the test. However, the objective is to perform as many correctly executed sit-ups as possible in the 60-second period.

FIGURE A–5   (a) Starting position; (b) up position.

(a)   (b)

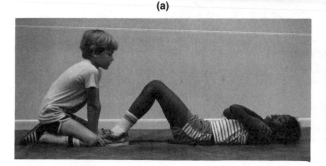
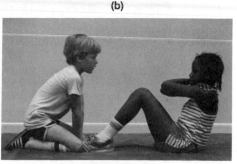

Suggestions.   It is important that the heels are placed a proper distance (12 to 18 inches) from the buttocks. Teachers may want to use a measuring stick to ensure that the proper distance is maintained. Partners can be used to count and record each other's score, but the supervising tester must carefully observe to ensure that the sit-ups are being done correctly. The reliability and validity of the test can be improved by providing sufficient instruction and practice in the correct sit-up technique prior to testing students. Be certain that the student's feet are in contact with the testing surface. This can be ensured by having the partner hold the other person's feet, ankles, or calves.

Scoring.   Record the number of correctly executed sit-ups that are completed in 60 seconds.

Interpreting test results.   Weak abdominal muscles are a contributing factor in the development of low back pain and associated problems. Students who score below the 50th percentile on this test item are encouraged to improve their abdominal strength and endurance along with low back, hip, and posterior thigh flexibility. This is especially critical for students below the 25th percentile. For those students, an individualized remedial program is warranted. Improved strength and flexibility in the areas listed above will aid in the prevention of musculoskeletal problems in the abdominal, back, and hip areas of the body.

SIT AND REACH (FLEXIBILITY OF THE LOWER BACK AND POSTERIOR THIGHS)

Equipment.   The sit-and-reach test apparatus consists of a specially constructed box with a measuring scale where 23 cm is at the level of the feet. Detailed instructions for constructing the apparatus are provided in Appendix B.

Description.   To assume the starting position, pupils remove their shoes and sit down at the test apparatus with their knees fully extended and the feet shoulder-width apart. The feet should be flat against the end board. The arms are extended forward with the hands placed on top of each other to perform the test. The pupil reaches directly forward, palms down, along the measuring scale four times and holds the position of maximum reach on the fourth trial. The position of maximum reach must be held for one second. The test apparatus and testing position are shown in Figure A–6.

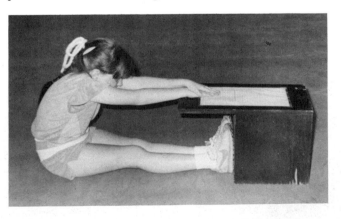

FIGURE A–6   Test apparatus and testing machine.

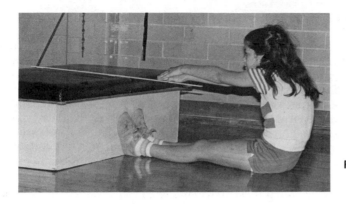

FIGURE A-7 Improvised apparatus for sit and reach.

Suggestions.   The reliability and validity of the test can be improved by providing sufficient time and instruction for warm-up. The warm-up should include slow, sustained, static stretching of the low back and posterior thighs. The test trial is repeated if (1) the hands reach out unevenly or (2) the knees are flexed during the trial. The flexing of knees can be prevented by having a monitor place his or her hands lightly across the knees.

It is recommended that an apparatus be constructed in accordance with the directions in Appendix B so as to ensure standardization of test procedures. However, if the apparatus in Appendix B cannot be made available, it can be improvised by using a bench with a metric ruler attached, as in Figure A–7. Regardless of the specific measurement device used, it is crucial that the soles of the feet be scored at 23 cm because the norm tables have been constructed on the basis of this assumption.

To prevent the test apparatus from sliding away from the student during the test, it should be placed against a wall or similar immovable object.

Scoring.   The score is the most distant point reached on the fourth trial measured to the nearest centimeter. The test administrator should remain close to the scale and note the most distant line touched by the fingertips of both hands. If the hands reach unevenly, the test should be readministered. The tester should place one hand on the subject's knees to ensure that they remain extended.

Interpreting results.   A score above the 50th percentile on this test item is considered a normal level of flexibility. Scores below the 50th percentile represent poor extensibility in at least one of the following areas: posterior thigh, low back, or posterior hip. Poor flexibility in these areas is a contributing factor in the development of musculoskeletal problems. Students who score below the 25th percentile have a critical lack of flexibility, and they should be provided with a remedial program of exercises.

It should be noted that it is normal for many boys and girls not to reach the 23-cm level during the preadolescent and adolescent growth spurt (ages 10 to 14). This is because the legs become proportionately longer in relation to the trunk during this period.

COMMENTS ON EVALUATING STUDENT FITNESS

Percentile norms are provided in Tables A–1 through A–12 for evaluating a student's physical fitness. The percentile rank represents the percentage of students who scored at or below the provided test scores. The larger percentiles represent higher levels of physical fitness.

The percentile norms provide the teacher with two general types of standards: (1) levels of physical fitness deemed desirable of all students and (2) levels of physical fitness excellence. These norms should be used to identify students who need a remedial program designed to meet their needs. The following guidelines are recommended:

1. A remedial individualized fitness program should be developed for all students who score below the 25th percentile on any of the fitness items.
2. Once a student has reached the 25th percentile, he or she should be encouraged to achieve at least the 50th percentile. The 50th percentile represents a level of physical fitness that most students can achieve with proper motivation and conditioning. This represents an average level of performance for the population with which the student is being compared.
3. Many students will be able to exceed the 50th percentile. The norms can be used with these students to define degrees of excellence in physical fitness achievement. Often the norms can be used to motivate the high-ability students.
4. A note of caution is needed for the skinfold test. It is desirable to have students seek low levels of body fat. However, when a student's skinfold score approaches the 90th percentile, additional weight loss is not appropriate because muscle tissue may also be lost. The loss of muscle tissue can have undesirable health consequences. Therefore, the 90th percentile should be considered the ultimate level of achievement on the skinfold test rather than the 99th percentile as is usually the case with most other fitness items.

NORMS

Table A-1   One-Mile Run for Boys (min/sec)

AGE	5	6	7	8	9	10	11	12
Percentile								
95	9:02	9:06	8:06	7:58	7:17	6:56	6:50	6:27
75	11:32	10:55	9:37	9:14	8:36	8:10	8:00	7:24
50	13:46	12:29	11:25	11:00	9:56	9:19	9:06	8:20
25	16:05	15:10	14:02	13:29	12:00	11:05	11:31	10:00
5	18:25	17:38	17:17	16:19	15:44	14:28	15:25	13:41

Table A-2   One-Mile Run for Girls (min/sec)

AGE	5	6	7	8	9	10	11	12
Percentile								
95	9:45	9:18	8:48	8:45	8:24	7:59	7:46	7:26
75	13:09	11:24	10:55	10:35	9:58	9:30	9:12	8:36
50	15:08	13:48	12:30	12:00	11:12	11:06	10:27	9:47
25	17:59	15:27	14:30	14:16	13:18	12:54	12:10	11:35
5	19:00	18:50	17:44	16:58	16:42	17:00	16:56	14:46

Table A-3 9-Minute Run for Boys (yds)

AGE	5	6	7	8	9	10	11	12
Percentile								
95	1760	1750	2020	2200	2175	2250	2250	2400
75	1320	1469	1683	1810	1835	1910	1925	1975
50	1170	1280	1440	1595	1660	1690	1725	1760
25	990	1090	1243	1380	1440	1487	1540	1500
5	600	816	990	1053	1104	1110	1170	1000

Table A-4 9-Minute Run for Girls (yds)

AGE	5	6	7	8	9	10	11	12
Percentile								
95	1540	1700	1900	1860	2050	2067	2000	2175
75	1300	1440	1540	1540	1650	1650	1723	1760
50	1140	1208	1344	1358	1425	1460	1480	1590
25	950	1017	1150	1225	1243	1250	1345	1356
5	700	750	860	970	960	940	904	1000

Table A-5 Sum of Triceps Plus Subscapular Skinfolds for Boys* (mm)

AGE	6	7	8	9	10	11	12
Percentile							
95	8	9	9	9	9	9	9
75	11	11	11	11	12	12	11
50	12	12	13	14	14	16	15
25	14	15	17	18	19	22	21
5	20	24	28	34	33	38	44

*Based on data from Johnson, F. E., D. V. Hamill, and S. Lemeshow. (1) *Skin-fold Thickness of Children 6–11 Years* (Series II, No. 120, 1972), and (2) *Skinfold Thickness of Youths 12–17 Years* (Series II, No. 132, 1974). U.S. National Center for Health Statistics, U.S. Department of HEW, Washington, D.C.

Table A-6 Sum of Triceps Plus Subscapular Skinfolds for Girls* (mm)

AGE	6	7	8	9	10	11	12
Percentile							
95	9	10	10	10	10	11	11
75	12	12	13	14	14	15	15
50	14	15	16	17	18	19	19
25	17	19	21	24	25	25	27
5	26	28	36	40	41	42	48

*Based on data from Johnson, F. E., D. V. Hamill, and S. Lemeshow. (1) *Skin-fold Thickness of Children 6–11 Years* (Series II, No. 120, 1972), and (2) *Skinfold Thickness of Youths 12–17 Years* (Series II, No. 132, 1974). U.S. National Center for Health Statistics, U.S. Department of HEW, Washington, D.C.

Table A-7 Triceps Skinfold for Boys* (mm)

AGE	6	7	8	9	10	11	12
Percentile							
95	5	4	4	5	5	5	5
75	6	6	6	7	7	7	7
50	8	8	8	8	9	10	9
25	9	10	11	12	12	14	13
5	13	14	17	20	20	22	23

*Based on data from Johnson, F. E., D. V. Hamill, and S. Lemeshow. (1) *Skin-fold Thickness of Children 6–11 Years* (Series II, No. 120, 1972), and (2) *Skinfold Thickness of Youths 12–17 Years* (Series II, No. 132, 1974). U.S. National Center for Health Statistics, U.S. Department of HEW, Washington, D.C.

Table A-8 Triceps Skinfold for Girls* (mm)

AGE	6	7	8	9	10	11	12
Percentile							
95	6	6	6	6	6	6	6
75	7	8	8	9	9	9	9
50	9	10	10	11	12	12	12
25	11	12	14	14	15	15	16
5	16	17	20	22	23	23	25

*Based on data from Johnson, F. E., D. V. Hamill, and S. Lemeshow. (1) *Skin-fold Thickness of Children 6–11 Years* (Series II, No. 120, 1972), and (2) *Skinfold Thickness of Youths 12–17 Years* (Series II, No. 132, 1974). U.S. National Center for Health Statistics, U.S. Department of HEW, Washington, D.C.

Table A-9 Sit-ups for Boys

AGE	5	6	7	8	9	10	11	12
Percentile								
95	30	36	42	48	47	50	51	56
75	23	26	33	37	38	40	42	46
50	18	20	26	30	32	34	37	39
25	11	15	19	25	25	27	30	31
5	2	6	10	15	15	15	17	19

Source: Reprinted by permission of the American Alliance for Health, Physical Education, Recreation and Dance, 1900 Association Drive, Reston, VA. 22091.

Table A-10 Sit-ups for Girls

AGE	5	6	7	8	9	10	11	12
Percentile								
95	28	35	40	44	44	47	50	52
75	24	28	31	35	35	39	40	41
50	19	22	25	29	29	32	34	36
25	12	14	20	22	23	25	28	30
5	2	6	10	12	14	15	19	19

Source: Reprinted by permission of the American Alliance for Health, Physical Education, Recreation and Dance, 1900 Association Drive, Reston, VA. 22091.

Table A–11   Sit and Reach for Boys (cm)

AGE	5	6	7	8	9	10	11	12
Percentile								
95	32	34	33	34	34	33	34	35
75	29	29	28	29	29	28	29	29
50	25	26	25	25	25	25	25	26
25	22	22	22	22	22	20	21	21
5	17	16	16	16	16	12	12	13

Source: Reprinted by permission of the American Alliance for Health, Physical Education, Recreation and Dance, 1900 Association Drive, Reston, VA 22091.

Table A–12   Sit and Reach for Girls (cm)

AGE	5	6	7	8	9	10	11	12
Percentile								
95	34	34	34	36	35	35	37	40
75	30	30	31	31	31	31	32	34
50	27	27	27	28	28	28	29	30
25	23	23	24	23	23	24	24	25
5	18	18	16	17	17	16	16	15

Source: Reprinted by permission of the American Alliance for Health, Physical Education, Recreation and Dance, 1900 Association Drive, Reston, VA. 22901.

Appendix B

SIT-AND-REACH MEASUREMENT APPARATUS *

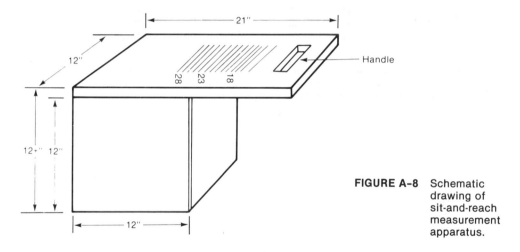

FIGURE A–8 Schematic drawing of sit-and-reach measurement apparatus.

CONSTRUCTION

1. Using any sturdy wood or comparable construction material (¾-inch plywood seems to work well) cut the following pieces:
   2 pieces—12 × 12 inches
   2 pieces—12 × 10½ inches
   1 piece—12 × 21 inches
2. Assemble the pieces using nails or screws and wood glue.
3. Inscribe the top panel with 1-cm gradations. It is crucial that the 23-cm line be exactly in line with the vertical panel against which the subjects' feet will be placed.
4. Cover the apparatus with two coats of polyurethane sealer or shellac.
5. For convenience, a handle can be made by cutting a 1-in. × 3-in. hole in the top panel.
6. The measuring scale should extend from about 9 cm to about 50 cm.

*From the AAHPERD Health-Related Physical Fitness Test Manual, with permission of the American Alliance for Health, Physical Education, Recreation and Dance, 1900 Association Dr., Reston, VA 22091.

Appendix C

TESTING PROCEDURES FOR SKILL-RELATED FITNESS SCREENING *

It is recommended that two days be used for testing:

DAY 1	DAY 2
Flexed-arm hang	Softball throw
Shuttle run	40-yard dash
Standing long jump	

FLEXED-ARM HANG

Equipment.   A horizontal bar approximately 1½ inches (3.81 cm) in diameter is preferred. A doorway gym bar can be used; if no regular equipment is available, a piece of pipe can serve the purpose. A stopwatch is needed.

Description.   The height of the bar should be adjusted so it is approximately equal to the pupil's standing height. The pupil should use an overhand grasp. With the assistance of two spotters, one in front and one in back of pupil, the pupil raises his or her body off the floor to a position where the chin is above the bar, the elbows are flexed, and the chest is close to the bar. The pupil holds this position as long as possible (Fig. A–9).

*Procedures from AAHPERD Youth Fitness Test Manual, Rev. 3rd ed. (1976). With permission of the American Alliance for Health, Physical Education, Recreation and Dance, 1900 Association Dr., Reston, VA 22091.

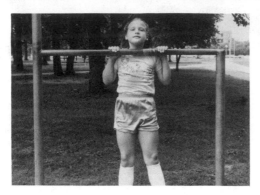

FIGURE A-9 Flexed-arm hang.

Rules:

1. The stopwatch is started as soon as the subject takes the hanging position.
2. The watch is stopped when (1) pupil's chin touches the bar, (2) pupil's head tilts backwards to keep chin above the bar, (3) pupil's chin falls below the level of the bar.

Scoring.   Record in seconds to the nearest second the length of time the subject holds the hanging position.

SHUTTLE RUN

Equipment.   Two blocks of wood, 2 × 2 × 4 inches (5.08 × 5.08 × 10.16 cm), and stopwatch. Pupils should wear sneakers or run barefooted.

Description.   Two parallel lines are marked on the floor 30 feet (9.14 m) apart. The width of a regulation volleyball court serves as a suitable area. Place the blocks of wood behind one of the lines as indicated in Figure A–10. The pupil starts from behind the other line. On the signal "Ready? Go!" the pupil runs to the blocks, picks up one, runs back to the starting line, and places the block behind the line; the pupil then runs back, picks up a second block, and carries it back across the starting line. If the scorer has two stopwatches or one with a split-second time, it is preferable to have two pupils running at the same time. To eliminate the necessity of returning the blocks after each race, start the races alternately, first from behind one line and then from behind the other.

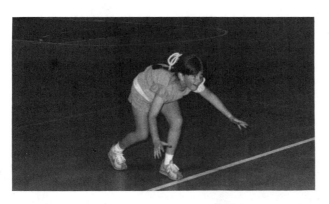

FIGURE A-10 Starting position for shuttle run.

Rules.   Allow two trials with some rest between.

Scoring.   Record the time of the better of the two trials to the nearest one-tenth of a second.

STANDING LONG JUMP

Equipment.   Mat, floor or outdoor jumping pit, and a tape measure.

Description.   Pupil stands with the feet several inches apart and the toes just behind the take-off line. Preparatory to jumping, the pupil swings the arms backward and bends the knees. The jump is accomplished by simultaneously extending the knees and swinging the arms forward (refer to "Jumping" section in Chapter 9 for a more detailed description).

Rules:

1. Allow three trials.
2. Measure from the take-off line to the heel or other part of the body that touches the floor nearest the take-off line.
3. When the test is given indoors, it is convenient to tape the tape measure to the floor at right angles to the take-off line and have the pupils jump along the tape. The scorer stands to the side and observes the mark to the nearest inch (or centimeter).

Scoring.   Record the best of the three trials in feet and inches to the nearest inch or centimeter.

SOFTBALL THROW

Equipment.   A football field or a comparable place on a playground. The necessary space will depend on the age and sex of the group performing the throw. Several regulation 12-inch softballs and a measuring tape. Small metal or wooden stakes may be used to mark throws.

Description.   Two parallel lines 6 feet apart are placed in the throwing area as restraining lines. The throw must be made from within this area. Scoring is facilitated if the field is marked off into additional parallel lines 5 yards apart. The student, using an overhand motion, throws the ball straight down the throwing area. The student can take several steps when making the throw provided the student remains in the 6-foot restraining area. Three trials are permitted and they are taken in succession. Only the farthest throw is marked by a stake. To facilitate things, students are told to stand by their stakes until several students have thrown. Measurement can then be made of several students' efforts.

Rules.   Participants must throw from within the space bounded by the two lines. Throw the ball overhand, for it will help the youngster's score to throw as straight as possible. After the last throw, participants run out and stand by their stakes and remain there until they have been scored.

Scoring.   The score is the best of the three trials measured to the nearest foot or meter.

Testing Personnel.   Two trained assistants are needed to administer this test item. One assistant will judge for fair trials and the second will mark the spot of the throws. These same two assistants can measure the throws and record scores.

40-YARD DASH*

Equipment.   Two stopwatches or one with a split-second timer.

Description.   It is preferable to administer this test to two pupils at a time. Have both pupils take positions behind the starting line. The starter will use the commands "Are you ready?" and "Go!" The latter will be accompanied by a down-ward sweep of the starter's arm to give a visual signal to the timer, who stands at the finish line.

Rules.   The score is the amount of time between the starter's signal and the instant the pupil crosses the finish line.

Scoring.   Record in seconds to the nearest one-tenth of a second.

*Modified from AAHPERD Youth Fitness Test Manual procedures for 50-yard dash.

INDEX